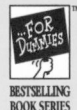

Conquering Childhood Obesity For Dummies®

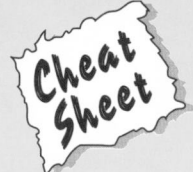

Healthy Food Substitutions and Suggestions

- Use plain yogurt in place of sour cream.
- Cut out egg yolks and only use egg whites — two egg whites are equal to one egg.
- Replace whole milk with skim or 1 percent in most recipes.
- In recipes that call for heavy cream for whipping, try 1 cup evaporated skim milk instead.
- Substitute skim-milk ricotta cheese for cream cheese.
- In recipes that call for 1 ounce of chocolate, use 3 tablespoons instead.
- Instead of using butter for sautéing, switch to canola oil, olive oil, or broth.
- Use applesauce or prune purée in place of vegetable oil in baking recipes.
- Use whole-grain flour and flour products, which provide a lot of nutrients and fiber, whenever possible.
- Trim the fat from any cut of meat before cooking it.
- Leave the skin on poultry to keep it moist while it's cooking, but remove the skin before serving.
- Use the low-fat varieties of your family's favorite dairy foods.
- Bake, broil, grill, or sauté foods instead of frying them.
- Cut out high-fat condiments like mayonnaise and salad dressings. Use vinegar or yogurt- or buttermilk-based dressings.
- Precut fresh fruits and veggies and store them in plastic containers for easy, healthy choices at snack time.
- Freeze bananas, grapes, strawberries, and berries to munch on by themselves or to use in smoothies or on cereal.
- Freeze fruit juice and fruit in ice cube or popsicle trays for convenient fruit servings.
- Flavor water with frozen fruit juice cubes or frozen fruit.

W9-AFI-602

For Dummies: Bestselling Book Series for Beginners

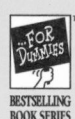

Conquering Childhood Obesity For Dummies®

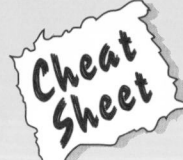

Cheat Sheet

Fun Ideas for Family Outings and Activities

- Walk a dog — yours or a neighbor's.
- Play tag or jump rope with small kids.
- Play volleyball in the pool.
- Find a not-so-high mountain or hill and set out for a family hike.
- Make visits to the park or playground part of your regular schedule. Remember to bring along Frisbees, balls, or bikes to add more interest to each outing.
- Encourage kids have races in the driveway (on foot) or around the block (on bikes). Give them a stopwatch to add some friendly competition.
- Encourage kids to organize an informal neighborhood baseball or football league, and let them use your front lawn for their home field.
- Allow older kids to get creative building bike ramps and jumps. (Inspect them for safety, of course!)
- Make sure kids have plenty of outdoor equipment to keep them busy, including a basketball hoop, rollerblades, bases for baseball or kickball, bats, balls, helmets — whatever they'll play with!
- If the kids want to go to a friend's house down the street, don't drive them. If you're concerned for their safety, walk with them.
- Don't hire someone to do your yard work; make it a family affair. Even the youngest kids can help rake or drag leaves to the rubbish pile.

Burning Calories During Exercise

The number of calories burned during exercise depends on height, weight, and *metabolic equivalent* (MET), which is a multiple of *resting metabolic rate* (RMR), a measurement of how hard your body works while remaining still. An MET of 3 means that your body is working three times as hard as it would if you weren't doing anything. You can gauge MET ranges as follows:

- 3 to 5 METs: Breathing fast but still able to talk
- 5 to 7 METs: Breathing hard but still able to talk a little bit
- More than 7 METs: Breathing so hard that conversation is impossible

The following is a list of activities that require a moderate amount of effort, roughly 3 to 6 METs:

- Walking
- Hiking
- Rollerblading
- Dancing
- Baseball
- Softball
- Swimming
- Basketball
- Gymnastics
- Skateboarding
- Mowing the lawn
- Shoveling snow
- Playing on playground equipment

A person weighing 150 pounds will, on average, burn approximately 250 calories exercising at a MET level of 3 for 60 minutes.

For Dummies: Bestselling Book Series for Beginners

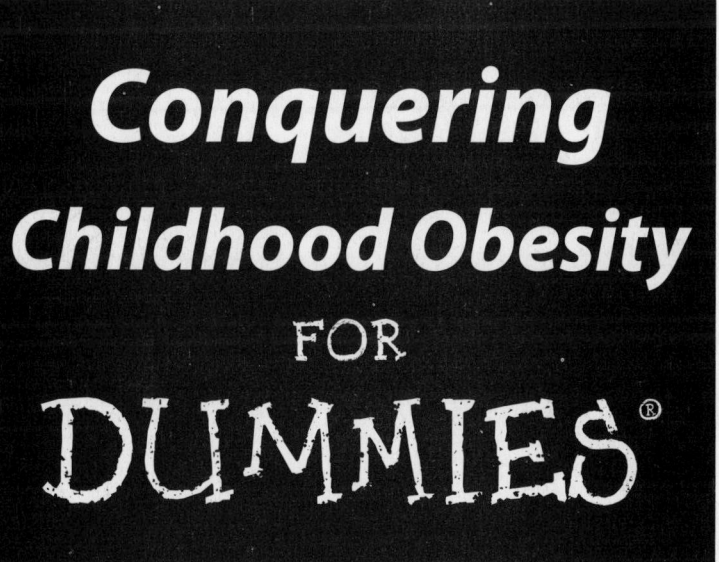

Conquering
Childhood Obesity
FOR
DUMMIES®

2007

JUL

CH

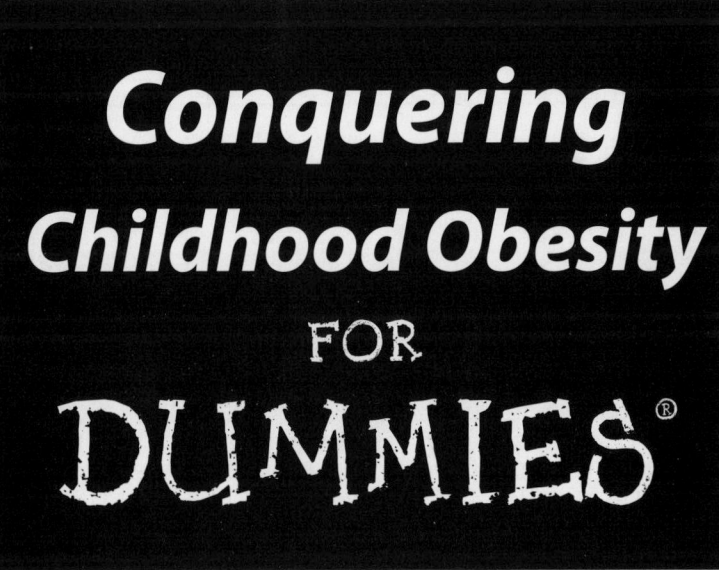

Conquering
Childhood Obesity
FOR
DUMMIES®

by Kimberly A. Tessmer, RD, LD
Meghan Beecher
Michelle Hagen

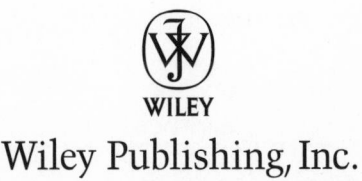

Wiley Publishing, Inc.

Conquering Childhood Obesity For Dummies®

Published by
Wiley Publishing, Inc.
111 River St.
Hoboken, NJ 07030-5774
www.wiley.com

Copyright © 2006 by Wiley Publishing, Inc., Indianapolis, Indiana

Published by Wiley Publishing, Inc., Indianapolis, Indiana

Published simultaneously in Canada

For general information on our other products and services, please contact our Customer Care Department within the U.S. at 800-762-2974, outside the U.S. at 317-572-3993, or fax 317-572-4002.

For technical support, please visit www.wiley.com/techsupport.

Wiley also publishes its books in a variety of electronic formats. Some content that appears in print may not be available in electronic books.

Library of Congress Control Number: 2006923948
ISBN-13: 978-0-471-79146-1
ISBN-10: 0-471-79146-6
Manufactured in the United States of America
10 9 8 7 6 5 4 3 2 1
1O/RW/QW/QW/IN

WILEY

About the Authors

Kimberly A. Tessmer, RD, LD, is a registered dietitian and freelance writer who currently owns and operates Nutrition Focus, a consulting company specializing in nutrition and weight management. She has authored numerous books and has written articles for several national magazines. Kim is a member of the American Dietetic Association and the ADA Practice Group "Nutrition Entrepreneurs." Kim resides in Cleveland, OH, with her husband Greg and daughter Tori.

Meghan Beecher is a Project Coordinator in the Childhood Weight Control Clinical Research Study at the University of Buffalo, a two-year study funded by a grant from the National Institutes of Health and run by Dr. Leonard Epstein, a leading expert in the field of childhood obesity. The study teaches obese children and their parents how to adopt a healthier lifestyle, which includes instruction about portion control, counting calories, and exercise. Prior to her involvement in the UB study, Meghan taught preschool and was also employed by the Montana Conservation Corps (a branch of Americorps), where she introduced adolescents to outdoor activities as a means of improving their lives. Because she is an avid runner, Meghan is well aware of the benefits of exercise and nutrition and was eager to find a career that would combine her love of children with her interest in health. When the UB study concludes, Meghan, a graduate of Xavier University with a BA in Social Work, plans on continuing in this field, educating children on the merits of a healthy lifestyle.

Shelly Hagen is the co-author of *Baby's First Year For Dummies* and has also authored eight books in the bestselling *Everything* series, including *The Everything Destination Weddings Book, The Everything Father of the Bride Book,* and *The Everything Body Language Book.* As a freelance writer and editor, Ms. Hagen has also performed extensive ghostwriting and book editing work, and has written features for *The Saratogian* daily newspaper. She has a degree in Literature from SUNY Empire State and lives in Saratoga Springs, NY, with her husband, Mike, and three sons, Sam, Hal, and Nolan.

Dedication

Kimberly Tessmer: To my beautiful new daughter, Tori, the light of my life!

Meghan Beecher: To my father, you have been an amazing role model my whole life. You have always supported me in all of my activities and life's challenges. You have set a perfect example as a father, a friend, a business man, and an avid morning runner. I am so grateful for the guidance you have given me throughout my life. To Will, from the very beginning you have been the support I needed to make significant changes in my life. Your trust and encouragement in me and my abilities means so much. Here's to the rest of our lives together.

Shelly Hagen: For my husband, the love of my life, who always knows that everything will work itself out in the end.

Authors' Acknowledgments

Kimberly Tessmer: Thanks to various dietitians that I counted on for their expert advice and opinions. Thank you also to The American Dietetic Association for their invaluable resources.

Meghan Beecher: Thank you to Leonard H. Epstein for giving me the opportunity to be apart of your important research and for having confidence in my abilities as a project coordinator. To Jennifer and Molly, you are not only my sisters but my friends, and you have helped me become who I am today. To Aunt Julie, you have set an example for all women as a wife, mother, aunt, friend, and guide. Thank you for all you have done throughout my life. To Maggie, my lifelong friend, for everything we have experienced together.

Shelly Hagen: Many thanks to Jessica Faust at Bookends Literary Agency for her assistance in getting this project up and running; to Tracy Boggier at Wiley for believing in this book and nurturing it on its way to reality; to Tim Gallan at Wiley, for his steady, even-keeled approach to editing (just my style!); and to Elizabeth Rea for all of her help during the final editing process. Thanks to Julie Negrin, Megan Brenn-White, and Cindy Guirino for their outstanding recipe contributions. I owe my co-authors Meghan and Kim more than a simple thanks; both are incredibly knowledgeable in their fields and so eager to help children lead healthier lives. Without them, this book honestly would not have been possible, and I am very grateful for their insight and assistance. Lastly, I need to thank to my husband, Mike, and my boys, Sam, Hal and Nolan, for their support and for being so patient when I'm working my way through a pile of research and first drafts. You guys are my #1s, always.

Publisher's Acknowledgments

We're proud of this book; please send us your comments through our Dummies online registration form located at www.dummies.com/register/.

Some of the people who helped bring this book to market include the following:

Acquisitions, Editorial, and Media Development

Senior Project Editor: Tim Gallan

Acquisitions Editor: Tracy Boggier

Copy Editor: Elizabeth Rea

Editorial Program Coordinator: Hanna K. Scott

Technical Editor: Mary Ann Graham

Recipe Testers: Keith and Kate Brown

Nutritional Analyst: Patricia Santelli

Editorial Manager: Christine Meloy Beck

Editorial Assistants: David Lutton, Nadine Bell, Erin Calligan

Cartoons: Rich Tennant (www.the5thwave.com)

Composition Services

Project Coordinator: Patrick Redmond

Layout and Graphics: Claudia Bell, Stephanie D. Jumper, Barry Offringa, Alicia B. South

Proofreaders: Laura Albert, David Faust, Leeann Harney, Techbooks

Indexer: Techbooks

Publishing and Editorial for Consumer Dummies

    Diane Graves Steele, Vice President and Publisher, Consumer Dummies

    Joyce Pepple, Acquisitions Director, Consumer Dummies

    Kristin A. Cocks, Product Development Director, Consumer Dummies

    Michael Spring, Vice President and Publisher, Travel

    Kelly Regan, Editorial Director, Travel

Publishing for Technology Dummies

    Andy Cummings, Vice President and Publisher, Dummies Technology/General User

Composition Services

    Gerry Fahey, Vice President of Production Services

    Debbie Stailey, Director of Composition Services

Contents at a Glance

Table of Contents

Introduction

What is it about overweight children that just breaks your heart? Is it that they sometimes have a hard time fitting in with their peers, or is it that they suffer from health problems that used to mainly afflict adults? Truly obese children used to be an anomaly in most schools; one or two were common, but you didn't see anywhere near as many severely overweight children as you see today. The increased number of obese children means that there are a lot of kids out there who have serious issues with food, lack of physical activity, and the emotional and physical conditions that result from being obese.

We wrote *Conquering Childhood Obesity For Dummies* not to say that, "Every child should be skinny, skinny, skinny!" We know that's not realistic (no more realistic than saying that every adult woman should weigh 110 pounds and have curves in all the right places — *please*). People come in different shapes and sizes; that's just the way nature works. What we're concerned with is the detrimental health effects that obese children face.

This book is all about making healthy lifestyle changes to improve the physical and emotional well-being of the obese child and her entire family. Studies have shown that a child does far better, both in the short and long term, if at least one parent is involved with her weight-loss efforts. And because healthy living never hurt anyone, we want to get your whole family eating more healthfully and making physical activity a part of their normal, everyday routines!

About This Book

What makes this book different from all the other weight-loss and diet books flooding the market is that it doesn't focus on weight loss. We're much more interested in helping obese kids feel better about themselves by improving their health. We're not working on the assumption that every child whose parents read this book is going to end up being thin. Some people are just programmed to be larger than their peers. However, cutting back on fat and increasing your child's activity level will lead to better health. When he feels better, he can do more, and the more he does, the better he feels.

This book isn't about eating specific foods on certain days in order to lose weight (in other words, this isn't a new-age diet book); rather, it's about breaking down the cycles of unhealthy living and replacing them with healthy habits.

What You're Not to Read

Assume that all the really super-important information in this book is found in the text itself and not in the *sidebars,* which are shaded gray boxes of information scattered throughout each chapter. Although we think the sidebars are incredibly interesting (naturally), we understand that many people don't want to be bothered with reading anything other than need-to-know information. (If you're interested in all facets of this topic, by all means soak up those sidebars.) Also, you can safely skip over information marked with a Technical Stuff icon. Like sidebars, these icons mark interesting information that isn't vital to your understanding of the text.

Foolish Assumptions

We assume that you're reading this book because you either have an overweight child or because you work with children and are concerned for their well-being. Either way, you need not be an expert of any sort to understand the information presented here. *Conquering Childhood Obesity For Dummies* isn't a medical text, nor is it a book about exercise physiology. When we do discuss anatomy and medical conditions, we stick to the bare minimum of scientific detail and break that down into language that's simple to read and understand. We assume that you don't want to have to read this book with a dictionary and a calculator in each hand; so you can assume that we don't overly complicate the subject.

How This Book Is Organized

This book breaks down into 5 parts and 19 chapters. We organized the information by following a chronicle of family involvement: First, you educate yourself on the issues surrounding the problem. Next, you get into the meat of how to solve the problem. You follow that up by troubleshooting any areas of difficulty, and you finish with some quick ideas for making the process as easy as possible.

Part 1: Understanding Childhood Obesity

The chapters in Part I focus on the underlying causes of obesity but also go into great detail about the physical and emotional effects of being a severely overweight kid. We address specific medical conditions related to obesity, how to handle bullies who torment your child, and how to initiate a healthier lifestyle in your home.

Part II: The Weight Is Over: Making Changes, One at a Time

In this part, we get down to the business of overhauling your family's lifestyle. We discuss how to encourage everyone to become more active, the essentials behind proper nutrition, what kind of foods are best for weight loss, and how to plan a menu and make your life a whole lot easier. We also talk about the healthiest ways to prepare food (and how to convince your family that the vegetables on their plate mean them no harm — really).

Part III: Managing, Troubleshooting, and Keeping the Weight Off

Changing your family's lifestyle around — and keeping it healthy — isn't always the easiest task. Problems such as weight gain, rebellion against the new system in the house, or simply falling back into old habits may pop up now and then. And, of course, your child is bound to face certain temptations at school and at friends' homes. We talk about all these issues in Part III and also include a chapter on how to determine whether your child may benefit from outside help.

Part IV: The Part of Tens

If you're familiar with *For Dummies* books, you know that the Part of Tens is often the quickest read and just the thing to keep you motivated on a busy day! The chapters in this part include fast, easy ideas for helping you to get your family on the healthy-living track and keep them there. Flip to this part whenever you need to remind yourself why you decided to take your family's health under control in the first place.

Part V: Appendixes

The Appendix offers 34 easy, low-calorie, low-fat recipes that not only taste good but are good for you. Your family will love them.

Icons Used in This Book

Each *For Dummies* book uses icons throughout the text to highlight information that's either so important that it bears repeating or doesn't really fit into the text but is worth reading about anyway. In this book, you find the following icons:

This icon draws your attention to timesavers and ideas for easing tensions and keeping your child and family on the right track.

This icon points out information we may have mentioned elsewhere that relates to the topic at hand as well as specific information that you should keep in mind as you address your child's weight problem.

This icon refers to issues that affect your child's physical or emotional well-being and therefore should be taken very seriously.

This icon highlights extra information that you don't really need to read in order to understand the text. Read it if you're so inclined, but if you're not in the mood, feel free to move on!

Where to Go from Here

Conquering Childhood Obesity For Dummies was written with the assumption that you want to be able to jump from chapter to chapter and section to section, reading only the information that most pertains to you and your situation. So go ahead and start in the section or chapter that interests you most. If you're just starting to look into the issue of childhood obesity and how to correct it, we suggest that you begin in Part I. On the other hand, if you're more interested in finding out about the best, most effective ways to overhaul your family's way of life, start with Part II.

Part I
Understanding Childhood Obesity

The 5th Wave   By Rich Tennant

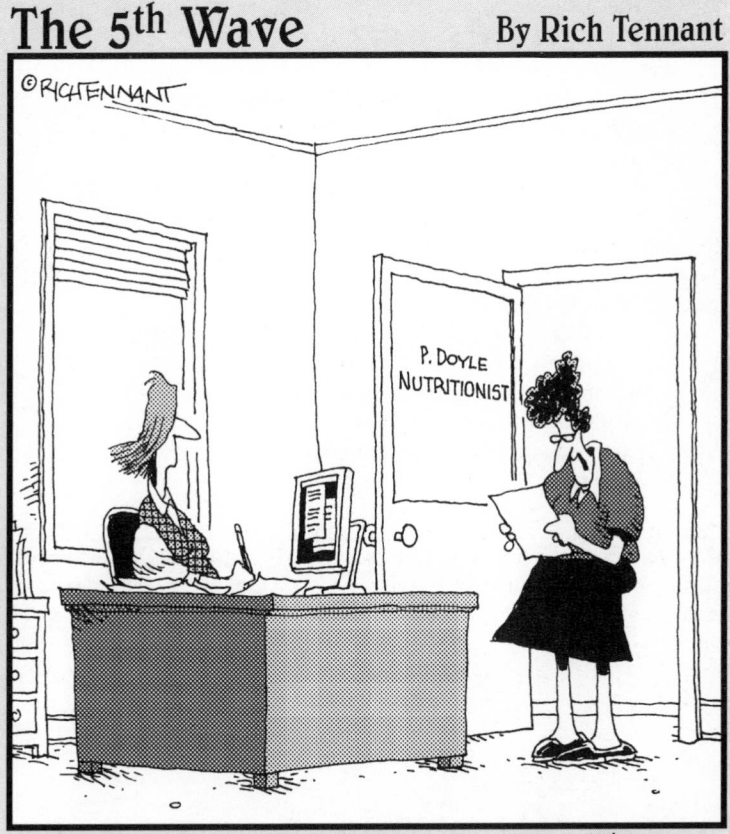

"The Dunsters would like to meet with you somewhere to discuss their son's weight problem. They're suggesting either Dinkle Donuts, The Slurp & Burger, or Pizza Jamboree."

In this part . . .

The numbers are in, and childhood obesity has been declared a public health crisis in the United States. Not only are obese children at higher risk for developing serious health issues that were previously only seen in adults, but they also tend to deal with heartbreaking emotional turmoil on a regular basis.

In this part, we talk about what's causing so many children to become severely overweight these days, and we also discuss the specific health risks these kids face. Throughout these chapters, we offer tips for creating a healthier home environment and for supporting your child as you start to make the changes that will result in better health for the whole family.

Chapter 1

Looking for Answers

. . . .

In This Chapter

▶ Nailing down the big causes of childhood obesity

▶ Changing your family's way of life

▶ Working through rough patches

. . . .

*I*f you've picked up this book and have made it to Chapter 1, we assume that you're interested in the topic of managing childhood obesity either on a personal or professional level. If you have kids or you work with kids (heck, if you see kids), you know that children these days are heavier than ever. Your kids' friends (and your friends' kids) are bigger, heavier, and less healthy than children were even 10 or 15 years ago. What's going on in this world that's causing this kind of weight gain?

Well, nothing's going on throughout the *world.* Childhood obesity (and obesity in general) affects wealthy, industrialized nations. The adult populations in third-world countries aren't worried about the ever-increasing size of their pants, nor are they concerned that their children are becoming too heavy. (In fact, these countries often have the exact reverse situation, wherein they're concerned about their kids having enough to eat.) In the United States, people have become accustomed to eating whatever they want, whenever they want, and eating too much of it. In addition, unlike their forefathers or friends in underdeveloped areas of the world, most Americans don't perform any sort of physical labor as a means of supporting their families. You'd think that would give everyone even more energy to exercise in the downtime, but apparently, everyone's all too interested in what's happening on TV. Sixty percent of adult Americans and 15 percent of American children are overweight. Neither children nor adults are using their stored energy (conserved from a day of sitting behind a desk or in front of the TV filling up on too many calories) to make themselves more fit.

Making oneself healthier usually involves two relatively simple steps:

> ✔ Cutting back on high-fat foods
>
> ✔ Increasing daily physical activity levels

You may be surprised to hear that although the consequences of childhood obesity are varied and complex, the causes and remedies of the condition are relatively simple. This chapter breaks the topic of childhood obesity down to address two main questions: Where did this problem come from, and what can parents do to help correct a child's weight issue (without making things worse)?

Gauging the Epidemic of Obese Children

With more and more kids getting bigger and bigger these days, doctors and other health professionals have to deal with diverse issues. Obesity isn't a condition that limits itself to weight, with the worst effect being low self-esteem. Childhood obesity can lead to some serious illnesses (like diabetes, high blood pressure, and heart disease) that can have long-lasting effects. So how bad is the problem of childhood obesity? We get to the bottom of that question in this section.

The widespread nature of childhood obesity

Thirty years ago, less than 5 percent of children were considered obese. Today's figures put the number of obese American children somewhere between 12 percent and 15 percent! That translates into millions of children, preteens, and teens suffering from very adult conditions like diabetes and depression related to weight gain.

Only a physician can make the official diagnosis of obesity. He or she does this by using height and weight charts along with BMI-for-age charts (see Chapter 5). These tools give the doctor a clear indication of

> ✔ How heavy a child is in relation to the normal weight for his or her age
>
> ✔ The types of interventions the doctor should recommend in order to improve the child's health

Although some areas of the country are touted to have larger populations of heavy adults and kids, childhood obesity isn't really a regional problem. The surgeon general has said that it's an epidemic affecting the entire country; he doesn't single out one specific state or city.

Changes for the worse at home

A large part of the childhood obesity epidemic is the result of some major lifestyle changes. Thirty years ago, back when a tiny percentage of children qualified as obese, there weren't 800 cable television channels to choose from. Video games were boring and low-tech, to say the least, and most people didn't even know what a computer was. Kids simply didn't have endless indoor entertainment options, so they played outside more often. They were active without even knowing it. It's simply what kids did back then!

Today, many kids are glued to some sort of screen much of the time. However, some kids aren't allowed to play outside because they come home from school to an empty house or to a babysitter who isn't quite up to the task of keeping the kids safe outdoors. Thirty years ago, in comparison, a large number of households had at least one parent who stayed home full time, who booted the kids out the door when they got on her nerves, and who prepared meals from scratch. We're not knocking moms who work full time outside the home nowadays. (Indeed, many homes depend on two full-time salaries just to keep things moving toward the black and away from the red.) Families are just far more dependent on fast food and convenience foods these days, both of which tend to be very high in fat, and both of which are believed to contribute mightily to obesity. (Chapter 7 has more detailed information on the drawbacks of the typical fast-food fare.)

With so many meals eaten on-the-go, families don't sit down to dinner together. People have forgotten how to eat for the sake of nutrition; instead, food has become part of entertainment (as when families eat in front of the TV) or a contest to see how fast one can finish an entire bagged meal (because she's running late and only has five minutes for dinner). People don't know what normal portions look like anymore, and they've forgotten how to slow down and evaluate the merits of what they're eating. (For more on family dinners, check out Chapter 11.)

Vending junk at school

In addition to the changes in the average home, many children also face the rigors of making healthy choices at school. In many school cafeterias, finding healthy options is difficult, especially if the school has allowed fast-food vendors to set up shop in the lunchroom. Vending machines have become so commonplace in schools that kids and parents hardly give them a second glance anymore; however, because these machines usually aren't stocked with apples and oranges but instead with soda and candy bars, even kids who want a healthy snack often find themselves out of luck.

What's to Be Done?

You can't fight the system, right? Kids are kids, and they're going to be exposed to ads for junk food and junk-food vendors their entire life. What's a parent to do?

Whether your child has a weight issue or not, you can't throw your hands up in the air and leave his health to fate. The human body — adult or child — is not programmed to subsist on a diet comprised mostly of fat and refined carbohydrates. Cavemen didn't eat French fries. The Pilgrims didn't visit the drive-thru window every evening. Native Americans didn't whip up milkshakes. And guess what? These populations also weren't obese.

Parents of obese children are often tempted to make a concerted effort to improve the child's weight and health, but most kids will try and fail if at least one parent isn't also involved in the regimen.

Easing into activity

Just cutting fat out of your family's diet is a huge step in the right direction. Adding physical activity is another important step. Exercise helps the weight come off faster and also helps keep it off. Plus, exercise has been shown to improve mental states and alleviate depression and anxiety, so it's good for the body *and* the soul.

We're not advocating that you start your heavy child off in some sort of marathon training program. Just get him outside to play. If he's little, play with him. If he's bigger, let him find his own playmates or encourage him to sign up for a sport. Of course, turning off the TV is an essential part of ensuring that your child's activity level increases, so be prepared for an argument — but also be prepared to stand your ground. For more on incorporating physical activity into your family's lifestyle, turn to Chapter 10.

Educating the kids

Your first instinct when faced with an obese child's health crisis may be to take the reins and make his meals, drag him outside for walks, and record his weight every single day. However, the best results in improving a child's health come from a parent leading the way but also allowing the child to make some of his own decisions.

Educating your child without dictating his every move makes him feel empowered to make the right choices when push comes to shove (for example, when he's at a friend's house and surrounded by high-fat treats). If he's been taking care of himself under your watchful eye, he'll be able to take care of himself in the real world, too. Chapter 12 contains ideas for educating your child on making the best choices when he's faced with not-so-healthy options.

Facing Trouble Head-On

If losing weight and keeping it off were easy, everyone would be super-thin. The fact is, making changes to your family's lifestyle takes time. It takes time to institute changes and time for the family to get used to them. It also takes time to start reaping the benefits of healthy living. Because this is a gradual, permanent change, it's not unusual for boredom and frustration to set in. During the adjustment period, you're your child's number one cheerleader. She needs you to remind her of the health benefits of losing weight, so be prepared to be patient with her.

Kids sometimes gain weight when parents think they should be losing. Your child may hit a plateau, when weight gain seems to come to a grinding halt for several weeks. At these times, everyone needs to keep their cool and stick with the new, healthy routines. Setbacks are normal, and despite the frustration, moving forward rather than settling into old habits is still the better way to go. For more on setbacks and remaining supportive, see Chapter 11.

If you suspect that your child would benefit from some sort of professional intervention, such as talking with a therapist or joining a support group for overweight kids, don't hesitate to find her help. Weight is an emotional issue that can leave permanent scars on a person's self-esteem. Improving her physical health is a wonderful goal; just make sure her emotional health is along for the ride. Chapter 14 contains advice on bringing in outside help for your child.

Chapter 2

The Growing Problem of Childhood Obesity

*1*t's no secret that today's children are different from the kids that roamed the planet a generation or two ago. Children today seem to mature faster in so many ways: They're smarter than we were at that age, they seem to be taller, and studies show that some kids even hit puberty at an earlier age. Although debate continues as to whether these changes are for better or worse, one trend is particularly disturbing because it encompasses so many potential long-term emotional and physical problems. You know what we're talking about: The trend towards obesity in children.

Statistics show that a significant percentage of children in the United States are obese, but what does *obese* really mean? And why is there a sudden spate of severely overweight children? Is your child part of that group? And most important, what can you do about it? In this chapter, we take a look at what's going on with kids today and talk about how our society has taken a turn toward inactivity that has resulted in adults and children alike packing on the pounds. We provide an overview of the dangers associated with being an obese child, and we also discuss how family life plays a role in the way your child eats as well as the way she spends her time.

As you read through this chapter, you may think to yourself, "This is too much! I can't help my child fix this!" Yes, you can. The first thing you have to do is take a step back and assess the situation your child is facing. Is she truly obese? Does she have a plethora of bad habits? Is she modeling what she sees in the home? A parent who's able to be honest about his or her child's problem is much more likely to be able to help that child correct it.

Is It Baby Fat or Something More?

Fat babies are cute. People want to snuggle them, pinch their cheeks, and tickle their plump bellies. Fathers beam with pride when someone remarks on the size of a huge baby boy and respond, "Yep, he's going to be our linebacker!" Mothers are only concerned that their big child doesn't know his own strength and will unwittingly crush the other children on the playground. In fact, if a mother expresses concern about a toddler's plumpness, she's often made to feel as though she's overly concerned with weight and/or appearance. She's assured (usually by the child's grandparents) that nothing's amiss and the child will grow into his weight.

Fortunately, many times these assurances are true. As children grow taller and simultaneously become more active, they tend to thin out. So when should a parent truly become concerned about a child's weight? Is a chubby infant a candidate for a baby aerobics class? What about a toddler or preschooler who shows no signs of limiting his food intake but who seems to be genuinely hungry? In this section, we discuss the criteria for differentiating between normal childhood chubbiness and childhood obesity. We also talk about the emotional pitfalls that obese children face and the reasons that make trying to correct bad habits as soon as possible so important.

Making the call: Is she obese or merely plump?

First things first: Infants and babies are never, ever diagnosed as being obese. Determining whether toddlers are truly overweight is difficult because they still have their protruding bellies. For older children, however, research has made clear that parents are often the last people to acknowledge their child's weight problem. A healthcare professional, on the other hand, is completely objective.

If your child's doctor is telling you that your child is obese, *listen*. He's not trying to be judgmental or mean spirited. He has seen the effects obesity has on the body, and he really has your child's best interest at heart — just as you do.

Diagnosing obesity

The one person who can make the diagnosis of true obesity is your child's doctor, who evaluates *adiposity,* a medical term for "how much fat a person has." There are several ways to assess adiposity, including the use of an MRI or an underwater scale, but these methods are expensive (and, some would argue, excessive).

Some physicians use calipers to measure subcutaneous fat at specific points on the body. Caliper readings are a really accurate way to diagnose the amount of fat a person has, but they're notoriously difficult to reproduce. The doctor may come in, do a measurement, and hand the calipers over to the nurse practitioner to confirm the reading . . . only to get a different measurement. So in terms of reliability and ease of use, calipers are great in the hands of a true expert but not so helpful when used by someone less skilled.

Measuring and comparing the distribution of body fat is another way doctors sometimes evaluate children for obesity, but again, this is a less-than-perfect science. Debate exists in the medical community as to which circumferences and ratios are most important in terms of obesity. For example, although it's widely accepted among doctors that belly fat is particularly dangerous in adults, this doesn't appear to be the case for children. (In short, more research in the area of children's body fat distribution needs to be done.)

Doctors most commonly use a chart called the *body mass index* (BMI) to make the differentiation between an overweight child and one who is obese. This chart, used for children and adults alike, measures the amount of fat a person carries around on his or her body frame.

You know that when you take your child to the pediatrician for a checkup, someone measures her height and weight and records the numbers on a chart, and the doctor turns to you and says, for example, "Susie is in the 90th percentile for height." Obese children tend to fall into the highest percentiles for weight, which can be deceiving because BMI uses height as one of the factors in calculation. So although your child may fall into a high weight percentile, she may not be obese if she also falls into a high percentile for height.

We cover BMI (along with other criteria used for diagnosing obesity in children) in great detail in Chapter 5, but for now, here's what you should know about the BMI chart:

- ✔ For adults, a BMI score of 30 or above indicates obesity.
- ✔ Children's BMI scores are evaluated according to their age.
- ✔ A child is considered obese if she scores in the 95th percentile for her age on the BMI scale.

The English formula for calculating BMI is:

[Weight (lb) ÷ Height (in) ÷ Height (in)] × 703

Whereas an adult has to hit the 30 mark on the BMI scale to be considered obese, an obese child's score is much lower. For example, a 6-year-old girl with a BMI score of 19.65 is considered obese because that score falls into the 95th percentile of BMI *for her age*. A child who falls into the 85th percentile (in this case, the 6-year old girl's BMI score would be 17.20) is considered overweight or at risk for becoming obese.

But why label kids as *obese* when they hit this point? When a child reaches the point of being severely overweight, it's time to do something about it, and a solid tool like the BMI scale allows both doctors and parents to say, "Look, this child is past the point of simply being a little too heavy. She's moving into critical territory with her weight, and we need to correct this condition before she develops dangerous health problems."

A doctor's level of concern may be directly associated with the child's age. An obese 6-year-old still has years of growing ahead of her and plenty of time to undo any damage that's starting to take hold inside of her body. An obese 16-year-old, on the other hand, is reaching the apex of her height potential and is at higher risk for carrying bad habits into adulthood. Depending on how long she's been obese, she may also be at high risk for developing health problems like type 2 diabetes, high blood pressure, asthma, and sleep apnea, all of which carry long-term risks of serious illness. (For more on these and other health problems, see Chapter 3.)

Super-Sized Babies: Born Big and Staying that Way

Some people question whether the increase of obese children is due to increased birth weight. The answer: Yes and no. Yes, birth weight can certainly affect a child as he grows, but no, an obese child doesn't always start life out in the 100th percentile for weight.

For the most part, physicians believe that most babies who are 12 pounds and over at birth are born to women with untreated gestational diabetes. Because the mother has too much glucose in her body during pregnancy, the baby receives too much glucose in the womb and grows well beyond everyone's expectations. Babies who measure in at or above the 90th percentile at birth (that is, they're larger than 90 percent of other babies who were in the womb for the same period of time, normally 38 to 40 weeks) are termed *large-for-gestational age*. Children who are this large at birth tend to stay large throughout childhood and adulthood.

Here's another twist to babies who aren't necessarily born big but who end up being too chubby within the first year: Doctors are struggling to treat a significant percentage of obese pregnant women. An obese mother may have other health issues, like diabetes or high blood pressure, that lead to premature births and/or *low birth weight* babies. (Yep, you read that correctly.) The fact that many of *these* children will, in time, become obese has far more to do with the environment they're raised in than their birthing experience.

Generally speaking, though, obese women tend to give birth to larger-than-average babies. These babies tend to remain large throughout childhood and adolescence and into adulthood. The factors involved may be genetic or environmental, but the end result is the same: These children are at higher risk for developing the long-term obesity-related complications and illnesses that we talk about in the following section and in Chapter 3.

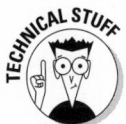

Statistics from the Center for Disease Control show that 30 percent of adult Americans are obese, and more than *60 percent* of adult Americans are at least overweight! It stands to reason, then, that many children are born to obese parents and the cycle of unhealthy lifestyle choices continues.

Studies have shown that babies who gain too much weight in the first week of life may actually reset their biological systems, making it easier for them to gain weight throughout their lifetimes. You certainly don't want to withhold food from a baby, so your pediatrician is your best resource for determining how much to feed your baby at any given point in time. Our point is that the trend toward obesity can start as early as the first few days of life; indeed, this research has indicated that excessive weight gain in the first week is far more likely to cause obesity later in life than excessive weight gain over the first several months of a child's life.

Physical and Emotional Dangers of Obesity

The reason that the trend toward obesity is so alarming to physicians is that excess weight can cause very damaging conditions — both physically and emotionally. And while the emphasis is on correcting and/or mitigating any permanent changes to a child's physical health, anyone who's ever been teased about their physical appearance can attest to the fact that the emotional scars can be just as painful as any physical hurt.

Aches, pains, and disease

Pediatricians see many serious health issues in obese children that used to be seen only in adults. Obese children have a higher risk of developing the following conditions:

- ✔ Type 2 diabetes
- ✔ High blood pressure
- ✔ Asthma
- ✔ Sleep apnea
- ✔ Rashes, fungal infections, and other skin conditions
- ✔ Early puberty in girls
- ✔ Delayed puberty in boys
- ✔ Orthopedic strains and fractures
- ✔ Heart disease (in early adulthood)

Chapter 3 goes into more detail about each of these conditions.

No one should have to worry about these conditions until adulthood, but they can start to develop as early as childhood. In fact, doctors are seeing more and more instances of type 2 diabetes and elevated cholesterol in children as more and more children become obese.

As for the worst of the worst, some of the most serious long-term side effects of type 2 diabetes include:

- ✔ Increased risk for heart disease and stroke
- ✔ Blindness
- ✔ Amputations

Some of the long-term complications of elevated cholesterol are an increased risk of heart disease and stroke. Combine a couple of these conditions, and a person can end up with very serious health issues. An adolescent who has both diabetes *and* high cholesterol, for example, has a much higher risk of developing heart disease than a teen who has one or the other. Unfortunately, because obesity predisposes people to developing these diseases, it's more common for an obese person to have more than one obesity-related disease.

Aching for acceptance: Emotional issues

As though the physical risks of obesity aren't enough, their peers put obese children through the emotional wringer each and every day. Overweight kids are easy targets for bullies, and unfortunately, even though we've done away with all kinds of overt discrimination in this country, a fat prejudice still exists and still is accepted among certain factions of the population.

Consider this: Obese adults face discrimination and outright nastiness from total strangers. (If you're severely overweight or obese, you can probably recall a time or two when someone had the nerve to judge you on nothing more than your physical appearance.) What are these strangers teaching *their* children, who are in school with *your* child? It's a hard, cruel world out there, but it's even worse for an obese child faced with taunts and name-calling on a daily basis. In Chapter 4, we talk more about the social issues and emotional wounds that overweight children face.

Self-esteem and isolation

Obese children are more likely than other kids to feel like they're on the outside of their peer social settings and, as a result, suffer from low self-esteem. Few children can tolerate being different from the other kids in their classes. Obese children look different, move differently, and have physical needs that other children don't (such as needing a larger desk, for example, or more time to complete a task in physical education class). Most kids want nothing more than to be accepted by other kids their own age. A child may feel like he stands out either because he's being made to feel that way by others or because he perceives himself as an alien being. Either way, the result is the same: The child doesn't succeed in social settings.

Problems during puberty

Obese girls tend to reach puberty earlier than other girls their age, which only adds to the problem of feeling like an outcast. When a 9-year-old faces weight issues *and* a burgeoning bosom *and* getting her period, she's dealing with some very adult issues at a very young age. Her friends are bound to look at her differently, as are adults. No one knows quite how to speak to a child who *looks* like a young woman.

Obese boys tend to go through puberty at a later age than boys who are of normal weight. While the other guys are starting to sprout upward and show signs of entering adulthood, obese boys are left wondering why their bodies are betraying them. Why aren't their voices getting deeper? Why aren't they shaving yet? A boy in this situation may wonder, "Isn't it bad enough being overweight without also being stuck in childhood?"

The teen scene

Obese children with low self-esteem tend to be stuck on the sidelines (at best) while their peers start going to dances and on group dates. It's not as though obese children don't take an interest in the opposite sex; they simply have fewer opportunities to test the waters, so to speak, and this setback further affects the way they view themselves as well as the way they're viewed by their peers.

Avoiding the Fat Lifestyle

Some obese adults and children truly believe that their weight problems stem from some sort of glandular problem, but this theory is true in a very small percentage of cases. Most of the time, obesity is caused by a synergy of two separate but equally powerful bad habits:

✔ Ingesting too much food (especially high-fat food)

✔ Leading a sedentary lifestyle

Being overweight and/or obese is usually what doctors call a *voluntary condition* — that is, the only reason for it is that a particular person has fallen into certain habits that have contributed to skyrocketing weight. But the fact that it's voluntary means that you can do something about it. Obesity isn't an incurable condition — it responds well to lifestyle modifications.

Kick the kids out!

Does your child *ever* play outside? Lack of physical movement contributes mightily to obesity.

Food is nothing more than edible energy. Calories are the measurement of the *potential* energy that a given amount and type of food contains. A body needs a minimum amount of calories in order to perform its basic functions, and the recommended caloric intake for this purpose varies according to age, body frame, and activity level. For example, a 22-year-old average-sized football player in training needs to ingest more calories than a skinny 35-year-old computer programmer who does little more than type all day long. The football player is younger, larger, and more active than the programmer, so he burns more calories and burns them faster.

Children's bodies need caloric energy in order to grow properly, but doctors often recommend restructuring the types of food an obese child gets her calories from. By eating healthy foods with fewer calories, your child will actually consume more food than if she were eating unhealthy foods with more calories, but the healthy foods will make her feel fuller sooner.

Because very few people take in only the bare minimum amount of calories that they need to operate each day, everyone needs to get their bodies moving in order to burn off the extra energy that's contained in food. In addition, children need to engage in physical activity to encourage the proper formation of bones and muscles. When a child never goes outside to play, a few things happen as a result:

- ✔ He gains weight. (No physical activity usually results in extra pounds.)
- ✔ He doesn't learn to interact with other kids.
- ✔ He doesn't discover how to use his imagination.

Obviously, the weight gain is the issue we focus most on in this book, but the other effects may also contribute to a child never wanting to go outside. If he sees other children playing a game he's never participated in, he may feel like the odd man out, even if he *wants* to join them. This feeling, in turn, makes him withdraw from the other kids even more and miss out on other activities. How does he console himself? With a snack and some time in front of the TV. It's a vicious cycle.

Do whatever you can to get your children outside every day, starting when they're babies. Make it a natural part of the day by calling it Outside Time, Playtime, Yard Time, or whatever sounds good to you. When they're very small, you can play games like tag or kickball or have simple "races" (where you let them win every time, of course). When they're older, you can encourage loosely organized sports in the yard, bike rides, or walks.

Even if you live in an area where winter hangs on for half the year, find some way to get those kids outside and moving. Take up skiing, go sledding (dragging that sled back up the hill takes energy!), or try ice-skating, hockey, or snowshoeing. Make activity a normal part of your kids' day, year-round, and you'll all lose weight.

If you live someplace where letting your children play outdoors is difficult or unsafe, find a nearby community center or a family program that offers children's activities. Many programs are available to youths at little or no cost.

Turn off the TV!

Given a free minute, most kids are glued to the television set. And they'll watch *anything*, which proves that their minds are turning to mush. (Kids used to be able to tell a good cartoon from a bad one. Not so these days. Put it on the air, make it talk, and most kids will watch it.)

Why TV is bad (as if you don't already know)

The telltale sign of a sedentary lifestyle is sitting around doing not much of anything; this type of nonactivity leads to weight gain because the person's not engaging in any physical activity that uses up the calories ingested over the course of the day. Studies have shown that watching a lot of TV

- ✔ Can actually lower *metabolism,* the body's way of effectively using calories for energy
- ✔ Encourages kids to snack without thinking about what they're eating

For some reason, kids are particularly drawn to snacking on high-fat, high-carbohydrate foods, like chips or cookies, while watching TV. Why this is the case is anyone's guess, but it's a good bet that those commercials hawking junk food have something to do with it.

TV viewing is like a perfect storm for weight gain. The very act of sitting down to stare at a screen causes metabolism to take a nose-dive while kids continue to take in more calories of the very worst kind. (Now, if your kids wanted to sit down and snack on a bowl of raw carrots, you'd still have the excessive TV viewing to contend with, but obesity wouldn't be as much of an issue.)

Why do people sit down in front of the TV with a snack, anyway? One reason is boredom. Watching TV day in and day out is *really* boring. (Many kids are so hooked on TV that they're completely immune to its entertainment value.) As a result of this boredom, some kids look for something else — anything else — to do while watching TV, and eating is the easiest activity when your mind is completely numb.

Also, if you haven't personally been exposed to children's television shows, sit down and watch with your kids some time. *A lot* of the commercials that air during children's programming are for food — and not healthy food. Chips, soda, cookies, yogurt loaded with sugar and cookie stir-ins, ice cream, various fast food restaurants. . . . Occasionally, you see an ad for milk, but you rarely see anyone pushing fruits and vegetables. Even the occasional public service announcements that try to educate young children on the virtues of eating a healthy diet are lost in the overwhelming deluge of ads promoting junk.

Simple solutions

No matter how long your children have been accustomed to snacking in front of the TV, make a new rule, effective immediately: No more eating while watching television. Taking away the background noise of cartoons and mindless shows forces the kids to consider what they're putting into their mouths and whether they're actually hungry.

Because TV is even geared toward babies these days, kids can easily fall into an all-TV, all-the-time routine. Add the old adage "Everything in moderation" into your daily parenting routine; a little TV watching isn't going to hurt your children, but spending hours upon hours in front of the tube may cause them to gain weight and, in any event, certainly won't do them any good, especially when they could be spending that time playing with friends.

Some households have the television on almost nonstop, so kicking a constant TV-watching habit can be as difficult as quitting smoking. Everyone has their shows that they watch every day or every week, but TV can become a physical dependence, a comfort, a member of the family. Do yourself and your kids a big favor by taking the following actions:

- ✔ **Limit the amount of television that your children are allowed to watch.** Pediatricians recommend that children under 2 years of age don't watch TV at all. After the age of 2, the recommendation is no more than two hours per day.

- ✔ **Enforce a no-snacking-while-watching rule.** Turn off the tube and concentrate on the food in front of you and the people around you. In Chapter 11, we talk about setting firm ground rules for mealtimes.

- ✔ **Make sure that you follow the new rules, too.** Studies have shown that kids are more likely to be hooked on TV if their parents are avid viewers. You can't really expect a child to accept a limit on her TV time if you continue to watch the tube 'round the clock.

- ✔ **Encourage your children to replace TV time with even a moderately active pastime.** You're likely to see big changes, both in their weight and in their attitudes, as they gain self-confidence and a renewed interest in life.

Do electronics truly cause weight gain?

You may be reading this chapter and thinking, "Well, I have one skinny kid and one overweight kid, and they *both* watch a lot of TV, so something besides the use of electronics must cause obesity in children." Certainly, not every child who spends too much time in front of the TV or computer is obese — but plenty are, or at least are headed in that direction.

The plain truth is that inactivity and excessive eating cause people to become overweight. Most cases of obesity aren't the result of glandular problems or inactive thyroids, and although obesity may have a genetic link (obese parents are more likely than thin parents to have children who are obese), environment plays a big role. Poor eating habits and inactive lifestyles are usually passed along from generation to generation. So can you blame TV for your children's weight problems? Not really, no. You have to look to yourself and your habits first . . . and *then* turn off those electronics.

Game over: Shut down the video games

You may have read the preceding section thinking, "My child never watches TV. He's off learning things on his computer." Although some computer and video games have educational components and are deemed "interactive," most are a far cry any sort of fat-burning activity. The problems linked with excessive TV viewing are echoed with video and computer games: They're sedentary activities. While playing these games, kids are apt to snack without thinking, and they're not outdoors interacting with other kids or getting rid of some energy.

Some doctors feel that video games are a little less harmful than excessive TV viewing as far as developing obesity is concerned. The theory is that computer and video games engage kids in activity that involves a lot of hand-eye coordination and other fine motor movements, and these kinds of motions utilize more caloric energy than simply sitting and staring at a TV screen. This theory may have some truth to it, but it's far from a solid endorsement of video games and computers.

In order to burn off a meaningful amount of fat and calories, a person has to be engaged in some sort of aerobic activity — something that raises the heart rate, uses the large muscles in the body, and gets the blood pumping. Video games just don't offer this health benefit.

Cut out the fast food

Suppose researchers were working in reverse and wanted parents to encourage their children to become obese. What would one of their very first recommendations be? Swing through the fast food drive-thru on a regular basis. Yep, that should do the trick.

To be fair, over the past few years, the fast food giants have made a real point of advertising healthier choices for adults. For the most part, they've done a fair job of providing nonfried foods, such as salads or grilled chicken sandwiches, for us older people. However, in most restaurants, kids' meals haven't changed. Fried Anything and Everything is still pretty much the meal *du jour,* along with the standard greasy burger. Throw in a shake or a soda to wash down the fatty food, and you've got instant weight gain — in a fun box with a toy!

Parents often don't think that feeding children fatty foods is going to do them any harm. Just because they're kids doesn't mean that their bodies can handle it any better than adults' bodies. Not only do children get fat on these meals, but evidence indicates that they can develop what cardiologists refer to as *fatty streaks* in the arteries. Fatty streaks are indicators of high cholesterol taking root and starting to do its damage — *in children!*

TIP

DDR is a-ok

Interestingly, one video game gets the thumbs up from doctors and researchers in the field of childhood obesity. It's called Dance Dance Revolution (DDR) and is so effective in getting kids off the couch and moving to the beat that at least one health insurance company is considering paying for the game for children who are diagnosed as being obese.

The game works like so:

1. A dance pad with arrows pointing to the front, back, and sides is laid on the floor and hooked up to a video game system.

2. The DDR disc is loaded into the game system.

3. Kids dance to the songs as animations on the TV screen light up the arrows to indicate which direction their feet should move on the dance pad.

4. The game keeps track of correct steps and missteps, and the dancer collects points accordingly.

This game gets kids dancing like wild people — they end up sweating bullets, trying to perfect the dance combinations. (A separate component can even be hooked up to include hand movements.)

The beauty of this game is that it's a good fit for almost any kid. Your son doesn't need to be an all-star athlete to get his groove on in the family room. The competitive nature of DDR also drives kids to want to continue playing — against friends or against the machine — and that *keeps* them moving. So far, the official preliminary studies done by the insurance agency look promising, and this game may well end up being a prescription for overweight kids.

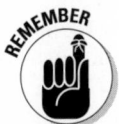
REMEMBER

The fast food giants are some of the biggest advertisers during children's television shows. These guys poke their heads right into your family room and tell your kids how great their food is. Your kids, in turn, beg you to take them, and *you* fall prey to these ads, too. Put your foot down and say, "No more fast food for *my* family!"

What's wrong with fast food

You know how the whole fast food habit gets started with kids: They want the toy in the kids' meal, and they eat the meal because it's there. Before you know it, they're bugging you for a kids' meal two or three times a week, and because it's so easy — and because you've finally found a meal that even your pickiest child will scarf down — you're only too happy to oblige.

Fast food is such bad news that it's hard to know where to begin. Here are the biggies:

✔ **Fast food is loaded with fat, cholesterol, triglycerides, and all sorts of things you don't want floating around and taking up residence in your child's body.** Not only do these compounds cause obesity, but they've also been linked with the development of heart disease and diabetes.

The fats that are most prevalent in fast food are saturated fats and trans fats — the kinds that are most likely to cause damage to the arteries (as opposed to unsaturated and monounsaturated fats).

✔ **You child can become hooked on fast food because it appeals to biological cravings for salt, sugar, and fat.**

✔ **The soda that usually accompanies a child's meal contains *no* nutrients, only calories from sugar that are easily converted into fat.**

✔ **Children who eat fast food on a regular basis (at least three times a week) are less likely to choose healthier foods like fruits, vegetables, milk, and whole grains when given the opportunity.**

✔ **Fast food feeds into the "super-size" mentality of larger-than-normal portion sizes, which can carry over into the home.**

Finding alternative restaurant food

In many cases, take-out restaurants are no better than drive-thrus where nutrition's concerned. Your local pizzeria may offer a salad or two, but a pizza crust that's made with lard and topped with extra pepperoni, extra cheese, and bacon is every bit as unhealthy as that double-bacon cheeseburger your teenagers love so much. And dishes like chicken parmesan and fish and chips are loaded with grease and fat. Just because something takes a little longer to cook than fries and a burger doesn't make it healthier.

Fortunately, many larger sit-down restaurants have turned the corner and offer kids healthier choices. Red Lobster is a great example of this trend. Their children's menu actually offers grilled fish served with raw veggies (and dip), a salad, or applesauce! That's quite an improvement over the standard chicken fingers and fries that are on almost every kid's menu everywhere.

In a sit-down restaurant, you can modify the standard child's meal and make it less fattening, but you have to know what to avoid in the first place. When you peruse a children's menu, eliminate the following right off the bat:

✔ **Fried mozzarella cheese sticks:** Although cheese is loaded with calcium, an essential nutrient for growing bones, most of the nutritional value of any food is lost the moment it enters the deep fryer. (Plus, that cheese in the middle is *not* of the low-fat variety.)

✔ **Chicken fingers, fried chicken, chicken nuggets, and popcorn chicken:** Although chicken is hailed as a low-fat meat, breast meat isn't usually used to produce processed chicken foods (like nuggets or patties). And even if it were white meat, after it's breaded and cooked in oil, it's just *fried* meat, which is high in fat no matter where it comes from.

✔ **Burgers with extra cheese, bacon, and mayo:** The burgers served in restaurants may be slightly lower in fat than drive-thru burgers, which makes them a marginally better choice than anything fried.

If a burger is your only option, encourage your children to leave off extra fattening toppings. If they have to have *something* on that burger, lettuce, tomato, pickles, ketchup, and mustard are some good low-fat choices. Also, adding veggies may satisfy an older child by adding more *zing* to the texture of a burger or sandwich.

✔ **Specialty drinks:** Your child opens the menu to find a milkshake layered with cookie pieces served in the world's tallest mug and topped off with whipped cream. Say no to his request for dessert-before-the-meal and encourage him to drink water or low-fat milk instead.

✔ **Fries:** Because childhood obesity has become such a far-reaching issue, many restaurants will honor your request to substitute a small salad or some type of fruit or vegetable in place of French fries that come with a kid's meal, even if these options aren't listed on the menu. Ask and you just may receive.

✔ **Dessert:** In many chain restaurants, servers are trained to push decadent cakes, sundaes, and pies on their customers. Desserts are usually big-profit items (along with appetizers), and because purchasing a round of ice cream boosts your bill, it also increases your server's tip. Just say no to dessert in restaurants and have some fresh fruit waiting at home.

Changing the dining-out habits of a child who has already firmly established what she will and won't eat can be hard. Young children tend to be much more malleable — that is, you can change their palates (their desire for certain foods) much more easily than older kids' because you're the boss, for one thing. If you say no to fried chicken, then the answer is no (and should remain no, no matter how much begging, whining, or crying goes on).

An older child may be interested in ordering from the adult menu, which generally offers more low-fat options or meals that are easily modified into lower-fat versions of what's listed on the menu. If your child is ordering from the regular section of the menu, check out which side dishes are included with a sandwich or meal. Grilled chicken with a side of fries is two steps forward and one step back.

If an adult meal is just too much for your child to handle, consider splitting a low-fat breakfast, lunch, or dinner. The portions served up in many restaurants are too large for many adults, so splitting a meal may work out perfectly for you and your child. Also, sharing is a great way for you to show her that you're also eating more healthfully.

For more advice on how to maintain healthy eating habits in restaurants and other places outside the home, flip to Chapter 12.

Eat healthy at home when time is limited

Every mother and father in the world — whether they work or stay at home with the kids — has, at one time or another, realized that there just isn't enough time in the day to do everything that needs to be done — including cooking.

Falling back on convenience foods

Today, countless precooked and frozen meal options make life easier. Deli counters and grocery store freezer cases full of frozen foods offer up fast and easy meal options that require no more work than turning the oven up to 400 degrees or punching a few buttons on the microwave.

These meals are often referred to as *convenience foods* because they're so easy to prepare. In fact, little or no preparation is required! You don't have to cut, measure, or season anything. If you can work the temperature gauge on the oven and operate the microwave, you're good to go.

Convenience foods are usually — but not always — frozen and may include:

- Casseroles
- Pizza
- Burritos or enchiladas
- Egg rolls
- Mini burgers
- TV dinners

Convenience foods tend to be high in saturated and trans fats, which translate into increased body fat and high cholesterol levels. Saturated and trans fats occur naturally in certain foods; however, most of the trans fats we end up eating are man-made by adding hydrogen to vegetable oil, which basically converts a liquid fat into a solid fat. For this reason, trans fats are also called *hydrogenated fats*. They're added to foods for two main reasons:

- To increase shelf life
- To make the taste more appealing to consumers

But so what? What's the deal with trans fats? Who cares if they help foods last longer and make them taste better? That's what we want! Well, along with "better" taste, you and your family get a healthy dose of a substance that contributes to elevated cholesterol levels and, subsequently, heart disease. These conditions can take root in childhood, especially in severely overweight and obese children.

Fat comes in different packages. Unsaturated, monounsaturated, and polyunsaturated fats tend not to be converted into body fat as easily as saturated and trans fats are. In addition, saturated and trans fats cause cholesterol levels to rise (even in kids). Trans fats are usually listed on food labels as *partially hydrogenated oils*.

High-fat convenience foods also tend to be high in sodium, which acts as a preservative and a taste enhancer. However, excessive sodium raises blood pressure and contributes to heart disease.

Finding convenient — and healthy — options

We're not saying that prepared meals aren't a godsend once in awhile. If you're working full time, two of your kids are involved in eight different activities during the week, and you're not even sure which kid you're supposed to pick up or where he or she might be at the moment, the least of your concerns is putting a balanced meal on the table. You're fairly sure that your children wouldn't eat it anyway! They prefer frozen lasagna over your home cooking, and the act of tossing a block of frozen noodles and cheese into the oven will *just* meet your tolerance for meal preparation this evening. We understand — honest. But healthy cooking doesn't have to be difficult or take hours on end.

Plenty of foods in the frozen-food aisle also qualify as healthy convenience foods. Frozen vegetables, for example, usually don't have any fat or salt added to them; frozen fruit is another healthy option, as are low-fat frozen meals (although these are often on the small side and may need to be coupled with salad or a separate side of vegetables). So we're not advising that you skip the frozen aisle altogether; rather, we advise that you take a closer look at what you select there.

If you just don't have time to cook dinner every night, consider cooking two or three big meals over the weekend and freezing leftovers for the week. Or browse cookbooks and surf the Internet for easy, low-fat recipes. Vegetable stir-fry, for example, can be very low in fat if you don't use a lot of oil from the get-go. It involves chopping and steaming veggies, but it's still a lot less involved than, say, preparing a huge turkey in the oven. Chapter 9 has more tips for preparing healthy meals in your kitchen.

Eat As I Say, Not As I Eat: How Parents Pass Along Bad Habits

To help your child lose weight, you can turn off the TV, make her go outside to play, encourage her to make healthier choices in restaurants, and start cooking low-fat meals for her at home. But if *you* don't change your own bad habits, your child is less likely to succeed in changing hers.

Studies have shown time and time again that an obese child needs intensive parental involvement in order to lose weight and keep it off in the long run. A big part of this requirement is due to the fact that parents control the purse strings and the family car and therefore also have a lot of control over the food that comes into the house.

If you push fresh green beans on your kids at dinnertime while you prepare a batch of frozen pizza bagels for yourself, they're going to have a hard time accepting your spiel about living a healthier lifestyle. And it doesn't matter if you're thin and your kids aren't. They need to see that you're committed to health, first and foremost.

Conquering obesity isn't about improving your child's appearance, although that may be a side effect of weight loss. Adapting to a healthier lifestyle is all about improving health, and that's something that every person, regardless of size or weight, should aim for.

Most obese children don't have glandular problems that cause weight gain, nor do they have thin parents; one or both parents usually have weight problems (and just to be absolutely clear, the parents don't have glandular problems, either). Even the parents' parents may have weight problems. One reason doctors have such difficulty nailing down the nature-or-nurture aspect of obesity is because it's probably a little bit of both. Some families may be predisposed to weight gain, but they also make poor lifestyle choices that lead to obesity and pass their attitudes about food and exercise on to the next generation.

Obese children tend to come from families in which:

- **At least one parent is significantly overweight or obese.**

- **Food is everything.** It's love, it's comfort, it's entertainment, and it's the topic of almost every conversation. As a result, life revolves around the next meal.

✔ **Television is a constant presence.** There may be a TV in the kitchen, the family room, and each bedroom, so no one misses out on more than five minutes of TV while they're at home.

✔ **Activity is regarded as a burden.** The thought of leaving the house to do something outdoors or at a community center seems overwhelming or like a waste of time.

Does this sound like your family? An obese child doesn't commonly appear in a family in which people are active, healthy meals are the norm, and everyone is of normal weight. Bad habits in the family contribute *significantly* to the development of obesity in children. Even if you've acknowledged your own weight issues and made a good effort to prevent your child from becoming overweight, children tend to copy their parents' behaviors. And if you don't have a handle on your own eating habits, you can't really judge how well your child is doing with hers.

If you have weight issues, educating yourself on the issue of obesity in general is the key to helping your child. This book will certainly help, but you may also want to:

✔ Read books that address adult weight problems.

✔ Join a weight-loss group, where you find out more about nutrition.

✔ Speak to your doctor about the best options for your own weight-loss program.

Schools Paying the Price for Obesity

Overweight children who are victimized by bullies are more apt to fake illness in order to skip school. Not only does this behavior affect the child, but it also affects the school. Consider this:

✔ Some states base their funding for schools on an acceptable level of attendance.

✔ Other states base funding on each school's performance on standardized tests.

✔ When a school has a high absentee rate, its funding is likely to drop.

"Well, so what?" you may say. "If the school isn't providing my child with the services he needs, why should I care if it gets its money?" You should care because the less money a school receives from the state, the less chance there is that anything will change and work to the advantage of overweight children. A school that's short on funding may not have a gym teacher, for example, or an outdoor play area that's suitable for kids. A school that's in dire financial straits is also more likely than other schools to fall prey to fast-food vendors who are more than eager to set up shop in any school cafeteria.

Schools that enter into contracts with fast food vendors make (and save) a great deal of money from the partnership. The fast food vendors, meanwhile, are more than happy to hook loyal customers for life. The best interests of the students and their health are lost in the shuffle.

Take a good look at your child's school to figure out whether it's a relatively healthy environment or one that's detrimental to its students' overall health. Here are some questions to ask as you examine the school and its practices:

- ✔ Does the school have a physical education program? How many times a week do students participate? What kinds of activities do they do? If your child is in elementary school, is there time (and space) for daily recess?

- ✔ Does the cafeteria have a fast-food banner hanging over the serving area? Are any healthy options offered, like salads, low-fat meats (a chicken breast sandwich, for example), and whole-grain breads?

- ✔ Are the walls of the cafeteria lined with vending machines stocked with soda and candy bars?

- ✔ What's the school's line on discrimination of any kind, including "fat discrimination"?

If you're not exactly the activist type, you may be wondering what good this type of investigation can do. Because your child spends most of her time at school, you need to know whether the school is helping or hurting your efforts to institute a healthy lifestyle with your family. You can talk about health at home until you're blue in the face, but if your child's unable to walk into that cafeteria and purchase a healthy lunch . . . you need to know that. If the school feels that bullying is something that kids should work out between themselves . . . you need to know *that.* If recess is nothing more than a time for youngsters to sit and play hand-held video games . . . you need to know *that.*

You're trying so hard to un-teach your child about *un*healthy habits. If she's hearing one thing at home and living the complete opposite experience at school, she may end up being confused at best; at worst, she may end up doing as the Romans do, so to speak, when she's at school, which will significantly impede her progress at home.

Mixed messages between home and school can affect your child's physical and emotional well-being. If she's in a mostly healthy environment at school, she'll probably fare much better in her quest to adapt to a healthy lifestyle. If she's facing obstacles every which way she turns (like if she really wants to go outside after lunch but instead is only given free time to read in the classroom, or if she has her mind set on choosing a healthy lunch but can't find one in the cafeteria), however, maintaining a healthy lifestyle will be harder — which is *not* to say it will be impossible. She may have to start packing her own lunch, for example, and you may have to make sure that she gets outside after school for more time than if she were also playing on the playground at school each day. The point is, the school environment affects her life substantially, and you need to see it firsthand in order to counteract any negative messages she brings home.

Chapter 3

Facing the Physical Effects of Childhood Obesity: The Damage You Don't See

As the parent of an obese child, you face a plethora of worries: Not only does your child deal with all sorts of emotional and social issues (like low self-esteem that stems from teasing), but he's also at high risk for developing serious, life-long physical ailments. The threat of these conditions is enough to keep you awake at night, worried for your obese child's life. The good news, however, is that many of these conditions are reversible or can at least be diminished if caught early enough.

Some parents are fooled by youth; they think that kids are resilient and that it's just not possible for something as commonplace as extra weight to do serious and sometimes permanent damage to a child's body. That kind of thinking is very dangerous, though, because it keeps parents from dealing with the gravity of their child's physical condition. So the first step in dealing with the serious physical effects of childhood obesity is acknowledging that they do occur with great frequency among obese children and that the sooner you can stop the problem, the more likely you are to mitigate the damage or reverse it altogether.

This chapter delves into the most common medical complications that arise from childhood obesity. Keep in mind that this chapter isn't intended to help you diagnose or cure ailments; only your child's doctor can do that. Rather, it's an overview of what can and does happen in the obese body on a regular basis. We shy away from using medical jargon as much as possible in the interest of keeping the information as easy to understand as possible.

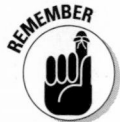

Perhaps the most frustrating part of these conditions is that they begin silently. Your child may not even realize when these ailments start to occur, so it's a safe bet that you won't, either. This chapter doesn't give you a particularly sunny view of what lies down the road for a child who remains obese. Is this information some kind of scare tactic? A bucket-of-ice-water-in-the-face wake-up call? Something to make you worry even more about your child? No. These are simply the facts.

Type 2 Diabetes

You probably know or have known someone with type 2 diabetes, and chances are, that person is an overweight adult. It wasn't until fairly recently that type 2 diabetes began popping up with some regularity in kids. And what do most of these kids have in common? You guessed it — they're obese.

But what *is* diabetes? How does it start? What does it do? Why is it such a dangerous disease? Basically, the condition results either from the body's inability to produce *insulin,* a hormone produced by the pancreas, or from the body's inability to use insulin properly. Insulin is necessary for breaking down sugar in the body and using its byproducts for energy. When sugar isn't metabolized properly, it builds up in the body, wreaking all sorts of havoc (which we get into later in this section).

A little background on diabetes

The two types of diabetes are

 ✔ **Type 1:** Occurs when the body simply doesn't produce enough insulin. Its onset is usually rapid and not related to weight gain; in fact, one symptom of this type of diabetes is weight *loss.*

Type 1 diabetes used to be called *juvenile diabetes* because it was once the only type of diabetes that doctors commonly saw in people under 30. Nowadays, type 2 diabetes is becoming so common among younger people that using the term *juvenile* to describe type 1 is misleading.

✔ **Type 2:** Occurs when a person has too much fatty tissue. In this environment, insulin just can't do its job correctly, which leads to a condition called insulin resistance; for that reason, type 2 is also sometimes called *insulin-resistant diabetes.* Due to the amount of food that they consume, obese children routinely rely on their bodies to produce an increased amount of insulin. One theory is that these kids' bodies just can't keep up with the demand, which is a pretty frightening thought considering children have to rely on their bodies for a long, long time.

Among kids, type 2 diabetes is most often found in obese adolescents and obese kids who have reached puberty. (Obesity can speed puberty along, which is why pubescent kids aren't always necessarily adolescents — at least not age-wise). Most of the obese kids who develop type 2 diabetes also have a family history of the disease. Some ethnic groups, including African Americans, Asians, Hispanics, and American Indians, are at higher risk than others for the disease.

Metabolic syndrome

In obese children who haven't yet reached puberty or adolescence, it's not uncommon to find what doctors call *metabolic syndrome,* a precursor to type 2 diabetes (and another condition that used to be seen mostly in adults). A doctor can diagnose metabolic syndrome if a child meets three of the following criteria:

✔ Obesity

✔ High blood sugar

✔ Increased blood pressure

✔ Raised levels of triglycerides

✔ Decreased levels of *high-density lipoprotein,* or HDL, the "good" cholesterol

Pretty alarming, yes? These conditions sound better suited to your old Uncle Sal, who's been eating sausages and smoking like a fiend for 50 years — not your child! The good news is that metabolic syndrome can be corrected and reversed through exercise, healthy eating, and weight loss; the bad news is that as soon as it progresses to diabetes, there's no going back.

Recognizing type 2 symptoms and complications

The health conditions that obese kids face are often insidious — they begin without much notice. Although your child may not have any sense of feeling unwell, symptoms of type 2 diabetes often include:

- ✔ Increased thirst and urination
- ✔ Blurry vision
- ✔ Increased appetite
- ✔ Constant tiredness
- ✔ Frequent infections, or infections or wounds that are very slow to heal

And what are the long-term complications of diabetes? Diabetes damages the blood vessels, which leads to:

- ✔ Kidney damage
- ✔ Eye problems
- ✔ Nerve damage
- ✔ Vascular disease

Common long-term complications of diabetes are varied and include blindness, amputation of the feet and legs, and complete kidney failure. (By *long-term,* we're talking about some of these conditions developing as early as the 20s or 30s if a person is diagnosed with diabetes in childhood.) Because the biggest risk factor for developing type 2 diabetes is obesity, stopping an obese child's weight gain as soon as possible is imperative. To get started, check out Part II of this book.

Good cholesterol?

In a nutshell, cholesterol comes in two varieties: LDL (low-density lipoprotein) and HDL (high-density lipoprotein). LDL is the "bad" cholesterol; it's what sticks to the arterial walls, causing blood clots and, by extension, heart attacks, poor circulation, and so on. HDL is the body's helper in that it helps to clear out those arteries, thus reducing one's chance of developing serious complications from cholesterol.

The latest recommendations on cholesterol are to not just lower the overall level but *increase* the HDL level. The easy way to remember which cholesterol is which is to look at it this way: You want *LDL* levels to be *low* and *HDL* levels to be *high.*

Up, Up, and Away: High Blood Pressure

Blood pressure technically measures the force of your blood pumping against the arterial walls. If you take a look at where that pressure comes from, you can say that blood pressure is the measure of how hard the heart is working. When a nurse straps that cuff on your child's arm and pumps it up, she's measuring his blood pressure. Normally, you're informed right then and there if the reading is high (indicating that the heart is working overtime). Children whose readings are marginal (on the high side) are often diagnosed with something called *prehypertension,* an indication that blood pressure may soon be out of control.

Increased blood pressure used to be seen primarily in adults but now is also a serious threat to obese children and adolescents. High blood pressure means that the heart is working harder than it should. Elevated blood pressure can be traced to a number of factors, like stress and certain kidney diseases, but being overweight is also a major cause.

Overweight and obese people tend to eat foods that are high in fat and cholesterol. When that food is broken down in the body, the cholesterol is deposited in the blood vessels, narrowing the passageways for blood to flow through. As a result, the heart pumps harder to get that blood through.

The serious ramifications of high blood pressure include an increased risk of heart disease, stroke, and kidney disease. Sure, these are serious ailments, but we're talking about children. These things just don't happen to kids, do they?

Well, with increasing regularity, they *are* happening to kids. Although the frequency of strokes, for example, in children is still quite low, the fact that these serious, adult-type ailments are striking obese kids *at all* is really frightening. Pediatricians are at a loss to compare these problems to anything they've seen in the past.

The danger of high blood pressure is that it does its damage over time. Even though your obese 10-year-old may seem to be doing well enough, he's at risk for developing serious complications as he gets older. When the rest of his friends are going strong through their early adulthood, your son's obesity and high blood pressure may catch up to him, and unfortunately, it's not all that uncommon to hear of an obese 30-year-old with heart disease. That's just too young for someone to be faced with a lifetime of illness.

Children who suffer from sleep apnea, a serious sleep disorder, also tend to have high blood pressure. We talk about sleep apnea as it relates to obesity in the "Sleep apnea" section later in this chapter.

Now for some good news about weight-induced high blood pressure: Even if an obese child's blood pressure is high enough to warrant medication, lifestyle changes can usually correct the condition to the point where the child doesn't have to stay on medication indefinitely. Eating healthy, low-fat foods and exercising, which increases blood flow and also helps to cleanse those arteries, can produce great results if the condition's caught and corrected early enough.

Strains and Pains

If a 100-pound person jumped up and sat on your shoulders, you'd notice, right? Aside from the immediate annoyance you'd feel toward whoever was taking up residence on your person, eventually your legs would feel tired, your knees might buckle, and you'd have to sit down (or toss the joker off his perch — or both).

The human body is only able to handle so much weight before joints, muscles, and bones start giving way. Because weight gain is usually a gradual process, it may seem reasonable enough to expect body parts to simply adapt to the extra pounds, but that's just not the way things turn out. Obese kids have an increased risk of:

✔ Decreased movement

✔ Fractures

✔ Joint deformities

✔ Joint pain

From decreased movement to fractures

Decreased movement is a big issue because obese children are often unable to move in all the ways that children should move. They're less likely to run and play sports because they find it too difficult to bend, stretch, and keep up with everyone else. Even the mundane activities of everyday life, like cleaning a bedroom, become impossible. And this inability to move properly leads to less movement, which makes the existing weight problem even worse.

Bones need weight-bearing exercise (which isn't nearly as involved as it sounds — walking is a weight-bearing exercise) to become strong and stay that way. When a person isn't able to strengthen bones through exercise, the bones actually become weaker, which makes them more prone to fracture. Fractures can further reduce mobility, which, of course, makes bones even more frail. The problem can build upon itself until a person is effectively immobile.

Simple physics also increase obese kids' risk of bone fractures. When these kids tumble, they bring their own weight down upon themselves. So if your daughter is 50 pounds overweight and she trips, it's like she has a 50-pound weight strapped to her back, pushing her into the ground with that much force. If she lands the wrong way on her wrist or her knee, you can imagine how easily the bone would break.

Loss of mobility is a problem that doctors take very seriously, and not just where obese children are concerned. The elderly, for example, are another population in which weak bones are a primary concern. The fact that children and elderly men and women share a common diagnosis is startling.

Joint points

Joint abnormalities are somewhat common among obese kids, but that doesn't make them any less serious. Conditions in the joints caused by obesity can lead to permanent deformity. Some of the more common joint problems include:

- ✔ **Bowing:** The knees and shins of overweight children obviously bear a lot of extra weight, so these bones may bow, causing pain and decreasing movement (which leads back to the preceding section).
- ✔ **Slipped capital femoral epiphysis:** In this hip condition, the ball of the hip joint doesn't develop properly, causing pain in either the hip or knee of an obese child.

Bone and joint pain can be the toughest obstacle to introducing an obese child to an exercise program. Exercise is sure to feel out of the question if your child's in pain whenever she moves. If your child suffers from bone or joint pain, non-weight-bearing exercises like swimming and cycling may be better options until she's lost at least some of the weight.

Back it up!

Back problems are an area of great concern with obese children. The spine is made up of joints called *vertebra* that are stacked on top of each other.

Excess weight causes them to compress, which results in back pain. This compression can lead to incredibly painful arthritic conditions of the spine.

Other back problems brought on by obesity include:

- **Degenerative disc disease:** Deterioration of the discs of the vertebra, leaving bone rubbing on bone
- **Sciatica:** Inflammation of the sciatic nerve running from the spine down the back of each leg
- **Spinal stenosis:** Narrowing of the spine, leading to increased pressure on the spinal cord

Obese children also tend not to have the best posture, which is something else that can bring on back pain and strain. Reminding your child to stand or sit up straight may help alleviate back pain.

If you know anyone who has suffered from back pain, then you know that it can be a debilitating condition. Taking the pressure off the vertebra before any permanent damage results is necessary for preventing years and years of excruciating pain.

Heavy Breathing: Asthma and Sleep Apnea

Obese children often experience labored breathing, and as a parent, you can only imagine how terrifying and frustrating it must be for your child to try as hard as he can and still feel as though he isn't filling his lungs sufficiently.

Asthma is a fairly common condition, and it can be brought on by a variety of triggers, one of which is obesity. There are a couple of theories as to how asthma relates to obesity. In this section, we talk about how obesity may bring on asthmatic conditions, and we also discuss sleep apnea, a condition marked by difficulty breathing during sleep.

Asthma and obesity

Asthma and obesity are both on the rise in this country, and there's some question as to whether obesity causes asthma . . . or asthma causes obesity.

The current thinking on the issue is that instead of being a trigger for asthma, obesity is a condition that it makes a bad situation even worse.

More and more kids are being diagnosed with obesity, and more kids are having a hard time with their lung function. Because these children are having a tough time catching their collective breath, they aren't getting much exercise — either by choice or because their parents won't allow it for fear of bringing on an asthmatic episode.

Wow. That's a tough position for a parent to be in. If your child is legitimately having trouble breathing because she has asthma, you obviously aren't going to send her off to the playing fields. And if she's also obese, you may be wracking your brain, trying to figure out how in the world you can help this child lose weight if she can't take 20 steps without her inhaler.

The 411 on asthma

To best understand asthma as it relates to obesity, you need a good, solid understanding of asthma on its own. Essentially, asthma causes a swelling of the lining of the airways. The muscles around the airways tighten, and the mucus produced clogs the airways and makes breathing difficult (and sometimes next to impossible). The following is a list of things that can trigger asthma attacks:

- **Allergens:** Cat hair, dust, mold, pollen
- **Stress:** Strong emotional reactions, like fear or shock
- **The elements:** Cold air, heat, humidity
- **Pollutants:** Smoke, smog, perfume, anything with a strong odor
- **Respiratory infections:** A bad cold, flu, sinus infection
- **Exercise:** Physical activity, particularly in cold weather

The role of obesity in triggering asthma

For decades, doctors have believed that people are either born with asthmatic tendencies or they aren't and that the right triggers have to be in place for someone with a genetic predisposition to the disease to actually develop it. (In other words, you may be born with asthmatic tendencies and never know it if nothing ever triggered an asthma attack.)

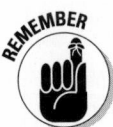

Recall that asthma causes a tightening of the muscles around the airways. Part of the new theory about obesity and asthma suggests that a significant amount of extra weight adds to the pressure exerted on the airways during an asthma attack. Another part of the obesity/asthma theory suggests that extra weight around the lungs may actually trigger an asthmatic episode because the excess weight narrows the airway passages, but, to date, this theory hasn't been proven.

What doctors know for sure is that adipose tissue (that's simply fat tissue, dressed in up medical terms) releases an inflammatory chemical called *interleukin* into the bloodstream and that this substance is found in elevated amounts in the blood of obese men, women, and children. Asthma symptoms result from an inflammation of the airways, so it stands to reason that someone with a genetic predisposition toward asthma *and* an excess amount of this inflammatory chemical floating around in the bloodstream would probably go on to develop asthma and that the asthma may only be exacerbated by the individual's weight problem.

Studies have shown that obese asthmatic children tend to have more severe reactions to triggers like smog and smoke; these reactions are most likely linked to increased levels of interleukin.

What else do doctors know for sure about asthma and obesity? Although many normal-weight children outgrow asthma by the time they reach their teen years, obese children are more likely to hang onto the condition through adulthood. Doctors aren't quite sure why this is so, but it's something they're seeing more and more frequently.

The final word on the connection between asthma and obesity in children is that it's a chicken-or-the-egg kind of issue. As of this writing, no one really knows which brings on which or if one condition makes the other one worse. Because both asthma and obesity are becoming so prevalent among kids, it's safe to say that research on these topics will continue and that, hopefully soon, a definitive link will be made between the two and improve treatment options.

Sleep apnea

Admit it: You still sneak into your kids' rooms at night just to make sure they're breathing. The parents of obese children sometimes get a shock when they realize their children aren't breathing, at least temporarily. *Obstructive sleep apnea* (OSA) is a condition that occurs in overweight children and adults and results in a person not breathing for ten seconds or more on a regular basis throughout the night. The person then wakes up gasping for breath and may or may not remember the episode in the morning.

OSA also affects older people and is usually associated with having a large neck. The neck is so full of fatty tissue that when the child lies down, the throat narrows, making breathing extremely difficult. Snoring is one of the classic symptoms of OSA (though not all people who snore have a breathing problem).

On the surface, OSA sounds scary — anything that causes your child to stop breathing, however temporary, is frightening. OSA and resulting sleeplessness can lead to some pretty grave social and health conditions, including:

- Constant fatigue
- Morning headaches
- Inability to concentrate and decreased attention span, leading to lower grades and poor judgment
- Hyperactivity
- Bedwetting
- Weight gain
- Depression

Sleep is incredibly important for children and adolescents; it's the time when their bodies grow and reenergize for what lies ahead the next day. And OSA often isn't limited to just one episode of gasping for air; some children awaken repeatedly throughout the night, every night, and don't remember anything about it (because they're *exhausted*).

When a child loses sleep on a regular basis, her body doesn't perform as it should. Metabolism slows down, which results in unused calories and, in turn, excess weight. Hormones are also thrown off balance, resulting in an increased feeling of hunger. Overall, OSA is linked to a definite decline in the enjoyment of life. How can a child have a productive day if she's fatigued and otherwise not feeling well? The findings that reveal that OSA can cause weight gain make this another vicious cycle that obese kids face: They're too tired to exercise but are physically unable to catch up on their sleep so that maybe tomorrow they'll feel (and do) better.

Even if your child isn't suffering any apparent daytime effects of OSA, the condition can lead to very serious physical ailments down the road, including high blood pressure and heart disease.

Fatty Liver

When we say "fatty liver," we're talking about an actual medical diagnosis; we're not insulting an oversized liver. The full name of this condition is *nonalcoholic fatty liver disease* (NAFLD), and it refers to the tendency of fat to accumulate in the livers of obese children and adults and people with diabetes.

So what does the liver do? A lot. Functions of the liver include:

- Absorbing fat
- Filtering toxins
- Regulating blood sugar
- Producing hormones and vitamins
- Storing minerals and iron

Wow! That's some organ!

While fatty liver in and of itself isn't all that harmful, its potential for destruction is big. NAFLD can cause inflammation of the liver, which can lead to scarring and other irregularities in the tissue. This damage can lead to a more serious inflammatory condition of the liver called *nonalcoholic steatohepatitis* (NASH).

Some doctors argue that all obese children should be tested for liver problems in order to stop the most serious damage before it goes too far. Ask your child's doctor about testing.

These liver conditions are diseases that progress very slowly, and the end results are rarely positive. Studies suggest that a child who develops NASH has a fairly good chance of going on to suffer from cirrhosis (scarring) of the liver later in life. The scarring blocks blood flow and pretty much shuts down the liver altogether. It's irreversible and very serious. Cirrhosis of the liver is also most commonly seen in long-term alcoholics, which gives you some idea of the damage that excess fat can do to the liver.

The concern here isn't that obese children are in immediate danger of developing a terminal illness of the liver; rather, the worry is that they're laying the groundwork for these ailments to more easily take root later in life. Liver disease is very hard to treat, let alone cure, so patients often end up on the list for donor livers (with varying degrees of success, of course). Liver donation is another worry within the medical community, because with the way obesity rates among children are climbing, it seems likely that in 10 or 15 years, the waiting list for donor livers may be filled with relatively young people.

Skin Eruptions

Yes, this chapter is called "The Damage You Don't See," and you can, of course, see most skin problems. However, at least one skin condition that's common among obese children stems from an *inner* physical condition. So you see, what we see isn't always the result of what we're seeing. (Confused? Read on.)

Pigment problems

Acanthosis nigricans is a skin condition characterized by markings around the armpits, neck, or groin. The marks are light to dark brown and look like flat velvet. Acanthosis nigricans doesn't affect only obese people, but in obese people, the condition's the result of elevated insulin levels.

What on earth do insulin levels have to do with brown marks on the skin? When there's too much insulin wandering around inside the body, it looks for a place to crash; the insulin goes in search of insulin receptors for this purpose, and it finds them in certain areas of the body (neck, armpits, and groin). Although acanthosis nigricans is a painless condition, it can be embarrassing. Sometimes a change in diet is enough to minimize its appearance; in other cases, a topical ointment may be prescribed.

When acanthosis nigricans appears, you know something's going on inside the body. Skin eruptions usually don't do any permanent damage (aside from acne, which can leave scars behind in thin kids *and* heavy kids), but they can be uncomfortable. Don't lose sleep over them, but do take your child for a doctor's visit.

Rashes

Obese kids are more susceptible than others to heat rash, an irritation of the top layer of the skin due to excessive perspiration. It doesn't need to be a hot, humid day in order for someone to break out in heat rash. Overweight people tend to perspire more than their thinner counterparts regardless of the environment, and sweat is the key player in this irritating rash.

Although rashes may seem like the least of your worries where your obese child is concerned, they're one more physical side effect of being overweight.

Fungus among us

Fungal infections can pop up in the skin folds of obese kids because fungi need a damp, warm environment in order to grow, and flaps of flesh do just fine. Fungal rashes are serious because

- ✔ They can be very painful.
- ✔ They can spread rapidly.
- ✔ They need to be treated with a topical antifungal. Soap and water won't do the trick, nor will any over-the-counter lotions or ointments.

If you suspect your child has a fungal skin infection, she should see her doctor as soon as possible.

All Backed Up: Digestive Problems

Kids love to tell jokes about constipation and dirty underwear. Digestive problems aren't so funny, though, when your child suffers from them on a chronic basis.

Obese kids are more prone to constipation than other kids because they're more likely to eat cookies, chips, and ice cream rather than healthy, fibrous foods such as fruits, veggies, and whole grains. If your child isn't eating enough (or any) fiber, his body will have a pretty tough time getting the remnants of the food moving through the intestines. Cleaning out the colon is fiber's main job and the reason why it's so important for good health. (Fiber also fills the stomach faster than sugar- or fat-loaded snacks do.)

Some of the side effects of constipation include:

- ✔ Nausea
- ✔ Gas pain
- ✔ Heartburn
- ✔ Painful straining in the bathroom (which can lead to hemorrhoids and fissures, which are tears in the rectal opening)

So, these may not be the most serious of all medical conditions, but chronic constipation can be very uncomfortable and cause depression (wouldn't you be depressed if you felt bound up all the time?); it also puts one at risk for developing colon cancer later in life. Cleaning out that bowel every day should be your child's goal! (Well, one of his goals.)

Not only are obese kids at a higher risk for constipation, but they're also more prone to *fecal soiling* (having an accident — large or small — in their underpants). As for why fecal soiling occurs more frequently in obese children, there's no solid answer, but it may be due to diet. Certain foods rich in sugar and grease can result in loose stools. The amount of food that an obese child takes in is substantial, and the substantial byproducts have to come out eventually.

Fecal soiling isn't considered a harmful condition, but certainly it can be a mortifying experience for a kid who's dealing with enough problems already. Kids may be too embarrassed to talk about it or ask for help. If you suspect that your child is having fecal soiling accidents, let him know he can talk to you without being embarrassed. Together, you can talk to his doctor and attempt to find a solution.

Heart Disease

You're an adult. If you're even slightly overweight, you've no doubt heard your doctor say, "Lose the weight!" But why? If you're not obese, and you're not at high risk for developing any of the ailments we talk about in this chapter, what harm can a few extra pounds do?

Heart disease is the leading killer of men and women in the United States. Damage to the heart and blood vessels can begin in childhood and is due to an unhealthy lifestyle! Although not all heart disease can be prevented, most of it can be. Being overweight puts a major strain on the heart and is one of the main factors in developing heart trouble. So if lugging around 15 extra pounds is reason for concern, carrying 50, 60, or 100 excess pounds is really reason to worry.

High cholesterol

High cholesterol plays a major part in the development of heart disease. We talk about HDL and LDL levels earlier in this chapter (see the sidebar "*Good cholesterol?*"), and we also discuss how cholesterol deposits itself on the walls of blood vessels. High cholesterol means that one has significant cholesterol buildup in his or her blood vessels. As blood tries to churn its way through the blood vessels, it gets caught on the cholesterol, causing a blood clot. Ultimately, the blood clot may finally break free and either travel to the heart and cause a heart attack or travel to the brain and cause a stroke.

What does high cholesterol and heart disease have to do with your obese child? The damage to the blood vessels can start in childhood! This is sometimes shocking news to parents who can't imagine that their child's arteries may look like those of a middle-aged man (and one who doesn't take very good care of himself, at that).

Strokes kill and impair 150,000 men and women every year. It's a condition that isn't always the result of being obese, but obesity significantly increases the risk of having a stroke.

Another condition that often begins in childhood and significantly increases an adult's chances of developing cardiovascular disease is *atherosclerosis,* or damage to the heart arteries.

Enlarged heart

When a cardiologist runs a risk factor score on an adult — a man, for example — to determine whether he's at high risk for heart disease, the doc very often takes a look at whether or not this patient has a condition of the heart called *left ventricular hypertrophy,* or what's commonly called an enlarged heart. (If the patient has an enlarged heart, that's not good news for him *or* his risk factor score.)

Now here's the frightening part: Even though this man is being evaluated as an adult, the enlargement may have begun in childhood, especially if he was obese. In some people, the heart fights back against resistance (narrowed blood vessels) it meets as it works to pump blood throughout the body by making itself larger. The heart doesn't know that it can't win this game by morphing into a monster organ.

Obesity and Development Problems

Take an informal survey of your own friends and colleagues and ask them what the most difficult time of their life was (excluding specific events like the death of a loved one or the loss of a job). We're willing to bet that a lot of your pals will say that junior high and/or high school were nightmare years, a time that they'd never return to even if they were given the chance and offered a million dollars to do so.

These years are hard for so many young people for different reasons, but when you think back on it, what was everyone dealing with? Puberty. Surely you remember it — feeling awkward in your new supposedly almost-adult body, dealing with the moodiness of shifting hormones, and wondering if anyone else was feeling the same way that you were. (Shudder.)

Early development in girls

Puberty for girls is occurring at younger ages these days. On average, girls start to develop one to two years earlier than their mothers did. What's causing these changes? You know the answer — obesity.

Just how obesity plays a role in the early development of puberty isn't crystal clear. However, obesity has been linked to a hormone called *leptin* that's found in fat cells. Research indicates that girls with high levels of leptin in their blood are entering puberty earlier than their thinner pals.

Are there any negative effects of early puberty? The jury is still out on the issue. It's possible that early puberty in girls may raise their risk for breast cancer in adulthood because they have increased levels of estrogen coursing through their bodies earlier and for a longer duration than their peers.

For the most part, the effects of early puberty in girls are mostly emotional. Being the first kid in the classroom to go through puberty — being not only obese but also the tallest and the only girl wearing a bra — is difficult, especially if all the other girls in the class seem to be light years away from making the leap. Different development is just another way that obese kids can feel different and separated from their peers.

Delayed development in boys

Interestingly, early studies have shown that obesity has the opposite effect on boys than it does on girls — that is, obesity may actually *slow* puberty in males. So where obese girls are feeling strange about being the first ones to develop breasts and tower over their friends, obese boys are often the shortest kids in their classrooms. While they listen to their friends' voices change and watch the other boys shoot past them on the growth charts, obese boys are left behind, feeling left out and different from everyone else.

Puberty and depression

Even though obese children may be relatively alone in their conditions (that is, they may only have a classmate or two in the same boat), dealing with the emotional highs and lows and the confusing physical changes of puberty at the age of 9 or 10 (for girls) is no easy task. It's hard enough for 12- and 13-year-olds. And being the last one to develop (as obese boys often are) also leaves a child feeling as though there's something wrong with him — why isn't he like his friends?

Obesity and puberty are two difficult conditions to deal with separately. Taken together, a child may come to feel depressed and isolated from his or her peers. We talk more about the emotional and social ramifications that puberty has on children in Chapter 4.

Making Changes: Time Is of the Essence!

Given all the terrible health problems your obese child could face, is there any good news? Should you just hang it up right now and forget about trying to help your child? The key word here is *could* — if the damage hasn't already been done, these conditions are, for the most part, preventable (where there isn't any genetic predisposition to an illness, like asthma, for example). And many of them are reversible. But as with the weight, the first priority is to stop the condition from getting any worse.

Avoiding cumulative effects

Most of the conditions we talk about in this chapter are like hurricanes at sea in that they get stronger with time, until one day you and your child realize that you're facing a crisis. The big storm comes blowing through, but unlike a natural disaster, it won't leave. With obesity-related health problems, you're left to deal with the ongoing damage.

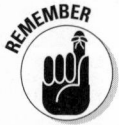

This chapter examines the long-term effects of diseases that can begin in obese children. This doesn't mean that every obese child will go on to suffer from these ailments. This information is more like a storm warning: If nothing changes, conditions are favorable for these illnesses to develop.

Because these ailments are, for the most part, preventable, it's an awful waste not to at least try to stop them from occurring. The benefits of heading trouble off at the pass are so plentiful, and the long-reaching effects of these conditions are so harmful that it's in your entire family's best interest to start *now.* Twenty years from today, you don't want to be watching your child struggling with obesity-related health conditions, lamenting the fact that none of you took the risks seriously when she was young.

As we say throughout the chapter, the damage starts early. Youth doesn't protect obese kids from suffering long-term health effects related to excess weight. Your child's doctor is the best source of information on your child's health, so pay him a visit, share your concerns, and listen to what he advises. There *is* no later. The damage done today only opens the door for more damage tomorrow, so help your child to cut it short.

Reversing adverse effects

In overweight kids, heart problems begin with elevated levels of cholesterol and a sedentary lifestyle. Cholesterol builds up in the blood vessels, raising blood pressure and putting your child at risk for developing blood clots, which put her at risk for all kinds of cardiovascular nightmares. However, if it hasn't gone too far, she can reverse some of this damage by increasing her activity and decreasing her intake of fatty foods.

The same thing goes for elevated blood pressure: A good diet and exercise go a long way toward counteracting the negative effects of obesity. As soon as your child gets on track, her heart function will improve, which means that her heart will pump more efficiently. If she's eating healthy foods and exercising, her LDL (bad cholesterol) levels will drop, and her HDL (good cholesterol) levels may rise, thus helping to clear out any narrowed blood vessels.

There's not a whole lot anyone can do about established diabetes, so prevention is really the key. Diabetes is such a serious condition with such varied effects and long-term complications that it's just best never to open the door to its arrival. Once established, diabetes can be managed through diet, exercise, and medication. Studies show that diabetics who adhere to their doctors' advice do much better in the long run than their diabetic counterparts who do nothing to improve their overall health. Doctors' advice most often includes losing weight, increasing activity, following a strict diet, and monitoring blood glucose levels closely.

Like diabetes, puberty is impossible to reverse. If your obese daughter has entered into puberty at an early age, her hormones are operating at an adult level. You can't undo her period or her breasts, but you can help her accept these changes and assure her that the other girls will eventually catch up. The same advice goes for boys experiencing delayed puberty.

Which of the other conditions discussed in this chapter are preventable?

✔ **Joint, muscle, and bone problems:** Fractures and bone deformities can cause lifelong pain. Losing weight and participating in weight-bearing exercise can help build bone density and promote bone health.

✔ **Sleep apnea:** Obstructive sleep apnea is caused by the throat closing in on itself. Losing weight shrinks the amount of fatty tissue surrounding the neck, thus preventing this problem.

✔ **Liver disease:** "Fatty liver," caused by an accumulation of fat cells in the liver, isn't a particularly harmful condition, but it can lead to more serious problems. Lose the fat, and you lose the potential for damage to the liver.

✔ **Skin problems:** Obese kids are more prone to rashes because the shape and condition of their bodies give bacteria and fungi a place to go to work. Increased sweating and folds of skin open the door to all sorts of infections. Losing weight and therefore changing the shape of the body is the most effective way to avoid common skin problems.

✔ **Constipation:** Adding fiber to the diet heads bowel trouble off at the pass.

This list includes almost everything we discuss in this chapter, so as frightening and depressing as this chapter is, it's all a prelude to this big message: These things don't have to happen to your child!

Considering that these ailments, at best, can make life miserable for your child and, at worst, can actually put your child's life in jeopardy, it makes perfect sense for a parent to want to put some plan into action. You want to stop the wheels of obesity and its related damage and steer your child toward a healthier life today. Just remember that change takes time. Losing the weight is well worth the effort, but it isn't going to happen overnight. Weight loss is a long-term commitment, and your child has to be willing to make some sacrifices in order to have a better, longer, happier life. This book can help, but your best resource where health matters are concerned is your child's pediatrician.

Chapter 4

Hurting from the Inside Out: The Emotional Effects of Childhood Obesity

In This Chapter

▶ Facing the damaging effects of bullying and discrimination

▶ Understanding the impact of emotional abuse

▶ Controlling abuse in sibling relationships

*I*n Chapter 3, we talk about the possible long-term physical consequences of children carrying around excess weight. In addition to health problems (or often because of these conditions), obese children's weight keeps them on the sidelines of life, quite literally: A severely overweight child is unlikely to be capable up keeping up with her thinner peers on the playing field. Worse, she may not even want to try; obese children are so often the objects of ridicule and finger-pointing at school and on the playground.

The type of torment that overweight kids face is different from what obese adults encounter for a couple of reasons: First, children are still discovering who they are, what they're capable of, and how they view themselves. A constant barrage of name-calling and teasing during these formative years can affect the way a kid feels about herself for the rest of her life. Second, unlike most adults, who are supposed to mature and accept one another as they age, children say what's on their little minds all the time. Most youngsters don't have a filtering switch, and even if little Susie asks your daughter only *once* why she's so heavy . . . your child has already faced the question from 50 other children.

The goal of this book is to help you help your child work toward better health and feel better about herself. We're not pushing the concept that all children must be stick-thin in order to be happy. But children have to feel well, both emotionally and physically, in order to feel good. This chapter addresses some of the emotional horrors that obese children face and gives you some tips to help your child steer her way through to better times.

Sticks and Stones? They're Nothing!

Everyone knows that the old self-esteem booster, "Sticks and stones may break my bones, but names will never hurt me" isn't true. It's a great concept, but try explaining it to an overweight preteen boy who's sitting in his room alone thinking about how he was teased in the school cafeteria last week. That vision is enough to just break your heart wide open, right? Why are other kids so cruel?

Although its small comfort to any parent whose child is suffering at the hands of peer emotional terrorists, your child isn't the first to go through this experience and, unfortunately, he won't be the last. Children are all about conformity, and your child isn't the only one being picked on. Kids who go after an overweight child also pick on someone from a different socioeconomic group, race, or even academic ranking; you name it, and it's fair game for some rotten apples out there.

What's really upsetting is that good apples are often influenced to treat peers badly, also. Most times, this type of behavior is nothing more than an attempt to protect themselves and/or conform to what everyone else is doing. It's the rare kid who can break free from the pack and truly not give a hoot about what the others are saying to or about him and his friends. Facing ridicule at the hands of a known bully is devastating enough for a child, and it's about a hundred times worse when his own friends turn on him.

In this section, we explain what your obese child may be facing in social situations and what you can do to help him stay strong.

Helping your child deal with bullies

If your child were one of a group of minority students in her school and someone tossed a racial epithet her way, you'd expect her teacher to step in and prevent it from happening again, right? And if your child were handicapped and a classmate constantly teased her about being in a wheelchair, you'd think that the school would find this type of behavior 100 percent unacceptable and take the bully to task, correct? Even though society's done away with condoning most types of discrimination, prejudice against overweight people still runs rampant.

The good news is that many school districts teach *character education* (compassion, acceptance of others, and how to stick up for other children) along with the three R's these days. However, some teachers (and schools) are better at nurturing these ideas than others. Teachers are only human, and they come with their own baggage, which may include very little tolerance for settling disputes between children when the letter of the law isn't involved (as it is in the case of a racial incident).

Even if your child has a wonderfully insightful and talented teacher, overweight kids who are picked on by their peers are often darned if they do, and darned if they don't — get the teacher involved, that is. If the teacher comes to your child's rescue on a regular basis, her classmates may label your kid a "tattletale" or a "baby." On the other hand, if your child doesn't report bullying, she may be setting herself up for further incidents. Bullies love a victim who sits quietly and takes the abuse, but they also love a kid who fights them, because then they feel completely justified in hurling insults at the child (in the name of self-defense).

Being the victim of a bully doesn't make kids tougher, nor does it teach them much about peer-to-peer relationships. Kids who are the victims of bullies:

✔ Tend to have low self-esteem and no self-confidence

✔ Often suffer from depression

✔ May develop nervous tics or compulsive habits

✔ Show signs of anxiety (such as having irrational fears or a general feeling of panic all the time)

✔ Have trouble sleeping

✔ May have thoughts of suicide

✔ Sometimes exhibit uncontrollable rage towards others

✔ Often have trouble with their schoolwork

Many of these effects can last well beyond the years when kids are actually being bullied, so it's safe to say that being tormented by a bully can have a profound, long-lasting effect on a child's life. It's even safe to say that being the victim of a bully can shape a child's life. (For more on the effects of bullying, see the section "How Emotional Abuse Hurts Your Child" later in this chapter.)

Understanding relational bullying

Bullying comes in many different forms. There's overt bullying — as in physical or verbal abuse or other physical acts of intimidation — and then there's *relational bullying,* which involves shutting the victim out of social groups and/or spreading rumors about the child.

If your child has been fortunate enough to escape being bullied or teased, she still may not be in the clear. Overweight kids often feel isolated from their classmates, who, studies have shown, perceive obese children as being less intelligent, lazier, and not as hygienic as the average kid. (Never mind the fact that your daughter may be smart as a whip, always eager to help around the house, and obsessed with keeping her desk as neat as a pin.) When kids intentionally ignore a peer or leave her out of group activities, that's relational bullying. It's not as obvious to the naked eye as someone beating your child up on the playground, but it's every bit as damaging to her self-esteem. Although relational bullying usually doesn't involve physical contact, it's meant to demean and intimidate the victim.

Relational bullying often takes the form of a classic passive-aggressive situation in which a child is left out of a group but isn't necessarily called names or teased. So where's the damage? The child feels invisible and not worthy of her peers' attention.

While it's debatable whether this type of bullying is preferable to your child being physically harmed by a classmate, it's just as harmful to her self-esteem. The one good thing — if there is a good thing — about physical bullying is that you know it's going on, you know who's doing it, and your child may have a legitimate recourse against the perpetrator (s). It's easier for a teacher or another adult to step in and stop physical bullying (although they don't always do it, of course).

Relational bullying is something that even the nicest, quietest kid in the classroom may be doing to your child (and what's worse, she may not even realize she's doing it at all!). Whereas many kids realize that overt bullying is wrong and would never dream of calling names or hitting a classmate, relational bullying tends to take on a life of its own, and before anyone knows what's happened, one or two children have been singled out. Unfortunately, because of the stereotypes associated with overweight people, obese children are an easy target for this type of social isolation.

Bullying is harmful to the psyche regardless of your child's age or gender, but girls seem to be particularly tough on obese peers during the teen years. Adolescent girls are more likely than boys to mock, taunt, or just ignore their overweight female schoolmates. And given that adolescents depend on peers to validate them (it's that conformity thing again), an obese teen girl who's teased by her peers on a daily basis is at high risk for depression.

An obese kid has to work twice as hard to convince his peers that there's more to him than a weight issue. He's often viewed as "the fat kid" — the one without any real feelings, interests, or goals in life. And the twist to this is that because overweight kids are so often teased, they're more likely to keep quiet in the classroom and to isolate themselves at recess or free time as a protective mechanism. No one gets to know your child because he's afraid of what may happen if he opens his mouth.

Taking action for your child

How can you help your child when she's being shunned and bullied by her classmates? It's always best for a child to try and work things out by herself first by ignoring unkind comments and walking away from the children who are making them. Many times, removing oneself from the situation is enough to stop cruelty in its tracks. However, when bullying escalates into a day-in, day-out, business-as-usual situation, you need to step in. You have a number of different ways to handle things:

- ✔ **If your child's teacher is someone you trust to help, take up the issue with him or her.** Good teachers are a special breed unto themselves, and they often come up with creative solutions that other people would never think of.

- ✔ **If the teacher isn't so great and the bullying is nonstop in the classroom, talk to him or her first, but be prepared to go to the principal if the situation doesn't improve.** Your child is at the very least entitled to learn in a nonthreatening environment.

- ✔ **Be there for your child, and continue with your weight-loss/health-improvement goals at home.** Offer your child loads and loads of support and plenty of opportunities to talk. Knowing that you're on her side no matter what happens outside of your home is exactly what she needs.

- ✔ **Let your child know that bullies are usually very weak people.** No one who likes themselves teases someone else. Also, remind her that bullies most often act only in front of their peers because they're seldom brave enough to act so badly all by themselves.

- ✔ **Encourage your child to stick with a group of pals.** Just as a bully is more likely to act when his buddies are in tow, he's somewhat less likely to attack if your child is with a group.

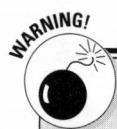

Cyberbullying

One of the worst kinds of relational bullying is *cyberbullying,* which is a growing problem in this technological day and age. Cyberbullies either post lies or gossip about their victims in chat rooms or on Web sites or they insult victims in instant-messaging (IM) sessions. The anonymity of this type of bullying means that it tends to get very ugly, very quickly. And tracking down a cyberbully can be very difficult, depending on how computer-savvy the bully is and how well you and/or your child know your own way around cyberspace. Most experts in the field of cyberbullying advise kids to simply ignore a one-time incident because responding to taunts or threats is likely to make the situation worse.

If your child is being bombarded with threats and insults, though, you should save and print all the messages you can and take them to your child's principal. School officials should be trained in combating this type of harassment, and many times, messages can be traced back to a specific computer. You can also contact the police if the threats are physical in nature (like someone telling your child she's going to be harmed).

To prevent this type of bullying in the first place, advise your child to only chat with known buddies and not to give out personal information to anyone who isn't already an established pal. Many times, kids are "baited" into chatting by acquaintances who then turn around and use the children's words against them.

✔ **Encourage your child to portray confidence, even if it's just for show.** Funny thing about that bully — he's quick to pick on a child who's always staring down at her shoes and walking with her shoulders slumped. He just may have second thoughts if his victim learns to stand up straight and stare him in the eye. A subtle difference in her demeanor can have big effects.

Discourage your child from returning taunts; instruct your child to keep herself civil and even-tempered. Bullies who open a back-and-forth dialogue with their victims often feel justified in continuing their tirades, and your child may even be blamed in the future for instigating trouble. Plus, there's a big difference between sitting quietly and taking the abuse, speaking up for herself, and getting lured into the bitterness that always results from trading insults with other people.

If the bullying problem is bad enough (that is, if your child is being hurt physically or tormented to the point where she refuses to go to school), *insist* upon an intervention at school. You want your child and the bullying ringleader to sit down and talk — that's all. The younger the kids, the more effective this meeting will be because younger bullies often only need to realize that the person they've been tormenting is a real, live person — and not a punching bag — before they call it quits. Parents and teachers should be present to lead the conversation and act as moderators.

Older bullies may be a little harder to convince, so you'll need the school on your side. Here's your angle: Your child has the right to learn in a nonthreatening environment; if the school isn't willing to take steps to create such an environment (by giving the bully a chance to knock it off or face detention or suspension), you'll be forced to take further action, in the form of hiring a lawyer who deals in discrimination. Period. Your child's well-being is at stake, so you really have no other choice than to take a course of action that's in her best interest.

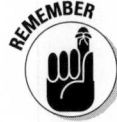

When bullying persists and you start getting all fired up, keep two caveats in mind:

- ✔ *Don't* threaten legal action until it becomes apparent that it's your last course of action.

- ✔ *Don't* threaten unless you mean it. The threat itself makes *you* a threat to the school district, and you'll be treated as such even though you're in the right.

You may feel as though it's only fair to give the school time to remedy the situation. Fair enough. Give the principal and the teacher a couple of weeks — maximum — to formulate a plan that's acceptable to you and your family, and be prepared to be given the bum's rush a few times. Be firm but polite, and *don't* give up on this. If the principal doesn't return your calls, clear some time to sit in the school office until she can see you. And if that doesn't work, speak to her boss and watch how fast she jumps into action. Remember to remain calm and polite, and document every communication between yourself and the school.

Maybe you feel like demanding change from your child's teacher and principal is taking things too far; the school certainly is looking out for your child, and anyway, kids are kids. What doesn't kill us makes us stronger, right?

Make no mistake about it: It may well be up to *you* to see that your child's school protects her emotional well-being. School administrators love to spout off for a crowd about their interest in child advocacy; the sad reality is that many times (though not always), the higher-ups are first and foremost *school* advocates (worried most about how test scores and negative gossip and publicity may affect their schools and, consequently, their jobs) and somewhere way, way down the line, they're concerned with the needs of each individual child.

And what about the notion that teasing acts as some sort of mechanism for developing a tougher skin? It's not true. Teasing often leads to:

- Depression
- Isolation
- Additional weight gain
- Anxiety
- Anger

Resolving bullying is a quality-of-life issue. The more your child is teased and bullied, the worse she feels about herself. And the worse she feels about herself, the worse her weight problem is likely to be. If she doesn't have any friends and is scared to leave the house, what else is she supposed to do besides watch TV and console herself with a snack?

Turning the tables: When obese kids become bullies

Here's an interesting twist to the bullying tale: Not only are obese children more likely to be bullied, but they're also more likely to turn the anger they feel toward other children and become bullies themselves. It makes perfect sense, if you think about it: How much isolation and taunting can a child bear before he starts hating everyone and wanting to hurt someone as badly as he's been hurt?

Mental health specialists see this type of behavior (abused becoming abuser) in victims of any sort of abuse. The victim has nothing to lose, nothing to look forward to, nothing to make him feel good about himself, and no one to turn to, so he lashes out. In obese children, this reaction is just as much a defense mechanism (as in "I'll hurt them before they can hurt me") as it is an action born of anger and depression.

So preventing your child from becoming a bully, too, is another very important reason for you to get involved and make sure your child's school is promoting a safe learning environment. We know, your parents never handled things this way. In your day, kids were expected to settle their own disputes, and parents often never knew a thing about what was really happening. Put that argument aside, and take a look at the world *right now*. Kids who are isolated from their peers often exhibit signs of severe depression, and the fallout can be extremely damaging in the long term, leading to a lifetime of poor self-esteem. School violence — often perpetrated by kids who've been bullied for years — and teen suicide have become things that parents cross their fingers and hope their kids don't get involved in.

Obesity and income: Chicken or the egg?

Researchers have found an inverse link between income and obesity in this country; that is, obese people are more likely to fall into a lower household income bracket. The studies don't explain why this is the case, though. Is it because obese people face discrimination in the job market and therefore aren't as likely as their peers to land high-paying jobs, or is it that healthy foods are just too expensive, so low-income families are forced to make less healthy choices at mealtimes? (In Chapter 8, we talk about this myth and give tips for shopping for healthy foods on a budget.) Or does it possibly go even deeper than that? Researchers are looking into the possibility that obese children have such low self-esteem that they're less likely to be overly ambitious in planning their futures, which makes them less likely to attend college and therefore less likely to end up in high-paying professions. The results aren't in, but this theory certainly makes sense from a logical point of view.

It's not your job to hold your child's hand all the way up through high school, but it *is* your job to make sure that the school does everything it can to provide a learning environment that's safe for your child and that doesn't make your child say things like, "I'd rather die than go to school." Because you can be sure of one thing: If your kid is being targeted, others are also suffering from the same type of injustice. That kind of environment breeds violence, and . . . yes, it's up to you to see that it stops here and now.

Facing fat prejudice

The torment that obese children face each day in school and on the playground is just a symptom of a much broader issue: Overweight people are fair game for overt discrimination, even in this day and age of supposed tolerance for everyone.

If you were walking down the street and someone made a derogatory comment about the color of your skin, bystanders would most likely be horrified. Some may even yell insults back to the perpetrator, defending not only your dignity but also civilized society, which doesn't tolerate such public displays of nastiness . . . except when it comes to overweight and obese people. If you were walking down the street and someone made a comment about the size of your thighs, not only would you feel ashamed, but also you probably wouldn't receive a whole lot of support from strangers on the street. The reason is simple: Overweight people are perceived to be lazy, unintelligent, responsible for their own situations, and therefore, no good.

In the section "Understanding relational bullying" earlier in this chapter, we describe how obese children are viewed by their peers, and the adjectives are exactly the same as the ones listed here. Weight prejudice is a societal problem, spanning all age groups. Logic would dictate that as the numbers of overweight children and adults increase, so would other people's understanding and tolerance. The fact of the matter is that things seem to be getting worse. Whether it's because society on the whole doesn't value politeness or because we don't encourage kindness between strangers, the fact is that overweight people deal with personal insults from complete strangers on a regular basis. This abuse is the emotional equivalent of walking along, minding your own business, and then stepping on a land mine, over and over again.

If you're overweight, you know what we're talking about, and you know how painful it is when someone catches you off guard with a nasty comment. In defense, perhaps your guard is up all the time or you have some nasty comebacks of your own. You know the toll this prejudice has taken on your own self-esteem, and you know you'd do anything to prevent your child from going through the same thing as an adult.

The fact is, she's already experiencing weight prejudice, and it will only continue. Whereas your boss, for example, is very likely to have a zero-tolerance policy for discrimination of any kind in the office (including weight discrimination, as lawsuits pop up all over the country), schools and the general world of kids aren't so well defined. You are your child's first line of defense and best source of information on the topic of weight discrimination; how you react to inappropriate remarks or behavior — whether or not you instruct her to follow your lead — speaks volumes about how you view yourself, your child, and the people you come into contact with. Make sure you're sending her the right message — namely, that it's not acceptable to judge *anyone* based on their weight.

Recognizing discrimination in the doctor's office

Many pediatricians (and heck, plenty of internists and other physicians who primarily treat adults) have come to view obesity as the health crisis that it is; they're compassionate and kind when discussing the issue of weight with their patients. However, some old-school doctors (which doesn't necessarily mean that they fall into an advanced age bracket) view overweight patients with contempt and believe that shaming the patient is the best way to get him or her to lose weight. If you've encountered this type of doctor, your blood is probably boiling right now; if not, your hair may be standing on end just imagining the damage this person could do to your child's self-esteem.

Because obese children are in a higher risk category for many illnesses (which we discuss in Chapter 3), they need to be completely comfortable speaking with their primary care doctors. Although the doctor should be looking for certain conditions commonly seen in overweight children, if your child is reluctant to report symptoms because he doesn't want another lecture about his weight, some conditions could go undiagnosed, at least for a time.

If your child is in elementary school, you probably hear every word that passes between him and the doctor. If you have an overweight teen, you need to be more vigilant about knowing how that relationship is faring. Don't expect your child to tell you everything that's said in the exam room, but do try to get a general feel for how much he likes — or dislikes — his doctor. And if you sense some tension in the doctor-patient relationship, find another doctor.

Studies have shown that obese women tend to have higher death rates from ovarian cancer than their thinner peers. One theory surrounding this finding is that obese women are less likely to visit their doctors on a regular basis because of medical fat discrimination. Ovarian cancer happens to be one illness that, if not detected early, is particularly lethal. The general gist of this finding can be carried over to your child's health: You don't want illness to get a stronghold in her, so make sure her doctor is thorough and compassionate enough that your child doesn't fear regular visits.

Accepting overweight people

One criticism we faced after deciding to write this book was that it could possibly *perpetuate* discrimination against obese children by suggesting that they can slim down easily and should start immediately. We were told that we should promote "fat acceptance" rather than tell parents how to help their kids lose weight.

Honestly, we're all for acceptance of *every* kind, and we couldn't care less about how much a person weighs or how well someone's pants fit. Childhood obesity isn't an aesthetic issue for us; we're primarily concerned with your child's physical and emotional health, and it's a fact that overweight kids tend to deal with a lot of adverse health and social issues. They certainly aren't alone — adolescence can be trying for thin kids, too — but obese children are at much higher risk for certain diseases. Poor health and low self-esteem can lead to major episodes of depression, anxiety, and isolation. It's bad enough that adults feel this way; it's a downright shame that so many kids experience adultlike illnesses and subsequent emotional roller coasters in their formative years.

Overweight *and* healthy?

Debate rages about whether people can be "fit and fat" or whether it's truly necessary to drop down to a particular weight in order to be healthy. Some kids will never be "thin," no matter how hard they try. Their body types and genetic predispositions just have them programmed to be larger-than-average people. Does this mean they shouldn't even bother trying, or can they remain heavy and just eat low-fat foods for good health?

The research on this topic has shown that it's better to be heavy and physically active than to be thin and lead a sedentary lifestyle. *However,* because being overweight can lead to other health problems, you should still consult your child's doctor and have her health evaluated. Just because your older child is heavy, active,

and healthy doesn't necessarily mean that your younger child will have the same luck with her health. Regardless of your child's age, obesity must be viewed as a risk factor in the development of certain diseases.

The good thing about being active is that it's often a remedy for certain physical ailments. The more your child moves, the better her health is going to be for it. Exercise is also a mood lifter. You've probably heard about how exercising releases hormones called *endorphins,* which make you feel good. So being active is great for the body and the mind, which, in turn, can lead to your child's increased self-esteem and enthusiasm about continuing to lead a healthy lifestyle.

How Emotional Abuse Hurts Your Child

Emotional abuse is very serious; name-calling and social isolation can result in lifelong feelings of unworthiness and self-doubt, even if an overweight child goes on to lose a substantial amount of weight. The wounds that go the deepest are usually the ones no one else sees.

In this section, we talk about some of the consequences of emotional abuse that overweight kids face; we also explore how missing out on some of the normal rites of passage of childhood may affect them in the long run.

Isolation

Social isolation can be a perpetual state. The average obese kid has a hard time breaking free of an "outcast" label, and it gets more difficult the older the age group. Being on the outside of peer activities often leads to depression and general anxiety; for example, a kid may become fearful of leaving the house, wondering who's going to insult or ignore him on that particular day.

Thanks to social isolation, self-esteem levels drop like a stone in the adolescent years, when the opposite sex becomes the main reason many kids bother showing up to school at all. Watching as her peers become involved in relationships, make plans for the weekend, and discuss their prom dresses all the while knowing that she won't be asked to join in the fun can be emotionally devastating for an obese teenager.

We don't want to give you the idea that obese or overweight kids are the only children who deal with social isolation, because that's just not true. The point is that this kind of isolation can affect the course of your child's entire life. Some kids find their own way in time; they either lose weight or just become more comfortable in their own skin and feel better about themselves. Other kids never get over these lonely, sad years. They may quit school, end up in dead-end jobs, and choose partners who treat them badly (because at least he or she is *there*).

How a child fares through difficult times such as social isolation largely depends on her support system at home. You need to be willing to talk, listen, or just sit quietly with a child who feels left out. Just as important, do what you can to help her feel better physically. The more successful she is at sticking to a healthy lifestyle, the better she's going to feel. This is true for several reasons:

- ✔ Physical aches and pains, in addition to social problems, can lead to depression. The more she moves, the better she'll feel physically, which may produce a great improvement in her outlook on life.

- ✔ The foods that are a large part of an unhealthy diet — sugar, in particular — can lead to mood swings and heighten feelings of anxiety and depression. Eating a more balanced diet should (eventually) help to balance out her mood.

- ✔ Exercise releases endorphins that put her in a good state of mind, at least temporarily (and that's a *start*).

- ✔ Sticking to a healthier lifestyle (regardless of weight loss) is an accomplishment in and of itself, and *that's* a great self-esteem booster.

When she's feeling good, it's time to encourage her to find a social outlet. It doesn't need to involve school; if she has a particular interest (art, reading, writing, animals, crafts — whatever), look for a group in your area with which she can sharpen her skills and get to know other people her own age. Settling into groups tends to be easier when everyone is gathered for the same reason — at least they all have something in common and something to talk about. And if she can learn to talk to people in a setting like this, her social skills — and her self-esteem — will get a bit of a boost that just may make things easier for her elsewhere.

Nose-diving grades

The emotional effects of being bullied — depression, anxiety, difficulty sleeping, low self-esteem, and diminished self-confidence — can have a negative impact on schoolwork. Anxiety, for example, often causes a child to worry irrationally, which decreases his ability to concentrate on anything. In addition, anxiety is emotionally *exhausting,* and your child may have no energy left over to devote to schoolwork after he's spent an entire week worrying about a tornado leveling your house (even though it's December and there hasn't been a tornado in your town . . . ever).

Anxiety over social standing at school can produce exhaustion, as well. And again, exhaustion leads to unfinished homework as well as an inability to concentrate. Grades start to slip when he doesn't do his reading for English class, and the teacher doesn't hide her disappointment when he's unable to answer a simple question. His report card arrives at the house, and you're dismayed to see that although your child is very bright, he's pulling Cs and Ds and negative comments from teachers.

Here's where the spiral that's tough to break free from starts. The lower the grades go, the lower his self-confidence dips, and he actually begins to believe that he *is* unintelligent and that he really *isn't* capable of doing any better. Studies have also shown that teachers may feed into (or buy into) the perception that overweight kids are less intelligent than their peers, either by calling on them less often in the classroom or by grading their papers more harshly than those of thinner students.

In addition, obese children who are victimized by bullies are more apt to feign illness in order to miss school (or, in the case of older kids, just skip class without bothering to fake the sore throat). Of course, obese children may have legitimate physical conditions (like asthma, for example) that keep them out of school more often than their classmates. But missed days in the classroom often translate into missed schoolwork and lower grades.

Teens who are suffering from anxiety, depression, and other emotional issues stemming from obesity may benefit from speaking to a school psychologist or therapist who's trained in dealing with overeating issues (which are generally grouped in with other eating disorders). Parents can help by remaining positive and supportive in the child's quest for a healthier lifestyle.

Mirror, mirror . . . I hate what I see: Low self-esteem

Every kid, regardless of age, shape, size, or attitude (if you have teenagers, you know what we mean), is lovable in some way. Each one has his or her own special abilities and talents, and each child is a shining star in some way. That's why it's so heartbreaking to watch kids go through phases of self-doubt and low self-esteem. Typically, adolescents are the prime targets for this kind of self-hatred, though more and more, younger children are experiencing low self-esteem, too. It makes sense for the average teenager to go through a period of finding out who they are (and who they aren't) and comparing themselves with their peers, trying to see how they measure up (literally and figuratively). With teenagers' raging hormones and changing bodies, this attitude shift comes as no surprise to parents, who remember their own days of gazing in the mirror and crying about what they saw.

Obese children sometimes fall into a special category of people with ultralow self-esteem. Given the emotions and physical effects of being an overweight youngster, it's difficult to imagine how scary life must be at times for an obese child, especially when diminished self-confidence is added to a serious weight-related illness, like diabetes.

How low self-esteem can make weight problems worse

For children who suffer from self-loathing (including those who aren't obese), every day looks bleak. They feel ostracized from their peers, they often feel physically unwell, and they honestly can't see a bright light at the end of the tunnel, even though you know that leading a healthier lifestyle will lead to better days. Kids are often unable to visualize where they'll be in a year; to them, that's an eternity.

Aside from being a dark cloud from which a child is unable to escape, low self-esteem can often make a weight problem even worse. When your daughter is feeling sad *all* the time, she may turn to comfort foods to see her through. Because weight loss takes a significant effort and a lot of time to produce visible results, she may also feel as though she has nothing to lose by eating more and nothing to gain by tossing out her favorite foods. And then when she overeats, she feels even worse about herself for not being able to break the unhealthy habit.

This kind of despair sometimes leads obese teens to risky behaviors, like drinking and smoking. Drinking, obviously, is a means of escape and of numbing those feelings of self-doubt and worthlessness. Smoking, on the other hand, is often rumored among teens to be a great way to lose weight.

(The argument goes something like, "Pop that cigarette in your mouth instead of food, and you're all set." Note how the risks of heart disease and cancer don't enter the conversation.)

Plenty of people actually have lost weight by becoming smokers, but it obviously isn't the best plan of action. You're trying to teach your child about making healthy choices that will see her through the rest of her life, so don't turn a blind eye to her new nicotine habit. A teen may mistakenly believe that losing weight by smoking is actually healthier than being obese. Educate her on the health risks associated with smoking, and *don't* accept it as a weight-loss measure.

Family matters

You may think that the increase in the rate of obese children and teens during just the last ten years would result in overweight kids being accepted for who they are, and as a result, obese kids wouldn't feel badly about their bodies. Unfortunately, even though the percentages of obese adults and children have risen dramatically, being obese is still grounds for becoming a social pariah. Other kids are cruel, and even teachers aren't always above being judgmental.

Several studies have been conducted to evaluate the self-esteem of obese children and determine whether lowered self-esteem among these kids is truly the result of being overweight or if it's just a natural phase of maturation. Researchers have found that children who had unconditional support at home were happier than other obese kids. Not surprisingly, kids whose families picked on them for being obese had the lowest levels of self-esteem. If a child is the subject of taunts and teasing at school because of his weight and he comes home to hear more of the same from the people who are supposed to love him, he's going to feel as though he has no one to turn to. *That's* despair, and that's just what a child with a weight problem doesn't need. Your child is more likely to adapt to a healthy lifestyle if he feels as though he has your support instead of fearing that he's going to disappoint you.

Make your house a safe haven for your child. No one is allowed to tease him about his weight, and no negative comments about his size are permitted. Every kid, regardless of weight, needs to be able to come home and just relax without fearing ridicule from family members.

Make it clear to your child that you're not going to judge; you're only there to *help*. Studies have shown that children who have a hand in developing a plan for a healthy lifestyle have higher self-esteem than kids whose parents put them on regimented eating plans. Obviously, age plays a big part in how much a child is capable of caring for himself, but the older the child, the more leeway you should allow him. Supervise, and don't step in unless you see some obvious errors in judgment (if, for example, your child plans a "healthy" breakfast menu that consists of sausage, bacon, and a bagel with cream cheese).

Resist the urge to do everything for your child, and instead teach him how to make himself healthier. You can do this by:

- ✔ Allowing him to have some input on the grocery list
- ✔ Encouraging him to help you prepare healthy meals
- ✔ Letting him choose the physical activities he's most interested in
- ✔ Not punishing him for the occasional slip-up

We talk more about making healthy food and cooking choices in Chapters 8 and 9, respectively, and about choosing fun physical activities in Chapter 10. Backsliding and resisting the urge to punish your child are discussed in more detail in Chapter 13.

Sibling versus Sibling

Most of the research done on childhood obesity shows that children who are significantly overweight most often come from families in which the parents are also overweight due to genetic and/or environmental factors (that is to say, the parents are either predisposed towards obesity, or their lifestyles have contributed to their weight problems, or both). As a result, it's not unusual for all the children in one family to have weight problems.

However, plenty of families exist in which only one child is heavy and the others are thin. And especially in this day and age of mixed families, you may have a couple of thin kids living with a set of thin parents, and an overweight half or step sibling who follows the genetic code of a parent living elsewhere. How can a parent deal with the weight problem of one child while keeping peace in the home?

All's fair in health at home

Many parents struggle with instituting a healthy lifestyle in the home if only one child is overweight. They feel as though it isn't fair to the other kids to deny them their favorite foods and treats, cut down on television-viewing time, and insist that everyone get outdoors and partake in some kind of physical activity just to accommodate the child who's obese.

If you're struggling with how all the kids in your house are affected by a healthy lifestyle, you have to restructure your way of thinking. An unhealthy lifestyle, which includes being sedentary and consuming too much fat, is unhealthy whether or not someone gains weight because of it.

Your thin child may appear to be perfectly fine and healthy, but if she's not eating foods that are high in essential nutrients, she may not be as healthy as you think. All children need to eat healthy foods and exercise in order to achieve their optimum levels of health. So it shouldn't come down to an issue of who's being forced to give up junk food and get outside to play because of whom — your entire family should be onboard *for health reasons.*

Still not convinced? You're thinking that you can still buy the treats for your skinny kids and just hide them from your overweight child? Don't do it! First of all, you only make your obese child feel like an outcast because everyone else can eat junk except for him. Even if you're supportive in every other way, making this type of differentiation between kids can have lasting and pro-found effects on the way your obese child views his place in the family. He may come to think of himself as "the fat one" or "the one with a problem."

Second, kids are kids. Imagine someone telling you that you can't eat your very favorite food anymore but everyone else in the house can. And because heaven knows you can't control yourself — there's one more blow to your child's self-esteem — the food is hidden from you. You know exactly what you're going to do: Hunt high and low for that treat until you find it, even if it means facing the disappointment of the family when they discover what you've done (yet *another* strike to your child's self-esteem).

When you go grocery shopping, assume that whatever you bring home is fair game for everyone in the household to eat. If it's not healthy, leave it right where it is — on the shelf.

Encouraging peace, love, and understanding at home

Children need to know that home is where they can be themselves without fear of cruel taunts and humiliation. Siblings are capable of being both best friends and worst enemies (sometimes going from one extreme to another in the span of two minutes!). No matter what the relationship is between your kids, teach them that cruel words hurt and that unkind exchanges in the home can be especially devastating, even if the person who's being made fun of doesn't show any emotion.

Because home is supposed to be the place where everyone lets their hair down, family is the first group setting in which people explore who they are; and no matter how old they get, they always fall into the same roles they played as children. The oldest child is often the boss of everyone else, and the youngest is sometimes viewed as the "flake," no matter what she achieves later in life. People are molded by how their families treat them in their early years.

The sibling who has been made to feel different — ugly, stupid, or fat — sometimes never forgives her siblings for casting her in that role. Obese children suffer enough at the hands of other kids; to come home and know that her own family sees her in the same light is incredibly hurtful. The child has no place where she can just be herself and feel unconditional love, and then the weight becomes even more of an issue because it prevents her from fitting in anywhere.

Should you force your children to love and respect one another and say only kind things when they speak to each other? (If you're laughing so hard at imagining that scene that you can barely see the words in front of you . . . we are, too.) We know that you can't make kids *like* their siblings. But you *can* enforce a no-nastiness rule in your house. It's no easy task, but you need to lay down the following laws:

- ✔ No one is allowed to call names based on physical characteristics or character traits (this includes monikers like "Elephant Ears," "Big Nose," and "Failure," as well as fat-inspired names).
- ✔ Privileges (or favorite toys) will be removed, one at a time and one for each offense, if you hear mean names being tossed back and forth. The privileges can be earned back when you start seeing respectful behavior.

Be prepared for your kids to break the rules, and be prepared to act when that happens. Also, don't be surprised when they're quite angry with you when you take away video games and computer privileges. But stick to your guns or the situation will never improve.

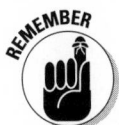

You have to follow the rules, too. You may call your forgetful child an "airhead" on a regular basis without even realizing it. Your kids will be more than happy to call you out on this behavior, so watch your own tongue.

If the kids are able to break away from name-calling, consider it a job well done. Don't go pushing for more just yet. Some siblings are just so different from each other that they really *don't* have a lot to talk about; however, enforcing the rules of respect eliminates a lot of potential problems, and you may find that, in time, the kids are willing to be civil to one another . . . and maybe even spend some time together of their own free will.

Sibling cruelty in social settings is especially devastating, so establish a firm rule forbidding this behavior, as well. The humiliation a child feels when his sister calls him a name on the school bus or encourages another child to do her dirty work (because she knows she'll lose computer time if she opens her mouth), for example, is unparalleled by any other feelings of shame in the universe. When an obese child's own family tears him to shreds in front of other people, other kids get a tacit green light to follow suit.

Part II
The Weight Is Over: Making Changes, One at a Time

The 5th Wave   By Rich Tennant

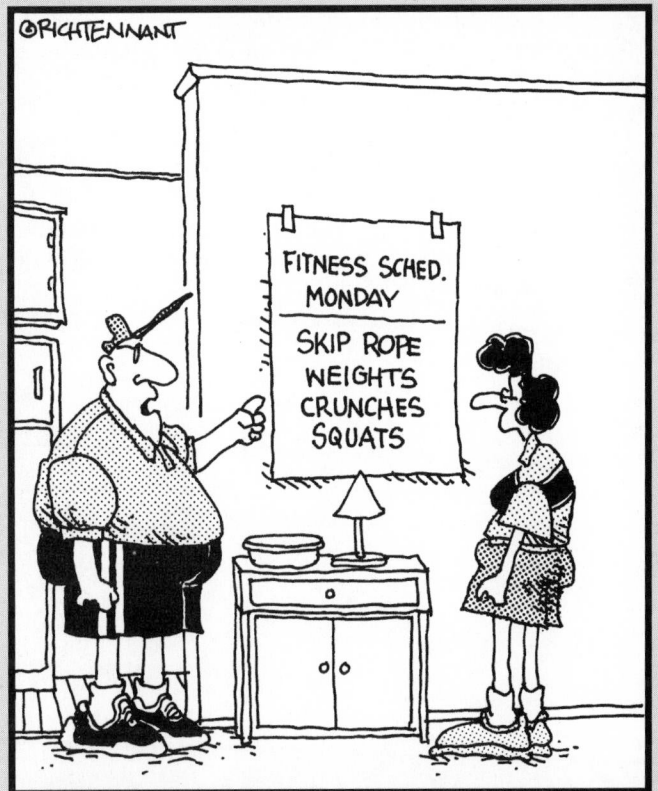

"I **AM** following the schedule! Today I skipped the rope, then I skipped the weights, then I skipped the crunches."

In this part . . .

An overweight child can only do so much for himself; he's very dependent on the rest of the family rallying around him and supporting his attempts to become healthier. In this part, we get down to the nitty-gritty — the specific changes that will ensure better health for everyone. These changes aren't difficult to make, but they take a certain amount of effort and dedication to the cause. If you're ready to help your child lose weight, you're ready to clean out the pantry and the family's unhealthy lifestyle. Out with the old, and in with the new!

Chapter 5

Assessing Your Child's Health

· ·

In This Chapter

▶ Determining your own biases concerning your child's weight

▶ Consulting with the pediatrician

▶ Diagnosing obesity with charts and other tests

· ·

How can you tell if your child is truly obese or merely overweight? One of the most remarkable things about the childhood obesity epidemic is that parents often don't recognize obesity in their own children. Regardless of the reason, the end result is usually the same: The child's weight goes unacknowledged as a serious health threat, and the condition worsens and worsens until the child starts developing secondary problems, such as asthma or diabetes. By that time, the child's health is in jeopardy, and parents feel as though they should have done something sooner.

Because obesity tends to be a household problem, parents of obese children tend to have weight problems themselves. If a parent has always struggled with her own weight but has never had any weight-related health problems, then it makes sense for her to look at her own heavy child and think, "He's just heavy like I was as a kid. My health was fine, and his will be, too." However, so much more is known these days about the long-term effects of childhood obesity that clearing up any doubt or confusion about a child's weight before disease takes hold in his body is the smart thing to do. When he's 25, he should be looking to a bright future, not lamenting the years of weight gain behind him that have left him with a lifetime of health problems.

Obesity has very specific criteria for diagnosis. In this chapter, we advise you on spotting some signs of obesity, and we discuss many of the diagnosis criteria so that you're well informed when you take your child to visit his or her doctor.

He Ain't Heavy, He's My Child

Missing the signs of obesity in your child sounds like an impossibility. After all, because obesity manifests itself in weight gain, you should be able to tell without a doubt just by looking at your child whether he's a little heavy or has a serious weight issue that may threaten his health.

You'd think it would be easy. In reality, parents often overlook their child's obesity for several reasons:

- ✔ If the parents are overweight, they may not be able to accurately judge their child's size and may underestimate it.

- ✔ Parents often think that their child is simply carrying baby fat well into his elementary school years.

- ✔ Adults tend to coo over fat babies, so a child who was plump in his first years of life may continue to be viewed as an adorable chubby imp, even when he's clearly not a baby anymore.

- ✔ Excess weight is sometimes misinterpreted as a sign of strength, especially in boys. Fathers sometimes look at their obese sons and remark, "That's my linebacker!"

On the opposite end of the weight issue, some parents are worried sick that their normal-weight, pot-bellied toddlers and preschoolers are headed for a lifetime of weight problems. So you need to know what's normal and what isn't.

Recognizing the signs of obesity

You really can't simply look at a heavy child and definitively say that she's obese, even though it may seem obvious to you. A child can have the following symptoms, all of which are commonly seen in obese children, but technically be merely overweight:

- ✔ Excess weight gain
- ✔ Shortness of breath upon exertion
- ✔ Sedentary lifestyle
- ✔ Orthopedic aches and pains
- ✔ Skin eruptions

In contrast, obese children often develop secondary conditions that are related to obesity, such as:

- Type 2 diabetes
- Metabolic syndrome
- Asthma
- Sleep apnea
- High blood pressure
- Delayed (boys) or early (girls) puberty

All these conditions are discussed in Chapter 3.

If your child has been diagnosed with one or more of the conditions listed and is markedly overweight, there's a good chance that she's obese, but *only a doctor can make that call.* Doctors use specific charts as diagnostic tools for childhood obesity. To help you better understand what the doctor is telling you about your child's weight, we break down this information in the section "Weighing In: Diagnosing Obesity" later in this chapter.

Talking to your child's doctor

At what point should you be concerned enough to discuss your child's weight with his doctor? If your child sees his pediatrician for regular check-ups, the doctor will alert you to any potential weight issues that your child is facing. If you're concerned about your child's weight, make an appointment with your child's doctor for a physical exam. Medical conditions other than obesity can cause weight gain, so play it safe, especially if the weight appears quite suddenly rather than gradually over a period of time.

If you're hearing from the doctor that your child's weight is cause for concern, take that warning seriously! Even in the face of a serious warning from a pediatrician, many parents simply don't believe that their child is obese. Chapter 3 talks about the physical ailments that are commonly caused by obesity; Chapter 4 discusses the emotional pain that obese children often suffer. Both can cause serious, long-term distress for a significantly overweight child, so the sooner you acknowledge the problem and start working to correct it, the better off your child (and your entire family) will be.

A child who has a weight issue needs to have a doctor that he's comfortable talking with. Obesity can cause some very serious health issues, and an obese child may end up spending a significant amount of time in the doctor's office. If your current pediatrician loves to lecture your child on his weight and you can see your child's discomfort whenever the topic comes up, it may be in everyone's best interest to find a more compassionate doc.

Weighing In: Diagnosing Obesity

There's no way to merely look at a child and determine whether he's obese. Doctors use specific diagnostic criteria to determine how serious a child's weight problem is and the likelihood of the child developing (or already having) weight-related health issues. Because it's always best to nip problems in the bud before they spiral out of control (health issues like diabetes, in particular, can be very difficult to manage), play it safe and let your child's doctor evaluate his weight.

If the doctor determines that your child isn't obese but merely overweight, he may recommend putting some preventive measures against obesity into practice in your home, such as a healthier diet and increased physical activity.

Differentiating between baby fat and a true weight issue

If your child is taller and larger than his peers or has a round, chubby face, it can be really tough to say whether that's his natural, healthy state of being or an indicator that he may be on the heavy side. It's a call for your pediatrician to make, using height and weight charts as his main diagnostic tools.

Babies are hardly ever diagnosed with weight problems, and they're never put on calorie-restricting diets. The same is true of toddlers. Small children need to eat enough calories to ensure proper development; a healthy diet provides enough calories for kids to grow at an appropriate rate. One exception: For kids under the age of 2, doctors usually recommend whole milk because it aids in development of the nervous system.

Understanding family history and other factors

When assessing your child's weight, one thing that a doctor takes into consideration is any factors that may predispose your child to becoming obese. These factors may include:

- ✔ **Family history:** A child who has at least one obese parent is more likely to become obese.

- ✔ **Race:** African Americans, American Indians, and Hispanics have a higher rate of obesity. Approximately one-quarter of the children from each of these minority groups are obese.

- ✔ **Lifestyle:** A sedentary lifestyle coupled with a high-fat diet is a recipe for obesity.

Obviously, family history and ethnicity can't be changed. However, lifestyle factors are usually very malleable if at least one parent is willing to jump in and contribute to making significant changes in the child's diet and activity level. When a doctor talks to you about making changes to your child's lifestyle, you need to already be in the mindset that your entire family will be taking part in a healthier way of life.

Evaluating height and weight

Doctors diagnose obesity by using a BMI (body mass index) chart, which we talk about in detail in the next section. In order to use the BMI, the doctor has to evaluate your child's height and weight in relation to children who are the same age as him. He makes this comparison by using a height and weight chart. There are several different height and weight charts; one is used for children from birth to 36 months, and another is used for kids from ages 2 to 20. Also, each chart is gender specific. Figure 5-1 shows a sample chart for boys.

When your child enters the pediatrician's office, he's weighed and his height is measured. These measurements are plotted vertically on the height and weight chart (age is plotted horizontally). The doctor gives you a report along the lines of, "Your child is in the 60th percentile for height and the 95th percentile for weight." What this means, simply, is that your child is taller than roughly 60 percent of kids his age and weighs more than 95 percent of those same kids.

Understanding body mass index (BMI) and children

When diagnosing obesity, the doctor takes the three components of the height and weight charts (see the preceding section) and plugs them into a formula for assessing BMI. The formula, in English measurements, is:

[Weight (lb) ÷ Height (in) ÷ Height (in)] × 703

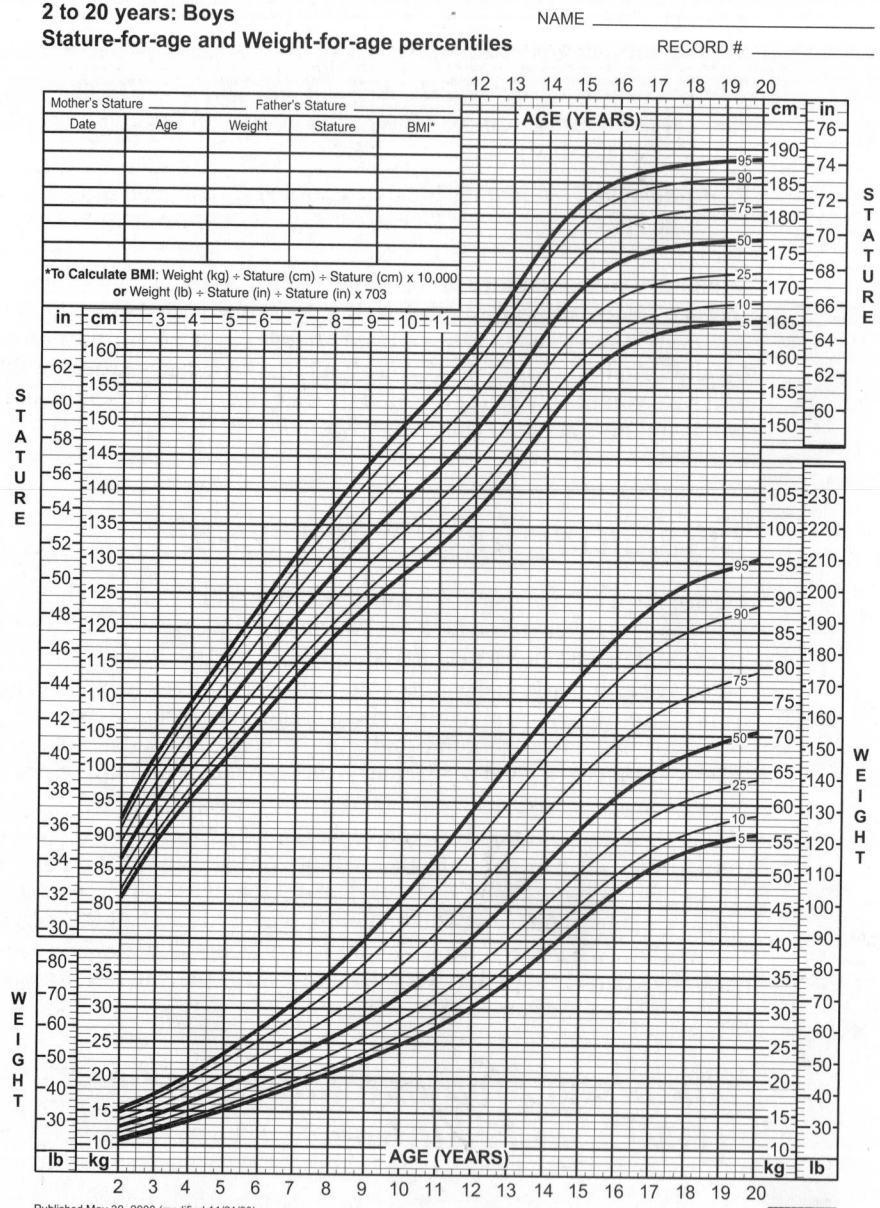

Figure 5-1:
A sample height and weight chart for boys ages 2 to 20.

Here's an example of how to use the BMI formula to figure out a child's BMI. Suppose a girl is 8 years old; 4 feet, 6 inches tall; and weighs 100 pounds. Plugging those numbers into the formula above tells you that this child's BMI is roughly 24.1. Simply calculating this child's BMI doesn't give an accurate indication of obesity, though. Because children are still growing, doctors use a special table for assessing their BMI scores that produces the *BMI-for-age score* (see Figure 5-2).

Plotting this child's age and her BMI number on the chart in Figure 5-2 shows that she's above the 95th BMI percentile for her age. But what does *that* mean, exactly?

If you're familiar with adult BMI tables, you know that obesity isn't a concern until someone reaches a BMI of 30 or more. However, evaluating BMI for children is different in that it takes into account the child's age, gender, and rate of growth. The Centers for Disease Control (CDC) breaks down the criteria for overweight children as follows:

- A child with a BMI-for-age greater than the 95th percentile is considered overweight.

- A child with a BMI-for-age in the 85th to 95th percentile is considered at risk for becoming overweight.

- A child with a BMI-for-age less than the 5th percentile is considered underweight.

Note that these ranges don't use the word "obese." The American Obesity Association (www.obesity.org), however, doesn't shy away from the term; it considers a child with an 85th percentile BMI-for-age overweight and a child with a 95th percentile reading obese.

The risk for obesity-related health issues increases along with BMI-for-age readings. Recent studies have shown that more than 50 percent of kids with a BMI-for-age over the 95th percentile had at least one obesity-related health issue, like diabetes or sleep apnea.

Along with these readings, your child's pediatrician can give you a healthy weight range for your child's age, height, and gender. Sometimes, the difference between their child's current weight and their ideal weight is what truly shocks parents into facing the magnitude of their child's weight problem.

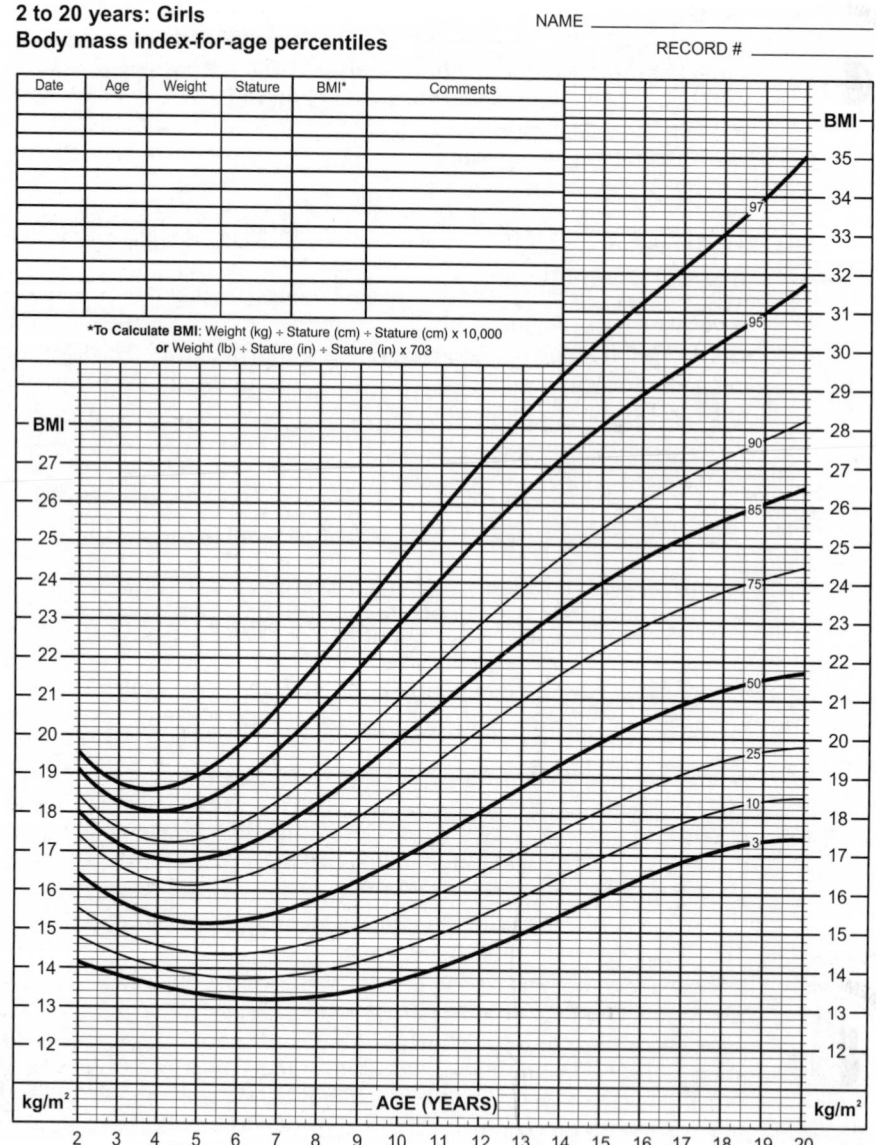

2 to 20 years: Girls
Body mass index-for-age percentiles

NAME _____

RECORD # _____

*To Calculate BMI: Weight (kg) ÷ Stature (cm) ÷ Stature (cm) x 10,000
or Weight (lb) ÷ Stature (in) ÷ Stature (in) x 703

Figure 5-2:
A sample
BMI chart
for girls
ages 2 to 20.

Published May 30, 2000 (modified 10/16/00).
SOURCE: Developed by the National Center for Health Statistics in collaboration with
the National Center for Chronic Disease Prevention and Health Promotion (2000).
http://www.cdc.gov/growthcharts

CDC
SAFER · HEALTHIER · PEOPLE™

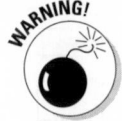

Although BMI charts give a fairly accurate reading of how overweight a child may be, they aren't perfect, especially where adults are concerned. A professional weight lifter, for example, can meet the BMI criteria for being overweight even though his extra weight is pure muscle. We talk about other ways to diagnose body fat in the following section.

Going beyond BMI to diagnose obesity

If you've ever been faced with weight-related medical tests, you know that several other procedures give more accurate readings of body fat than a BMI chart does. If an obviously overweight child scores a high BMI-for-age reading, a doctor will assume that the extra weight comes from body fat and not muscle. Despite its limitations, BMI is by far the most common method of diagnosing childhood obesity because it's quick, easy, cheap, and fairly accurate.

Other tests that can be used for diagnosing obesity include:

- **Hydrostatic water test:** A person is submerged in water and weighed.

- **Dual-energy X-ray absorptiometry (DEXA):** One X-ray with two energy levels scans the entire body and gives a reading of the amount of body fat. This test is commonly used to assess bone density.

- **Bioelectrical impedence (BIA):** An electrical impulse is sent throughout the body to assess the amount of water contained in the body. A higher amount of water generally translates into more lean tissue.

- **Calipers:** A trained professional uses this instrument consisting of two moveable, curved legs fastened at one end to assess skin-fold thickness at various points of the body. Calipers give an accurate reading when used correctly; unfortunately, they're often used incorrectly.

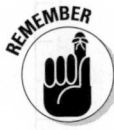

If these tests are performed, they're usually done on adults. The hydrostatic water test and DEXA are both costly tests to perform and aren't widely available. BIA and calipers are both used in some health clubs but usually aren't seen in a pediatrician's office. Doctors can easily make obesity diagnoses by putting together their observations of children and their BMI-for-age readings, so those are the criteria pediatricians usually rely on and consider when recommending options for correcting the condition.

Waisting your child's time?

For overweight adults, the risk for conditions like heart disease and diabetes is thought to increase with waist-to-hip ratio (WHR), a measurement calculated by dividing the waist circumference by the hip circumference. Men with a WHR of 0.9 or lower and women with a WHR of 0.8 or lower are considered to be in the safe zone; adults with a WHR of 1.0 or higher are in a high-risk category for developing weight-related illnesses.

While WHR may be a worthwhile tool for assessing an adult's risk of illness, it's not used on obese children. Studies have shown that it doesn't accurately reflect a child's level of health; when a child reaches adolescence, however, WHR is a more useful diagnostic tool.

Discussing the family's lifestyle

Your child's pediatrician probably won't stop at diagnosing your child with a weight problem and recommending that you do something about it. He'll want to get a good feel for your family's lifestyle and for the factors that may have contributed to your child's weight gain. He may ask about your child's:

- ✔ **Diet:** What types of food does your child typically eat over the course of a day? Would you say that she eats a large amount of food?

- ✔ **Eating habits:** Does she sit in front of the TV and eat or take a bag of chips up to her room before bed?

- ✔ **Activity level:** Does she enjoy getting outside with friends? Is she interested in sports?

- ✔ **State of mind:** Does she seem concerned or depressed over her weight?

- ✔ **Physical well-being:** Is she feeling well, generally speaking, or does she complain of various ailments that may be related to her weight?

Be prepared to answer these types of inquiries — and be honest! The doctor already knows that a child usually doesn't become obese in the absence of unhealthy lifestyle factors. In other words, there's no use trying to sugarcoat your answers, so to speak. The more forthcoming you are about your family's lifestyle, the better equipped the physician will be to help your child.

Taking additional tests

The doctor may want to do a full physical exam to evaluate whether your child is at risk for obesity-related health issues or if she may already be battling a condition or two. Some tests the doctor may recommend include:

✔ **Blood screening:** He may want to test your child's insulin level to rule out diabetes. He may also evaluate her cholesterol levels.

✔ **Cardiac evaluation:** Heart rate, blood pressure, and cardiac output (how much blood the heart puts out per minute) tend to be elevated in obese children, putting a greater strain on the heart, so all three may be tested.

✔ **Orthopedic evaluation:** Obese children may have malformations in the bones or ligament and muscle strains from carrying around excess weight.

✔ **Examination of the skin:** Because overweight and obese children can suffer from various skin eruptions (discussed in Chapter 3), the doctor may recommend treating them as soon as possible so they don't worsen.

Chapter 6

Overhauling the Family's Lifestyle

In This Chapter

► Exploring your own attitudes toward food and exercise
► Making easy changes for big results
► Convincing kids that weight loss is possible

*P*arents often wonder if their child's weight gain is due to an underlying medical condition. Does the child have a glandular problem, for example? Has his or her metabolism shut down for some reason? What else, these parents reason, could possibly cause an otherwise healthy child to become obese?

There very well may be some sort of genetic component that contributes to weight gain, but in most cases, obesity in adults and children alike is due to an unhealthy, inactive lifestyle. Although certain genetic factors may make weight gain more likely, lack of exercise and a high-fat diet are two variables that give a person an added push toward obesity. These habits are usually passed on from one generation to the next so that overweight or obese children grow up without knowing that there's a different way of doing things, that healthy foods and exercise are staples in many households.

Kids also pick up on their parents' attitudes about food and weight. Your child knows whether your relationship with food is a love/hate or love/love situation, and what's more, his own attitudes are shaped by what he sees and hears at home. Getting to the bottom of those feelings concerning food can reveal how unhealthy habits got established in the first place, which may be an eye-opener for how to break those habits in the future.

Obviously, a child can't learn healthy habits unless his parents teach him; that's where you come in. Even if you grew up in a house where unhealthy habits were the order of the day, even if you've never led anything resembling a healthy lifestyle, it's not too late for you to turn things around if your intentions are in the right place. A healthy lifestyle focuses on preventing weight-related illness like diabetes and heart disease; it's *not* about losing weight in order to look like a model. Even though the initial changes to the family's diet and activity levels can be made over a relatively short period of time, the results take longer to show themselves. For that reason, it's important for everyone to have a realistic idea of what these healthy changes are all about and what they can realistically expect from their efforts.

Recognizing How Your Own Actions and Attitudes Affect the Family

Before you can begin to help your child on her quest toward a healthier future, you have to first be able to assess your own relationship with and attitudes toward food and physical activity. On the surface, it would seem as though your eating habits and level of daily physical activity only affect one person (yourself); however, that's just not so. Parents are the ultimate role models for their children, especially in the kids' earliest, attitude-forming years. The fact of the matter is, when a child develops a relationship with food that goes *way* past basic nourishment, the end result is often an eating disorder of some kind, either related to overeating or undereating.

Passing the buck . . . and your own attitudes about food

The relationship you have with food can be complex. You need food to survive, but you may love it, hate it, or feel indifferent toward it — or feel every which way about it depending on the time of day, year, or the particular phase of life you're in at any given time. For example, when adults are experiencing particularly stressful times, it's not unusual for them to experience weight loss or weight gain, which means that people often either eat more or far less than usual when they're feeling pressured.

Emotions obviously come into play here, and they may affect the hunger cues you feel. Someone who's horrifically depressed, for example, may not feel hunger pangs at all and may actually forget to eat, resulting in weight loss. By the same token, depression can make people feel more hungry than usual or turn to certain so-called comfort foods even when they aren't hungry. Weight gain is often the end result here.

You needn't be extremely depressed to have a relationship with food that's rather askew, although having an unhealthy relationship with food can certainly lead to depression. Depression is an extreme example of how the mind can either turn people toward food or turn them away from it. This section focuses on determining whether your own eating habits are born of genuine hunger or whether you eat based on external factors (which is often the case in families where obesity in an issue).

Obsessing over food

Food has become nothing short of an obsession; instead of depending on food for survival, people have broken food down into so many subcategories that it's often the one thing the entire day revolves around. What did you eat for breakfast? Who's ordering lunch? Where are you going to eat dinner? Do you have anything for dessert at home?

Just for comparison's sake, think about how past generations viewed food. It was a means to nourish tired bodies after they spent the day working in the fields or factories. You can bet that the laborer who spent the day breaking his back in a steel mill wasn't really thinking about whether he was going to have chocolate cake that evening; if he thought about food at all (and he probably only gave it some thought when his stomach started rumbling), he thought that his next meal was the fuel he needed to keep him going. That's a relationship born of sheer necessity.

These days, most people have no worries about securing their next meal, nor do they work at physically demanding jobs that make food an essential source of energy. They can stop off at the grocery store on the way home from work or breeze into a restaurant and literally order someone to bring heaping plates of food to them. While people still need food for nourishment, it's become something of a luxury, too. No one *needs* chocolate cake, for example, in order to see them through the day.

Food is everywhere. Ads for fast food show up on TV and billboards, and you can't drive more than a mile in many areas without seeing a fast-food restaurant, and in urban areas, sit-down restaurants are everywhere. As a population, we can't seem to get enough food! And the statistics of overweight and obese Americans (some 60 percent of adults in this country are at least overweight; 30 percent are obese) seem to bear this out.

Social eating

In addition to the ubiquitous ads and restaurants, many social functions revolve around food. When was the last time you had a morning meeting without coffee cake, bagels, or Danish? When was the last time you invited someone over for a visit without setting out cookies or brownies? Maybe your family has a tradition of a huge Sunday family gathering with a buffet that looks like something straight off a cruise ship.

You're thinking, "Of course we do this kind of thing. It's tradition; it's polite; it's simply what's done." Sure, it's polite to feed people, but food doesn't have to be the *focal* point of almost every gathering. That's exactly how many people end up becoming overweight in the first place. It's engrained in your mind that passing up a treat a host or hostess offers is impolite, so you probably end up *eating* everywhere you go. Unfortunately, when you get away from eating three square meals a day, snacking your way through the morning, afternoon, and night is a piece of cake . . . er, as easy as pie . . . well, you get the idea.

Emotional connections

For some people, a connection to food may start with depression or be caused by depression — it's kind of a chicken-or-the-egg–type scenario: Where did this whole unhealthy relationship start? The end result is that these people become dependent on food as a means of calming their nerves and making them feel safe. Many obese people describe overeating as a way of filling up an emotional emptiness they feel, but the sense of serenity is only temporary. Overeaters often feel regret over their unhealthy eating patterns, and that regret is only exacerbated by the depression they feel over their weight.

Is food an addiction?

Is it possible to be addicted to something we need for survival? Isn't that a slight exaggeration? No, it's not. It's one thing to think about food, prepare a menu for the week, or even look forward to a favorite meal. It's quite another to plan your entire day around food and think about it almost constantly. Food addiction is thought to have a biological component — that is, the body craves certain elements or compounds contained in particular foods. In Chapter 7, we discuss the theory that fast food has some rather addictive components, such as caffeine and sugar; that same theory is the basis for food addiction, except that it extends to include all sorts of foods and the feeling of being completely out of control where food is concerned.

According to this theory, food addiction is every bit as real as a chemical dependence on drugs or alcohol. Cutting back on certain foods may result in withdrawal symptoms, such as irritability or a general sense of malaise. Like other addictions, help is available for people who feel as though they can't kick their unhealthy eating habits on their own. A therapist who's experienced in treating eating disorders may employ cognitive or behavioral therapy in order to help someone with this disorder.

The cycle goes on: Depression may cause withdrawal from social contacts (often because obese people fear rejection or are embarrassed by their size, or both), and isolation makes food all the more attractive. Food can't reject overtures of friendship, and food sticks around for as long as one needs it to be there. The immediate satisfaction food gives seems irreplaceable. It's not unlike a smoker's addiction to nicotine — the smoker knows smoking's an unhealthy habit with serious health consequences, but the body (along with the mind) has this uncontrollable craving for another cigarette.

Giving kids the wrong idea

You may think that issues like social eating and depression apply only to adults, but they affect kids in several ways:

- Kids take in everything and look to their parents as examples. If your child watches one or both parents eat throughout the course of the day (in addition to or in place of regular meals), he'll follow suit. A small child in particular doesn't know the first thing about healthy and unhealthy habits. He assumes that whatever his parents do is right; thus, if you snack on a package of cookies to pass time in front of the TV, he'll follow your example.

- Households rarely have more than one set of rules concerning food, so if you have unhealthy eating habits, it's very unlikely that your child is eating low-fat, low-sugar, high-fiber meals when he's hungry.

- Ever hear that expression, "If mom's not happy, no one's happy"? Kids feel their parents' emotional pain. If you're depressed, it's affecting your child in some way. He may feel distant from you, or he may even think that he's caused your sadness. If he sees that you're "medicating" yourself with food, he's likely to use this form of comfort when he's feeling blue.

Some parents have the absolute best intentions and try desperately not to pass their eating habits on to their children. However, leading by example is the only method of truly breaking this cycle. In other words, you simply can't continue to eat a high-fat and/or high-sugar diet and expect your children to accept their veggies and lean meats at mealtimes. We know that breaking life-long (or at least long-term) habits is hard, but in order to instill in kids the best ways to stay healthy, parents have to live a healthy lifestyle, too.

Studies have shown that obese children do far better in their long-term weight loss goals if at least one of their parents is involved in creating a healthier lifestyle in the home.

Analyzing what goes in your grocery cart

Because parents are almost entirely in control of the food that comes into the home, they're also in charge of overhauling the family's eating habits. You can assume that anything that you buy is fair game for the entire family, so don't buy candy for your spouse if your child's trying so hard to eat healthier foods; it's a temptation that's best left in the store.

Some items that have no place in a home that's undergoing a health makeover include:

- **Fried foods:** Fresh or frozen, they're high in fat and don't belong in your fridge or freezer.

- **Most convenience foods:** Pay attention to food labels (see Chapter 8) so that you don't bring home almost-prepared foods that are high in sugar and/or saturated fats.

- **Sugary treats:** Part of this whole healthier-living process is discovering how to enjoy foods in their most natural states. An apple is a good dessert, for example, because it's low in fat and naturally sweet. Eating lots of refined sugar can make fruit taste sugarless, by contrast, and that's not the direction you want to go in.

- **Refined carbohydrates:** When the natural fiber is stripped from flour, the body has a tough time metabolizing it. Whole grains are best; they're high in fiber (which is very filling) and nutrients.

- **High-fat dairy:** Whole milk, whole-milk cheeses, ice cream, and whipped cream are all high in fat. Buy skim milk and low-fat counterparts as alternatives.

- **High-fat condiments:** Mayonnaise, salad dressings, and tartar sauce can all catapult otherwise low-fat meals into the fat stratosphere. Use vinegar, olive oil, or lemon instead.

- **Processed meats:** Pepperoni and sausages are usually high in fat. Read those nutrition labels on meat products and look for lower-fat versions of these foods.

Many juices, popsicles, cereals, and yogurts — all favorites of the typical American child — fall into one or more of the categories listed above.

If you're thinking that we've pretty much wiped out your grocery list, you may be wondering what we expect you to feed your family. Low-fat, low-sugar foods, of course. Foods that are in as natural a state as possible (like fruits, veggies, and whole grains) come power-packed with vitamins and minerals and also fill up the stomach so that your child will be far less hungry, say, an hour after eating an apple than she would be an hour after eating a candy bar. For more advice on making good choices when food shopping, turn to Chapter 8.

You may have a hard time making the switch from buying the kinds of foods that your family has enjoyed for so many years to buying healthy foods only. (Fortunately, in practice, it's *very* easy these days to find low-fat alternatives in almost every grocery store in this country!) To make the transition as quick and painless as possible, pick a day to clean out the pantry and fridge, tossing the last vestiges of unhealthy foods. Don't keep one bag of chips around for an "emergency." If it's in the house, somebody's going to find it and eat it. If unhealthy snacks are nowhere to be found, truly hungry family members have to settle for a low-fat alternative. And if they're looking for snacks because they're bored . . . well, sometimes going to the pantry and discovering their favorite treats aren't there is just the thing that breaks kids (and adults) of unnecessary snacking habits.

No life-threatening event will ever be solved by tearing open a bag of fried potato slices; if that were possible, emergency rooms would keep chips under lock and key. The worst that's going to happen when the treats are gone is that the family will express their displeasure. They'll live through that kind of disappointment — *without* an emergency chip infusion.

Curing your exercise allergies

Eating healthier foods is only one part of instituting an overall healthier lifestyle in your home. Setting an example of physical activity is the other essential part of this equation. For parents who loathe and despise exercise, this can be a bit of a sticking point: They're willing to encourage their children to become more active, but they aren't quite willing to get involved in exercise themselves. Why should they, they wonder? They work all day; they're exhausted; they have no energy or desire to become super-fit, so what's the point?

Recall that children pick up on their parents' attitudes. Your child no doubt already knows how you feel about physical activity, especially if you've dropped comments like these in the past:

✔ "I'm allergic to exercise."

✔ "Exercise makes me cranky."

✔ "It's impossible for me to exercise."

Of course, there are some people for whom exercise may actually be impossible. However, many people who claim that they can't exercise usually have the wrong idea of what exercise is all about. A significantly overweight woman who has led a sedentary lifestyle for the past ten years may not be able to run a mile, but she can take a walk. Perhaps she could ride a bike or even do some water aerobics. Barring any true physical debilitation diagnosed by a doctor, overweight people can find some form of low-impact activity to help them on their way to a healthier lifestyle. (And to date, no one has been diagnosed with an actual case of an "exercise allergy.")

Is getting active going to be easy? No. But the fact that becoming more active isn't easy when you're overweight yourself sends a very powerful message to your child: *This is hard work. I didn't particularly want to do this, but it's important enough to my health that I am doing it. And if I can do it, so can you.*

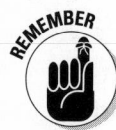

Exercise doesn't always result in a person becoming ultrathin or super-fit, but it almost always leads to better health, especially in people who have high blood pressure and high cholesterol levels (two conditions that are fairly common in overweight adults and kids).

Adults should check with their doctors before beginning exercise programs, just to rule out any potential problems. Even adults who are in a healthy weight range should heed this advice because health issues can occasionally pop up seemingly out of nowhere.

When your child sees that you're making a concerted effort to exercise in order to improve your health, he's going to think that *this* is the right way to live, simply because it's what you're teaching him through your actions. Keep in mind that kids don't exercise in the same way adults do; they *play*. Encourage him, and help him find an activity or two that he enjoys and that he can participate in on a regular basis (at least four to five times a week). The more fun his physical activity is, the more likely he is to think of it as playtime and not as some sort of torture. You can find tips for helping your child in this regard in Chapter 10.

Weighty judgments

The ways in which parents judge others by their weight influence how kids view the world. If you're overweight, you no doubt already know that a fat prejudice is unfortunately alive and (un)well in this country. But ask yourself this: Do *you* judge thin people based on their appearance? Be honest. When a thin model or actress is on TV shilling for a car manufacturer or a cosmetics company, do you find yourself thinking (or saying) things like, "She's so stupid" or, "She's not even talented; they just hired her because she's thin" or, "Why doesn't she eat something once in a while?"

Judging people based on their appearances isn't right, and many times, those judgments end up being inaccurate, but it's human nature to draw certain conclusions between a person's personality and his or her appearance. Whereas overweight people are often judged to be lazy, dumb, and unhygienic, very thin people are sometimes judged to be vain, egotistical, and unhealthy.

When you say things like, "She's so skinny, I hate her!" or, "She's so thin, she looks like a cadaver," you're teaching your child to judge a person based on how he or she looks. You may also unwittingly pass along the idea that thin people are bad people. This kind of blanket judgment can affect your child's relationship with other people. If a thin classmate approaches your daughter and her first reaction is, "She's thin, so she's probably mean," where do you think *that* relationship is going?

On the flip side, if you're one to go on and on about how you wish you were as skinny as so-and-so, if you're always talking about weight (yours and other people's) and looking at life from a perspective of weight loss or weight gain, you're essentially telling your child that the only thing that matters is weight and appearance. For example, comments like these are not at all unusual:

✔ "I saw my cousin last night. She gained 20 pounds! Oh, and she won some big award at work, but you should *see* how heavy she is!"

✔ "My sister lost her job and her husband left her. She was so depressed that she lost 20 pounds. At least she *looks* really great."

These very realistic comments are examples of how many people think that weight loss cures everything and weight gain diminishes achievements. These aren't the kinds of messages that children should be learning. And although you can't do a whole lot about the advertisements that your kids are exposed to on a regular basis or the things they hear at school, you *can* make sure you're communicating healthy messages about weight at home. And what are those messages?

✔ Weight isn't the ultimate issue; *health* is.

✔ People come in all different shapes and sizes.

✔ A person's appearance is not necessarily a reflection of his or her personality.

Maybe you were teased by thin kids when you were younger; maybe your child has experienced the same kind of cruelty, and you both think you have every right to dislike skinny people. Turn that thought around: What if an overweight child teased you? Would that affect how you felt about all heavy people? Probably not, especially if you've always been heavy yourself. People tend to fear (or outright dislike) people who look different from themselves. Remind your child (and yourself) that *everyone* is different and that you can't group people and their personality traits together based on general appearance.

Judging a book by its cover isn't right, but how on earth do your feelings about Ms. Model affect your child's weight? Even if you have a kid who argues with everything you say, your point of view on major issues comes through loud and clear. For the most part, your views dig themselves into your child's very impressionable mind, and she's very likely taking whatever you say and turning those words into her very own feelings on any given issue. When you berate skinny people, she may think to herself, "Who'd want to be thin?" If you're obsessed with becoming thin, however, she may worry that she'll never meet *your* ideals for body weight.

Little Changes, Big Long-Term Results

So what does overhauling your family's lifestyle really entail? Do you have to hire a personal chef, make room for a home gym, and bring a personal trainer into the family fold? Wouldn't it be easier to move everyone out to the wilderness where you'd be forced to build your own log cabin and grow your own food?

If you've been thinking about uprooting the family and leaving society behind *anyway,* then by all means go right ahead. But if you're looking to stay right where you are, improve your family's health, and *not* lay out a fortune in the process, then we have great news for you: Big health benefits can come from changes that are relatively easy to make. Cutting fat out of the family's diet, reducing calories and portion sizes, and finding ways to increase physical activity are the main ways of improving health.

Cutting back on fat and calories

Theoretically, all you need to cut fat out of your family's diet is some knowledge about fat itself and the will to follow through on your best intentions. Here are some tips for keeping fat to a minimum:

✔ **Learn to read food labels.** Know the difference between saturated (unhealthy) and unsaturated (acceptable in moderate amounts) fat.

✔ **Buy foods in their most natural state whenever possible.** Fruits, veggies, and whole grains are all naturally low in fat and high in fiber.

✔ **Look for low-fat alternatives.** Don't buy whole-milk products; choose skim or fat free.

✔ **Avoid fast food.** Most of it is loaded with saturated fat.

✔ **Check out school lunches.** If you're seeing a plethora of meals with high-fat contents (or worse, there's a fast-food vendor in your child's cafeteria), pack your child's lunch at home.

✔ **Don't let fat sneak in at snack or dessert time.** You're trying to teach the family that healthy foods are best; don't make an exception like, "We'll eat healthy all day long, but we'll have pie for dessert." You'll be sending a mixed message.

These are ways to keep the fat out of your house; however, the best foods for weight loss pack the one-two wallop of being low in fat *and* sugar. Low-fat foods can *still* have a high-sugar content, which can contribute to weight gain. Sugar is high in calories, and calories that aren't used for energy are stored as fat. An obese child only needs 1,200 to 1,500 calories a day; to meet that goal, low-sugar, low-fat foods are your child's best bet. When you're actually setting out to make low-fat meals, you can find more-specific cooking tips in Chapter 9.

Making exercise a part of life

The family that plays together gets healthy together. Start changing your family's lifestyle to include healthier options by going on family outings. Outings get everyone out the door *and* introduce exercise in the form of a fun activity that everyone can do — young, old, heavy, or thin. The outings you plan (at least at first) should be based on what your family enjoys most. Walking, swimming, hiking, biking — these are all good activities for families who are just making their foray into the world of physical activity. Remember to pack a healthy snack and water for everyone!

Although an activity should be fun for everyone, it should *not* be centered around food! If the whole family wants to go bowling, for example, that's certainly better than sitting home and watching TV. But if you end up with a pizza, a pitcher of soda, and a basket of fries, that's not good. For this reason, heading to the great outdoors where the only food present is the low-fat fare you've packed yourself is usually better.

Making exercise a regular part of everyone's day takes effort. Start by limiting the time your family spends in front of the TV, computer, and video game console. Electronics have become such a part of life that families often don't realize how much time they spend staring at those screens.

You can't expect family members to spend every minute that they aren't watching TV exercising, but in order to get them doing *anything* active, you have to lead by example. So cut back on your own TV viewing. Go outside with them. Stock your garage and yard with fun games. Some toys that can get your child playing outside include:

- Bike
- Rollerblades
- Basketball hoop
- Scooter
- Skateboard
- Jump rope

Make sure, of course, that you take safety into consideration by providing helmets and adult supervision where applicable.

Younger children usually need a parent to get them outside and play with them; older kids are more likely to want to play with kids their own age. You can make a difference here by encouraging your child to invite active kids over. (You know, some children love to play outside and others like to park it in front of the TV all day long.) Getting your child to exercise and be active will be much easier on you if he has a pal or two to play with outside. On the other hand, allowing him to invite over a friend who refuses to do anything even remotely active may be a big pain in the neck for you. You shouldn't start banning lifelong friends who are otherwise not objectionable little people; you just have to make it clear that you have new limits on electronic playtime when these friends visit.

Stick to your rules limiting TV watching and outdoor activity even when friends are visiting. Your child needs to realize that there's no going back and that the healthier lifestyle rules are in effect no matter who comes into the house.

Chapter 10 contains more advice for making exercise an enjoyable activity for the entire family — rain or shine!

Yes, You Can!

Most cases of obesity are caused by overeating and underexercising. Flipping unhealthy habits around are the keys to better health. There's no magic pill or hoops to jump through. Achieving weight loss and health goals is possible for every family, regardless of how many times you've all tried without success. Think of it as an opportunity to change the future.

If you and/or your child did well on a health-improvement program in the past and then lost your focus and fell back into bad habits, that's not failure! It's proof that you *can* do it. You just need to take it farther than you did the last time and make those lifestyle changes *permanent*.

We're not advocating what experts call "yo-yo dieting," a pattern of weight loss followed by weight gain, followed by weight loss, and so on. Over the years, yo-yo dieting can take a toll on the body and lead to serious health issues. It can also result in stubborn weight gain that doesn't respond to healthy lifestyle modifications.

Losing weight is possible!

But it takes determination, effort, and the right mindset. Changing your family's point of view about diet and exercise is essential in this whole process. An obese child, for example, probably knows only one way of life — the one he's leading right now. When a kid has been raised with unhealthy habits, he simply has no idea that there's any other way of doing things. An obese child may not realize, for example, that:

✔ Turning off the TV and video games adds a whole lot of playtime to the day.

✔ Eating dinner with the TV off gives everyone the opportunity to talk about what happened at work or school.

✔ Playing outside is a terrific way to make new friends.

✔ Trying new activities teaches him a lot about himself and his abilities.

✔ Substituting low-fat, high-fiber foods for high-sugar, high-fat snacks makes him feel fuller, longer.

✔ Making permanent lifestyle changes takes time, but the results are worth it!

Obviously, a child who's never known a different way of life isn't going to make these realizations on his own. A healthier lifestyle starts with at least one parent displaying a healthier outlook on life, one that starts with not having any illusions about weight loss and how hard or easy it's going to be. Changes to the grocery list and activity level are, *theoretically,* not so difficult to make. Leaving the cookies in the grocery store, opting for fruits and vegetables as snacks, learning to bake or broil foods instead of fry them, and taking a walk several times a week are nothing compared to, say, cooking gourmet meals with exotic ingredients and training for a marathon. We're talking about starting with *little* changes, which make all the difference in the world.

Losing heart with the whole healthier living process is common when a child (or family) expects too much, too soon. Emphasize to everyone that this is a slow, steady process, that these are permanent changes, and that there's no going back. You can help everyone stay committed by not wavering from your stance and by showing your positive attitude. For example:

- ✔ Don't give in to requests, pleas, or demands for high-fat and high-sugar foods.

- ✔ Don't allow TV to remain the focal point of every day.

- ✔ Don't shame or yell at kids when they're less than enthusiastic about a healthy meal or playing outside.

- ✔ Do encourage family outings and outdoor playtime.

- ✔ Do experiment with healthy foods and new recipes.

- ✔ Do get the kids involved in the cooking.

- ✔ Do use positive reinforcement, such as complimenting your child on his efforts and acknowledging his progress.

Successful weight loss is all about getting to the roots of the weight problem — eating too many unhealthy foods and leading a sedentary lifestyle — and treating them like they're weed roots. You can't go halfway; you have to get rid of them so that they can't get a stranglehold on the family again!

Sticking with the changes

Making changes to your family's lifestyle is a major accomplishment in and of itself. If you've cleared the junk food out of the house, found some healthy recipes to try out, and discovered ways to get the kids out the door and playing in the yard, kudos to you. Those are major steps in the right direction.

Hopefully, your family has been accepting of these changes. Depending on their personalities, kids may be excited or . . . less than excited.

Helping kids see the long-term goals

Obviously, working with a child who *wants* to become healthier is much easier than working with one who doesn't; however, sometimes even children who are eager to start a healthy living turnaround become less and less excited as time goes on. Kids want immediate results, so if something isn't going to happen in a short period of time, they may have serious doubts about whether it will happen at all. Depending on age, a child honestly may not have the ability to rationally say to herself, "If I just stick with it, I'll feel so much healthier three months from now." Three months is a long, long way off as far as she's concerned.

If your child's losing interest in the healthy living plan, find ways to point out how major things take time. Remind her of the seasons, for example, and how, in the dead of winter, it seems as though it will never be spring. When it's freezing outside, it's hard to believe that the cold will eventually disappear and everyone will be outside running around in shorts. And yet spring *does* show up every year. Change just takes time.

Teens are a different story. They have a better handle on the passage of time; however, they also often want instant gratification. Your teen may benefit more from keeping a weight-loss journal that provides a visual aid of her progress. As often as she needs to, she can refer to the journal and see that she's indeed making progress. Perhaps the weight loss is slow-going (for best results, it should be), but as long as she can see that her efforts are paying off, she's more likely to remain strong in the face of boredom or frustration with the new lifestyle.

Dealing with resistance

Convincing a kid to make healthy changes is a little different when she's opposed to any changes in her way of life. Can you drag her outside and make her play with you? If she's small enough, yes, you can (as long as you're pleasant about it); a younger child is dependent on you to lead the way, and because you're still the boss of this child (no matter what she may say or think), you absolutely can plan outings with and for her. Heck, that's your responsibility.

A teen who's resistant to change is another matter, however. Because older kids can be notoriously defiant and rebellious, you don't want to push her too much or you may make matters worse. You don't want to create a battleground over her weight issue or she may very well continue to overeat just to spite you and show you that she's in control of her body. Instead, she needs to be the one to take the initiative. You're playing a supporting role, so the best thing you can do for a teen in this situation is lead by example. Keep the junk foods out of the house, and live your own healthy lifestyle. When she's ready, she'll come around, and if she sees that you actually know what you're talking about (having changed your own unhealthy habits), she'll be that much more interested in what you have to say. For more on this topic, check out Chapter 13.

Chapter 7

The Basics of Good Nutrition

In This Chapter

▶ Decoding the FDA food pyramid

▶ Substituting healthy foods for less healthy choices

▶ Figuring out how much food is just enough

▶ Getting used to *new* favorite foods

▶ Kissing fast food goodbye

*I*nitiating and maintaining a healthy lifestyle in your home begins with knowing something about nutrition. Nutrients give everyone in the house a boost and make them feel well enough to begin participating in physical activities, a vital part of weight loss and healthy living.

Aside from helping one gear up for physical outings, nutrition plays an important part in the day of a growing child. Many studies have shown that kids who skip breakfast don't perform as well in school as their pals who take the time to eat in the morning. Kids need

✔ Calcium for developing bones and teeth

✔ Vitamins and minerals in order to grow well

✔ Good hydration to keep their organs in tiptop shape

✔ Protein for muscle development

In addition to eating a healthy diet, children need to learn how to balance that diet by including food groups of all sorts. This is where the United States Department of Agriculture (USDA) food pyramid can be a big help; it contains realistic recommendations of the kinds of foods everyone should work into their daily diet and how much of these foods they should be eating. In this chapter, we talk about everything nutrition, from the food pyramid and typical sources of fat in the diet to calorie counts and fast food.

Understanding Nutritional Requirements: Look to the Food Pyramid

In January 2005, the USDA responded to criticism of its old, standard food pyramid by launching an entirely new, interactive pyramid (see Figure 7-1). The main goals of this new program are:

✔ To spread the news that one eating plan isn't right for every single person

✔ To provide clearer, more specific information for each individual person according to his or her age, weight, and gender

The Web site (www.mypyramid.gov) that accompanies this new program provides helpful, realistic recommendations and information about how your individual eating plan stacks up against the government recommendations. You can type in all the food that you and your child have eaten in the last 24 hours, and the site analyzes its nutritional values and lets you know (with a series of happy or sad-faced icons) how you're doing.

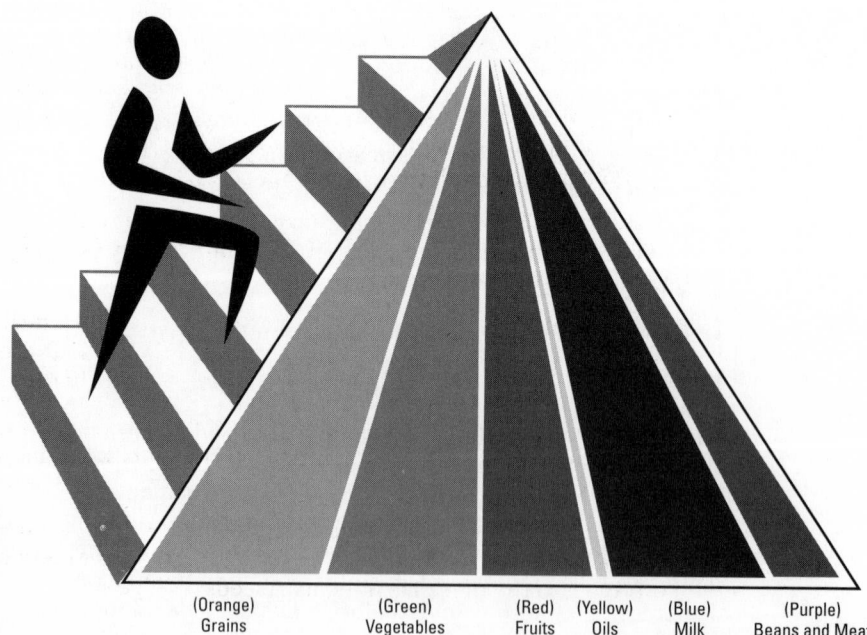

Figure 7-1: The revised USDA food pyramid.

(Orange) Grains   (Green) Vegetables   (Red) Fruits   (Yellow) Oils   (Blue) Milk   (Purple) Beans and Meat

The latest incarnation of the food pyramid is more in touch with middle America, taking into account that . . . well, most people just didn't *get* the old pyramid, which seemed to have a whole lot of food listed willy-nilly. The pasta and grain group, for example, recommended 6 to 11 servings per day but didn't tell you specifically what kinds of breads and grains you should be eating — or how much. (Eleven whole-grain rolls sure seems like a lot of bread to ingest day after day!) The revised pyramid, in contrast, breaks recommendations down into how many specific measurements (ounces or cups) of a food group you should be shooting for each day — and it makes these recommendations based on age and gender. Now *that* makes sense!

Look at all the pretty colors: What the pyramid means

The recommendations contained in the new food pyramid are based on *daily caloric intake,* which means that one serving size doesn't fit all. Based on a daily caloric intake of 2,000 calories, here's what the colors of the food pyramid translate into, foodwise:

- ✓ **Orange: Grains.** The recommendation is 5 to 8 ounces of whole grains per day.

- ✓ **Green: Veggies.** The recommendation starts out at 2½ cups each day for a person who consumes 2,000 calories daily, and the amount is raised or lowered with individual caloric intake. In addition, the USDA recommends regularly choosing from different veggie groups (specifically, leafy, orange, dark green, legumes, and starches).

- ✓ **Red: Fruits.** The recommendation is 2 cups per day of a variety of fruits; choose fresh, frozen, canned, or dried, but go easy on fruit juices, which tend to be packed with sugar.

- ✓ **Yellow: Oils.** The pyramid makes a distinction between healthy fats (like those from fish and nuts) and unhealthy fats (like those from butter and lard). The recommendation is to choose sparingly from healthy fat sources.

- ✓ **Blue: Milk/Dairy.** The recommendation is 3 cups of low-fat or fat-free milk or dairy products each day.

- ✓ **Purple: Beans and meats.** The recommendation is to choose lean meats, use healthy cooking methods (no frying!), and work different sources of protein into the diet (like nuts, fish, seeds, and peas).

The revised pyramid gives a general recommendation for daily caloric intake and then advises monitoring weight to see how that recommendation is working out. If your child seems to be gaining weight, you should cut her calories down a bit more. When we talk about daily caloric intake for obese children later in this chapter (see the section "Counting Up the Calories: How Much Should My Overweight Child Be Eating?"), we advise going a bit lower than 2,000 calories per day, which puts your child in the same general ballpark as the above recommendations, but we stick by the recommendation that monitoring weight is the only way to know whether your child's daily intake is adequate or if it's too much.

In addition to specific nutrition recommendations, the revised USDA food pyramid also includes:

✔ **An emphasis on activity:** The little person on the side of the pyramid is climbing the pyramid's steps. The new program recommends at least 60 minutes of activity per day for kids (on most days).

✔ **Recommendations for working various foods into your family's diet:** Throwing carrots at the kids each night isn't enough, according to the pyramid. Instead, you should shoot for green veggies on one night and orange veggies the next night in order to get the most benefit from healthy foods.

✔ **A de-emphasis on sugar:** Although the old pyramid also advised using sugars sparingly, the revised pyramid specifically advises against sugar-laden drinks, like many fruit juices and sodas. (Hooray, we say!)

✔ **An explanation of healthy fats:** Fish oils, for example, are a good source of essential fatty acids, but butter is simply a source of fat. This pyramid makes the distinction clear.

The Web site for the revised food pyramid, www.mypyramid.gov, includes helpful links to other sites (such as the President's Challenge for physical fitness, in the event your family members want to make a friendly competition out of becoming fit). It also has loads of helpful tips for preparing healthy foods and snacks as well as an entire page of interactive games just for kids!

Putting the pyramid to good use

Taking the recommendations from the food pyramid under advisement is the first step in knowing what kinds of foods should show up at mealtimes in your home. A healthy plate has two things going for it:

> ✔ It has foods representing all the major food groups (which are repre-
> sented on the food pyramid by the different-colored stripes).
>
> ✔ The portions are under control.

A discussion about the appropriate types of food must also address portion
sizes. Simply put, many people eat too much food and don't even know what
a normal-sized portion looks like anymore. A single serving in a restaurant is
very often enough to feed at least two people or enough to be eaten by one
person at two separate sittings; however, because huge portions have become
the norm when eating out in this country (and because so many people eat
out so often for various reasons), we seem to have forgotten that leaving the
table feeling ready to burst isn't normal or healthy.

Structuring a healthier lifestyle for the family includes redefining how much
food is enough to get each body through the day without depriving it of fuel
for its most basic functions and physical activities. Anything more than that
results in weight gain. We talk more about portion sizes in Chapter 9.

Fat Is As Fat Does: Recognizing the Fat in Your Family's Diet

When you're gathering information and knowledge about nutrients and nutrition, you can't really go halfway. It all snowballs until you know more than
you ever expected. When you begin to understand how a couple of nutrients
benefit or negatively affect the body, you also find out about the effects of
other nutrients. Nutrition may seem like a complicated topic, but we can
assure you that it really isn't. All you need is a desire to learn and a willingness to commit yourself to becoming more informed. You don't need an
advanced degree in medicine to comprehend this information!

Avoiding fat

You can't initiate and maintain a healthy lifestyle in your home if you unwittingly
undermine yourself by making uninformed nutrition choices. Consider this scenario: You plan a lovely dinner for the family, making sure to include something
from each of the food groups: chicken, broccoli, whole-grain rolls, and milk to
wash everything down. At first glance, this meal sounds very balanced and
healthy. But what's this — you're serving *fried* chicken? Broccoli with cheese
sauce? Butter slathered on the roll? Whole milk with chocolate syrup?

Fat in baby and toddler diets

The one exception to cutting down fat in your household is if you have a baby or toddler. Small children need some fat in their diet for the development of their central nervous systems, which is why youngsters who aren't breast-fed drink formula or whole milk (both of which are good sources of fat) for the first two years of life. Breast-fed infants get an adequate amount of fat from their mother's milk.

Most pediatricians recommend formula for the first year of life, supplemented with a healthy, balanced diet. Doctors don't recommend putting toddlers on an all-fish-fry diet, as this would provide kids with far more fat in their diets than is healthy. Chances are, kids will get a sufficient amount of fat from the foods they eat, even in the healthiest households.

This meal, which was headed in the right direction, has taken a nose dive with the addition of a whole lot of fat, which the USDA food pyramid recommends using "sparingly." (The same advice goes for sugar, by the way, which is why that glass of milk would have been a healthier choice if it were skim and plain.) Fat is practically the central nutrient of the meal, and regardless of what you're serving — whether it's low-fat meat, fish, or vegetables — if you add a not-so-healthy dose of fat to it (by frying it, smothering it in a fatty sauce, or dousing it with a high-fat condiment), you're undoing the health benefits of that food.

Adding fat to meals really is *that* bad for the body, whether that body's heavy or thin. Not only can excessive dietary fat lead to the development of obesity and all its associated health risks (outlined in Chapter 3), but it also can lead to elevated cholesterol levels, which in turn can increase a person's risk of cardiovascular disease. In addition, fat can cause damage to some of the internal organs (the liver, for instance, and the intestines), even if a person isn't overweight.

Making healthier food choices

A healthy food covered with fat is no longer healthy. There's really no exception to this rule. Excessive amounts of fat negate the healthy qualities a food has to offer, and this rule applies to eating foods in combination with one another, as well. For example, upon entering your favorite fast-food establishment, you may peruse the menu and settle upon a grilled chicken salad, which is a great choice. The chicken gives you your protein, and the veggies pack a nutritional wallop loaded with vitamins and minerals. Heck, you even decide to go with the low-fat dressing in order to keep the salad 100 percent healthy. Great work!

Ooh, but then you spy the milkshake that you really need to have. That qualifies as dairy, right? And the French fries? One more veggie can only mean more goodness for you at this meal!

Things were going really well until the shake and the fries appeared on your tray or in your bag. Technically, the shake may qualify as a dairy product (although more and more, fast-food milkshakes are made from man-made products and don't include any milk at all), but it also provides a whole lot of fat and refined sugar. And the fries? They don't have even *one* redeeming quality, even though they started out as healthy spuds.

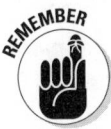

With fried foods, not only is fat absorbed into the food, but the frying process itself is thought to increase the risk of certain kinds of cancers. No matter the food (vegetable, fish, meat, cheese — whatever), once it hits the oil in the deep-fryer, it goes in a food group that doesn't merit its own space on the food pyramid: Fat on a Platter. It's even worse than eating plain fat, so avoid it at all costs.

Other misguided attempts at nutrition may include:

- ✔ **Candy-coated fruits:** A raisin shouldn't be covered in chocolate; it's sweet enough on its own. And even though allowing your kids to dip their apple slices in caramel isn't the end of the world, the apple is much, much healthier on its own. Plus, you don't want them to get the idea that fruit is only edible when it's covered in sugar.

- ✔ **Super-sweetened yogurts:** The lowest-fat varieties of fruit-flavored yogurts provide your child with a healthy serving of dairy. Hint: These yogurts usually aren't the ones that are shocking blue or neon green in color, nor are they the yogurts with the stir-in candy pieces.

- ✔ **High-fat dressings and condiments:** Dipping carrot sticks into chunky blue cheese dressing may sound like a great after-school snack (and isn't nearly as bad as substituting Buffalo wings for the carrots), but it provides your child with far more fat than you've bargained for. (And the cheese in the high-fat dressing is definitely not the best way to work dairy into your child's day.)

- ✔ **Chips:** Potato or corn, fried chips aren't healthy. If your child loves the crunch of a chip for a snack, give him a baked snack instead, like pretzels, which are much lower in fat than their fried counterparts, or try corn or rice cakes. Both are low in fat and calories. And by the way, potato chips don't qualify as veggies.

✔ **Too many servings, or too-large portion sizes:** Too much of anything isn't good. Although healthy foods like fruits and vegetables have a high fiber content and are therefore quite filling, it's still possible to consume too much of them, especially if your child is accustomed to large portion sizes. Excess calories cause weight gain, whether those calories come from fruit or chocolate!

Making the occasional error doesn't spell disaster for your child's weight-loss or maintenance goal, but repeating several mistakes for a long period of time could be the reason your child continues to gain weight despite your best efforts. It's in your best interest to educate yourself regarding the major facts about nutrition and to keep yourself informed, especially as new products hit the grocery store shelves. Take an interest in how food is prepared and how that food will be used (or stored) in the body.

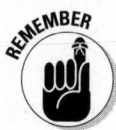

When you get a handle on the basics of nutrition, the rest falls into place. For example, when you begin planning your weekly menus to include all the basic food groups, you'll start thinking in a new way: "Does this food fall into the protein or fat category?" or "Is this condiment a spice or a fat?" (Spices can be used with a liberal hand; fats, as you know, are used sparingly.)

Counting Up the Calories: How Much Should My Overweight Child Be Eating?

The human body only needs so much fuel in order to maintain its most basic functions. Food provides this fuel in the form of calories, and everyone needs a minimum amount of calories per day. Recommended caloric intake varies according to age, gender, and activity levels; some bodies simply need more fuel than others. When too much food is consumed and the additional caloric fuel isn't used for bodily functions or physical activity, the extra fuel is stored as fat.

The recommendation for daily caloric intake for obese children is 1,500 to 1,800 calories per day. When the child reaches a healthy weight range and incorporates activity as a normal part of his day, you can start adding calories back in, little by little (100 to 200 calories at a time), until he achieves a healthy maintenance level.

Weighing in regularly when adding calories back into the diet is important for assessing how many calories are *too* many.

Getting your vitamins from the foods you eat

As you discover more and more about the basics of nutrition, you may become more interested in specifics, like which vegetables offer the highest amounts of a particular vitamin. A lot of this information tends to become individualized from family to family. For example, if your family has a long history of poor eyesight, you may be most interested in finding vegetables packed with vitamin A (like carrots), which is beneficial for the eyes. Or if your family is sick from October to April every year, you may be interested in providing them with megadoses of

vitamin C in its natural form (citrus fruits are a good choice here). Rest assured, feeding your family a balanced diet consisting of all the major food groups is usually enough to ensure good health all around.

Research has shown that vitamins from their natural sources (food) tend to provide more benefits than those taken in pill form. So eating healthy has a dual benefit: It's a low-fat way of life and one that may prevent illnesses like the common cold, too!

An obese child is usually overweight due to excessive eating (even though genetics may play a role and make him more prone to weight gain). Excessive eating leads to excessive caloric intake. Therefore, decreasing portion sizes automatically decreases caloric intake and produces major results in the weight-loss area. Combining physical activity with a reduction in his daily caloric consumption is the key to success.

The average school-age child needs between 1,600 and 2,500 calories each day (depending on age, size, and activity level). The average obese child's caloric intake far exceeds these margins, which leaves a surplus of fat and stored energy. Cutting calories back until a healthy weight range is achieved doesn't sound like an easy task; in fact, we know that it's going to take a lot of effort and determination on your part as well as on the part of your child. However, this technique really does work, and it's not harmful to your child.

Rather than keeping a rigid record of caloric intake, try first cutting your child's food intake back to include only the daily food group recommendations for a child his age. (You can easily find these recommendations on the food pyramid Web site.) Hit the major food groups, and encourage whole grains and fiber, which are very filling.

A sample menu with plenty of food

When we talk about cutting back on fat and sugar in order to lose weight and lead a healthy lifestyle, we're not really talking about eating tiny quantities of

Dietary fat versus body fat: They're not the same, but they're related

Dietary fat is very dense in calories, so the more fat your child eats, the better the chance that it ends up stored in her body as fat. Body fat, meanwhile, has a biological function: insulation from the elements. For this reason, fat is always looking for more unused calories to grab and hold onto. Unfortunately, this function of body fat was much more useful to our ancestors, who performed manual labor all day long and were routinely exposed to the elements, than it is to us in this day and age.

food; we're talking about choosing the *right* kinds of food. To demonstrate a day's worth of food following these recommendations, this section contains a sample menu of low-fat, low-sugar meals and snacks.

The following menu plan is appropriate for a female child between 7 and 9 years of age who engages in 30 to 60 minutes of physical activity daily. Calorie needs change depending on a child's age, gender, and physical activity. Check out www.mypyramid.gov to find out what your child's calorie needs are and what foods are needed to plan a healthy, well-balanced diet for him or her.

✔ **Breakfast** (1 Grain, ½ Fruit, ½ Milk/Dairy)

- 1 cup Cheerios cereal
- ½ cup fat-free milk
- ½ banana, sliced

✔ **Lunch** (2 Grains, ½ Vegetable, ½ Milk/Dairy, 2 ounces Meat)

- ½ cup baby carrots
- 1 ounce pretzels
- Turkey sandwich:

   1 flour tortilla

   2 ounces turkey breast

   1 slice low-fat American cheese

   2 slices tomato

1 lettuce leaf

1 teaspoon mustard

✔ **Snack** (1 Grain, 1 Milk/Dairy, 1 Meat)

- 1 slice whole-wheat bread
- 1 tablespoon peanut butter
- 1 cup fat-free milk

✔ **Dinner** (1 Grain, 2 Vegetables, 1 Milk/Dairy, 2 ounces Meat, 1 Fat)

- 2 ounces grilled chicken with barbecue sauce
- 1 cup mixed greens salad
- 1 tablespoon low-fat salad dressing
- 1 cup steamed green beans
- ½ cup cooked brown rice
- 1 cup fat-free milk

✔ **Snack** (1 Fruit)

- 1 small apple

Total: 5 ounces Grains, 1½ cups Fruit, 2 cups Vegetables, 3 cups Milk/Dairy, 5 ounces Meat, 1 Fat; 1,600 calories.

Am I shortchanging my child?!

You may be asking, "Are 1,500 calories per day enough for my child? Is my child going to starve?" Absolutely not. In order to lose weight, your child needs to eat enough food to maintain her bodily functions and no more. In her overweight condition, her body has so much stored fat (which, remember, is stored energy) that cutting back her caloric intake to the point of simply maintaining her bodily functions doesn't have any adverse effects. The body simply turns to the stored fat for energy.

This is not a starvation diet! In fact, this diet isn't about dieting at all; it's about *understanding food.* How much food is necessary to survive? How much extra food is your child consuming each day? How is that affecting her body? How does cutting back on food make her feel physically? These are questions that obese children never give a moment's thought. For them, overeating is a way of life, and it has nothing to do with food's true purpose, which is to keep the body up and running.

Your child may not be happy about the change, and, no doubt about it, she'll be hungry when you first make the switch from unhealthy to healthy foods (and portion sizes) in your home. But a lot of her reaction is due to the fact that:

- ✔ **She's used to eating certain types of foods.** Greasy foods and sweet foods are thought to have a calming effect on the brain, which makes them almost addictive to some people.

- ✔ **She's used to eating while doing certain activities, like watching TV.** Viewing a show without her usual snack may make her downright irritable.

- ✔ **She's used to eating larger-than-normal portion sizes.** Her stomach is accustomed to being overfilled, so even if she's eats enough food to keep her functioning, her stomach won't feel full.

A child whose meals follow the food pyramid recommendations gets not only plenty of food but also foods that give her lots of energy to boot. A healthy, balanced diet makes engaging in physical activity, which is also vital to weight loss, much easier.

Managing mealtimes and hunger

Studies have shown that obese people tend to eat because of external factors instead of responding to the body's natural cues of hunger, like stomach rumbles and contractions. For example, if your child is accustomed to setting herself up in front of the TV just before bedtime each night with a bowl of ice cream and a glass of soda, there's a good chance that she's not actually hungry, especially if she just ate dinner an hour or two earlier. But the ice cream and soda is her evening routine, so she's attached to it; it's the way she winds down after a long day.

There's nothing wrong with routines, of course. Children thrive on them, but when routines include food — especially high-fat and/or high-sugar foods — you can almost bet that weight gain is the end result. Every person (children *and* adults) should learn how to listen to their body's cues for hunger and eat only when they're legitimately hungry. This awareness is the first step in controlling the amount of food — and how many calories — your child consumes each day.

If your child just isn't hungry at 6 p.m. when you're ready to put a healthy dinner on the table, don't make her eat. Even though having family dinners several times each week is a good routine, it's also a flexible one. A child who isn't hungry should still come to the table with everyone else; however, if she doesn't feel like eating, don't make her sit through the entire meal. Let her talk with the family for a few minutes, and when she's ready, allow her to wrap her plate and put it in the fridge for later. Gathering around the table is less about the food and more about being together and catching up on each others' days. Most important, the family dinner is about *not* mindlessly consuming food — and calories — in front of the TV. We talk more about the importance of family meals in Chapter 11.

One of the worst best-intentioned moves that parents can make is forcing a child to eat simply because it's mealtime. However, you don't want your child to start skipping meals, either, because that isn't healthy. So have her come to the table at the dinnertime. If she isn't hungry right then and there, wrap her plate up and put it in the fridge for when she *is* hungry.

Farewell Forever, Favorite Foods?

The most distressing part of adopting a healthier lifestyle is saying goodbye to the old one. Putting a stop to family moments that have revolved around food for as long as you can recall may seem downright impossible. Sunday dinners, holidays, spur-of-the-moment gatherings, your nightly chats over pie and ice cream . . . you name it, and it's a tradition in someone's family. Occasionally indulging yourselves in a celebration that includes sweets or a hot dog or two isn't the end of the world (that kind of all-or-nothing thinking is as dangerous as giving into cravings at every turn); the trick is to see these times as special events and *not* as everyday occurrences.

Healthy food is always the better choice, kids!

If you can't imagine telling your kids that healthy foods are best without them laughing in your face, you're not alone; moms and dads everywhere have this same problem. But getting through to the overweight child on this topic is especially important. It's one thing to talk *at* the kid about healthy choices; it's another thing entirely to have him understand why you've changed how you do things in the kitchen.

Accepting a new, healthy eating regimen takes time and a lot of effort. Don't trick yourself into thinking that your kids are going to be just tickled pink when you refuse to serve up their beloved chicken Parmesan and garlic bread smothered in mozzarella cheese. Unhealthy goodies are all they've ever known, after all, and they may cling to their old favorites like a rock climber on a sheer mountain face.

Convincing your child that a healthy diet isn't a study in deprivation is a helpful first step in helping him accept this new way of life.

Visualizing the differences

Because fat and sugar are so densely packed with calories, your child can actually eat larger quantities of low-fat, low-sugar foods for the same amount of calories. In addition, the larger quantities of food (and fiber) make your child feel full in a way that high-fat, high-sugar foods can't (at least not in single servings of these foods).

For example, the average candy bar has about 300 calories, give or take a few. What kinds of healthy snacks can your child substitute for roughly the same number of calories?

- 9 cups of air-popped popcorn
- 6 small apples
- Almost 90 pretzel sticks (not the larger pretzel rods)
- 2 large pieces of whole-wheat bread
- 100 grapes
- 75 baby carrots
- 300 blueberries (230 calories)
- 3 cups of oat-ring cereal with milk (360 calories)

Do you think your child could really eat 100 grapes or 75 carrot sticks, or even 9 cups of popcorn? Obviously, he's going to feel full on these foods well before he reaches the caloric equivalent of the candy bar (which is good because these portions aren't exactly ideal and should only be used for comparison's sake).

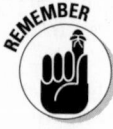

When we talk about cutting back on fat and sugar in order to lose weight and lead a healthy lifestyle, we're not really talking about eating tiny quantities of food; we're talking about choosing the *right* kinds of food.

Leading the way

Convincing your child that healthy food is best is *your* job. Start by educating yourself about healthy foods, and then educate your child. When you're making his sandwich in the morning and he's whining about not having white bread, tell him *why* you're giving him whole wheat. Explain why you're packing him a tuna sandwich rather than salami. Let him know why low-fat milk is a better choice than whole milk and why you're tossing an orange in his lunch box for dessert rather than cookies.

Kids are much more apt to give into a healthier lifestyle if they see that you're leading the charge! For that reason, it's as important for you to follow through on your own words and instructions in your own life. Demanding that your child eat whole grains while you continue to eat your own refined carbohydrates because you just hate the taste of whole-wheat bread is setting a poor example. So is ordering fried chicken for yourself in a restaurant while you order grilled chicken for your child. You have to live the life before you can sell it to your child.

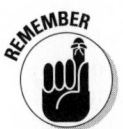

Even if only one child in your household is overweight, everyone should follow the same set of healthy rules. The change is about good health, first and foremost, and bad habits are bad for you, no matter what your weight.

Educating your child about the effects of being obese is also an effective tool. You don't want to scare your child, of course, but because serious health issues are common in obese children and adults, your child needs to know what he'll be up against if things don't change in your household.

Learning the ropes in the kitchen

Encourage your kids to get in the kitchen and make their own healthy snacks as well as help you when you're preparing meals. Not only is food prep a great learning tool, but it also gives kids a feeling of being in control. If the only foods in your house are healthy choices, then you don't have to worry about them making unhealthy snacks, no matter how unappetizing some of their healthy combinations may look to you.

Don't say a word if your child chooses to make a healthy snack that seems unpalatable to you. Exploring food is as much a part of growing up as growing hair long or wearing pants with holes in the knees: Kids need to establish their food likes and dislikes on their own, or they may never be able to make healthy decisions for themselves. Observe and keep an eye on portion sizes, but otherwise . . . mum's the word.

Getting used to the taste of nonfried foods

In recent years, the recommendation for weight loss has moved away from *dieting* (that is, temporarily giving up high-fat, high-sugar foods in order to achieve weight loss) toward redesigning one's entire lifestyle.

To people who are very entrenched in their eating habits, conventional dieting can seem like the lesser of two evils when compared with changing everything about the way they — and their families — have been eating (and probably *not* exercising). However, reworking an unhealthy lifestyle is the *only* thing that works for permanent weight loss and improved health! We know that it isn't easy for you to make a blanket statement to the family along the lines of, "Well, we can never, ever, ever have fried foods again. Sorry." For one thing, you're likely to be met with rebellion; for another, it's not exactly a true statement. A more accurate statement is, "We're going to start eating grilled, baked, and broiled foods on a regular basis."

Your kids probably won't like healthy foods, at least not in the beginning. What do you do when your child refuses to eat your low-fat dinner, saying that he hates the taste? Eat the food on your own plate, and put his plate in the refrigerator for later. If the only foods in your house are healthy options, you don't have to worry about him sneaking a cookie or a piece of candy. Consistency is the name of the game when you're introducing the family to new tastes and textures. Be firm, don't give in, and don't make separate meals. (For more on healthy meals and picky eaters, check out Chapter 9.)

New foods may taste strange to your kids (and to you) at first. Introduce foods that they'll find most palatable first — no sense giving them ammunition to work with by serving up a healthy dish containing a food no one has ever liked, fried or not. For example, if your family has always refused to eat fish of any sort, don't serve up tuna steaks during your first week of healthy eating. You want to keep their spirits high and get their palates to accept nongreasy, nonsugary foods first; then you can branch out with meals.

Here area some other tips for getting those taste buds in gear:

- **Have a positive outlook:** You're the leader of the pack, but that doesn't mean that you won't have your own moments of weakness. Do your best to keep in mind that all your efforts will pay off for every member of the family — even if they don't like what you're serving for dinner tonight.

- **Keep a journal:** Note the new foods you try and your family's reactions. When you've found several meals that are acceptable to everyone, making your weekly menu will be easy. You'll also have an easier time experimenting with new recipes using staple items, like chicken or pasta.

- **Watch the snacks:** Your kids certainly need an afternoon snack, but don't let them load up too much — even on healthy items like fruit. You want them to be hungry enough to at least *want* to eat their dinner. (On the flip side, if they fill up on snacks, they won't have much motivation to try out your new recipe.)

Your family will get used to the taste of healthy foods as long as you're willing to stick with your resolve to buy and serve only healthy foods. Cooking low-fat, healthy foods is all about changing your family's palate (the foods that they crave and accept at mealtimes). After they get used to low-fat, low-sugar meals, you may find that fried and sugary foods actually give your family members stomachaches!

Don't forget to compliment your child for being a trooper in this whole process. It's not easy for a kid to fall into step in a healthy lifestyle, so when you see that he's doing well and keeping up a positive attitude, tell him how proud you are — regardless of whether he's lost any weight. Having the right attitude is the toughest part of accepting a new lifestyle; if he has a good outlook, the rest is more likely to fall into place.

The Lures and Dangers of Fast Food

Fast food is bad for your child and your entire family. Stop buying it. (Is that the end of the story? Oh, *hardly!*)

We understand — really, truly, sincerely comprehend — that fast food is the ultimate godsend on a busy weeknight when you've worked a full day and the kids are going in different directions. At the end of a busy day, you feel as though you can't commit to any dinner that isn't already prepared and bagged up for your convenience.

Although completely understandable, these still aren't good enough reasons to feed your family the typical drive-thru fare. In this section, we talk about why eating fast food has become so common, why it's so unhealthy, and why cutting out this habit completely — especially in families with weight issues — is so important.

Fa(s)t food: What you crave

Recently, many fast-food chains have started offering their customers healthier options, like salads and grilled chicken sandwiches. Heck, you can even find bottled water in a lot of places these days. So if you're really in a pinch, you can definitely find a healthy option or two for your kids. You'd think we'd lay off fast food for this reason.

Well, you'd be wrong. The problem with fast food is that so many people crave and consume the unhealthy items on the menu, which far outnumber the healthier options. And the reason that people crave these foods, according to some researchers, is because they're loaded with addictive compounds, including:

- ✔ Sugar
- ✔ Fat
- ✔ Caffeine
- ✔ Refined carbohydrates

Thinking that there may be addictive compounds in fast food isn't such a big leap in logic. If you don't just love your morning coffee but actually *have* to have it or else your entire day is ruined, you know the feeling of having a chemical dependence. This addiction isn't as serious as heroin or nicotine addiction, but it's still real. Caffeine and sugar tend to act on the body by providing a burst of energy; fats and carbohydrates tend to have an opposite, more mellowing (sometimes tiring) effect. Combine these substances in one sitting on a regular basis and your child's body doesn't know *what's* going on; all it knows is that it wants these substances and wants them *now*.

Some critics of the fast-food industry have gone so far as to suggest that restaurants know exactly what they're doing by pushing unhealthy foods with addictive compounds: They're creating a nation of addicts who truly feel a physical craving for burgers, shakes, and fries. Whether you believe that there's a true intention to hook people on fast food is your own call, but you can't deny the argument that a regular fast-food habit can be very hard to break.

Addictive qualities aside, the average frequent fast-food customer may expect weight gain, heart disease, and/or diabetes after consuming a diet high in fat and sugar for several years. Although an exception to this rule may exist somewhere (like someone who's eaten huge burgers every day of his life for the past ten years and looks and feels fit as a fiddle), most people who eat fast food on a regular basis can pretty much expect that their weight will climb and their overall health will decline.

Kids and fast-food meals

The average kids' meal at a fast-food place contains:

- ✔ Burger: 280 calories; 13 grams total fat; 4 grams saturated fat
- ✔ Small fry: 240 calories; 13 grams total fat; 2.75 grams saturated fat
- ✔ Small soda: 270 calories; 30 grams sugar

Good fat, bad fat, and really bad fat

It's no secret that most fast-food items are high in fat. However, what many people don't know is that not all fat is created equally, and before you can truly understand how bad fast food is for the body, you have to know a little bit about the chemistry of fat. (And we promise, it's a *very* little bit of chemistry.)

All fat consists of chains of carbon atoms with hydrogen attached. The number of hydrogen atoms attached to the carbon determines what kind of fat the molecule is and how it will be used in the body. For example, monounsaturated and polyunsaturated fats each have a hydrogen atom attached but also have a space open for a molecule other than hydrogen to attach itself. These fats aren't *saturated* with carbon.

The saturated fat molecule, meanwhile, has hydrogen atoms attached at every open spot. While mono and polyunsaturated fats can be used elsewhere in the body (depending on what kind of element attaches itself to their open area), saturated fats can never be anything but fat. That's why saturated fat tends to raise *cholesterol levels* (a measurement of fatty deposits inside the arteries; these deposits can lead to heart attacks and strokes).

Trans fats (also called *hydrogenated fats*) are a type of saturated fat usually manmade in a process called *hydrogenation,* which adds hydrogen to the chemical makeup of unsaturated fats. This process was initiated in order to make fat more stable and give foods a longer shelf life. You can think of saturated and trans fats as solid fat; shortening, for example, contains both types of fats. Now imagine that kind of substance floating around in your bloodstream, through your arteries. Trans and saturated fat are far more likely than unsaturated fat to start raising blood cholesterol levels, clogging up the works and leading to heart disease and strokes in adults.

Trans and saturated fats are believed to lower HDL (high-density lipoprotein), which is the "good" cholesterol, and raise LDL (low-density lipoprotein), which is the "bad," artery-clogging cholesterol. HDL may actually help to lower LDL, but only if the HDL measurement in the blood is higher than the LDL. (Which it definitely won't be if you're eating lots of saturated and trans fats.)

The really scary thing about saturated and trans fats is this: With childhood obesity on the rise, more doctors are doing research into the damage that the youngest bodies sustain from eating a diet too high in fat. They're finding that kids in elementary school are already showing signs of high cholesterol!

The U.S. Food and Drug Administration considers trans fats such a serious health risk that as of January 1, 2006, food manufacturers are required to list the number of grams of trans fats per serving on their nutrition labels. Fast-food places aren't required to list their nutritional counts on every hamburger wrapper and French fry container that crosses their counter, but they're supposed to make that information available to the public. Some places keep their pamphlets out in the open, whereas others only hand them out to customers upon request. Most of the bigger chains also list nutritional information on their Web sites.

This one meal adds up to 790 calories, 26 total grams of fat, and 30 grams of sugar. You know what's missing, though? Vitamins, minerals, and fiber.

Also, 790 calories is on the high side for one meal (and the smallest "complete" meal you'll find in a fast-food place, at that), especially when we're talking about limiting calories to about 1,500 to 1,800 per day for obese children. You can do better than this kids' meal for your child. She could have a plate of grilled chicken, salad, and a baked potato and consume far fewer calories, fat, and sugar! Or try one of the recipes in Appendix A of this book. For example, the Salmon Patties and Mini Black Bean Burgers are interesting, tasty, and healthy substitutions for fat-laden drive-thru fare.

What you can do: Dust off the burners

When was the last time you prepared a meal with fresh ingredients? If you can scarcely recall making a meal from scratch, you're not alone. In this day and age of parents working full time and single parents doing *everything,* it makes sense that the fast-food industry should step in and help us out where we most need it — at mealtimes.

But fast food is what you make of it, and *you* can prepare meals for nights when the family is on the run. Chapter 9 offers tips for preparing and freezing meals ahead of time for nights when you know everyone will be taking off in different directions. All you need to do is find a way to transport those servings, and even that's simple: Pack food in small plastic containers and bring along plastic utensils for eating in the car or at the game. (Loading up your cabinets with the right equipment makes *any* meal portable! Check out Appendix A for ideas for healthy take-along meals, like Creamy Carrot Soup or Turkey Burgers.) Add bottled water, and you've just replaced your family's normal fast-food dinner with something healthy.

No, it's not as easy as ordering at the drive-thru speaker, but it's far better for your family's health. After you've made your own version of fast food a few times, you'll see that it really isn't difficult and your family *can* eat healthy foods just about anywhere!

Chapter 8

Planning Your Menu and Shopping

● ●

In This Chapter
▶ Working on a shopping list
▶ Involving the kids in healthy meal planning
▶ Buying healthy without going broke
▶ Understanding the layout of the grocery store
▶ Reading nutrition labels

● ●

*G*iven a choice between having a maid, a nanny, or a cook, plenty of parents would choose the cook, especially as their children get older and more independent. As a parent, you're eventually freed from the chains of diapering and constantly picking up toys, but you *always* have to feed the kids. Planning meals that are acceptable to the entire family isn't always an easy task even under the best circumstances because children are wont to change their tastes without consulting the person working so hard to prepare their meals (that would be you). It can be especially trying, however, to convince a child who's accustomed to eating sweet, greasy and/or salty foods that fresh produce is a better choice. (Heck, it can be difficult to coax an *adult* into eating a more healthful diet!)

Switching a family from eating almost nothing except fattening foods to a healthy diet can be so frustrating that parents are left bewildered, disheartened, and without hope. (How is it that your sister, your neighbor, or your best friend manages to feed her children grapes and apples while your kids pull the old gag-and-faint-on-the-floor routine when presented with a lovely fruit plate?) Is it possible — really, truly within the realm of reality — to entice your family into better eating habits? The answer, of course, is yes, but you can't do it without some planning.

Conquering your child's weight problem begins at home with the creation of weekly menus and solid grocery lists featuring healthy foods. This chapter offers tips for preparing to feed your family more nutritious foods and also includes advice on how to get the kids involved in (and maybe even excited about) this new venture.

Eating Right Requires a Plan!

Turning your family's eating habits around requires diligence and dedication. What's at stake is a loss of physical mobility, a loss of health, and a loss of self-esteem in your obese child. In fact, the situation is pretty dire because your child only has one body to see him through the many, many years ahead.

Mobility, good health, and positive self-esteem play a huge part in the lives of happy people, but unhealthy eating habits can diminish or destroy these factors. When you think about it, it would be a shame *not* to jump in and play referee between your family and fatty foods, right?

Taking charge of the food that comes into the house isn't actually all that difficult (at least theoretically), especially if you have small kids — after all, you're the boss. You're the keeper and manager of the food funds and the guardian of the gate. Stand tall and repeat the mantra, "No junk shall pass through these doors."

Correcting your family's eating habits is made much more difficult when you happen to be a junk-food junkie yourself. Taking the cupcake from your toddler's hand is easy; tossing it in the trash may not be. To this end, a solid grocery-shopping plan is a must. If the cupcakes aren't in the house to begin with, you spare yourself and your family the temptation any time the pantry door opens.

Making a List and Checking It Twice: What to Shop For and Why

A lot of parents aren't keen on the idea of hitting the grocery store armed with a page-long list and loading up the cart until it overflows. "Too much of a bother," they say. The grocery store isn't going anywhere; it's easy enough to pop in on a day-to-day basis to pick up dinner fixings, and hey, it's even easier to swing through the burger (or taco) drive-thru after picking up staples like milk and bread. And why should parents fight the crowds at the market when some fast-food joints offer healthy-ish choices?

Well, for starters:

- ✔ **Preparing a list forces you to take inventory at home.** What do you need? What's been lingering in your cabinets and refrigerator drawers? Out with the old, in with the new (and fresh)!

- ✔ **Having a list in hand actually saves time.** If you hate the grocery store, it could be because you often feel lost wandering the aisles looking for items that you may or may not need. It could also be because you're there every other day, stressing over what to make for dinner.

- ✔ **Preparing food in your home is always cheaper and healthier than buying fast food.** In fact, the healthy choices in the drive-thru are often the most expensive items on the menu! For example, you may pay close to $4 for a grilled chicken sandwich at your favorite burger place, but you can buy *several* chicken breasts for the same price at the grocery store.

Fair enough, you say. Perhaps making a commitment to visit the grocery store on a weekly basis is more cost-efficient. But what should you be buying if your main goal is to promote healthier eating habits in your home? By and large, the foods that you end up feeding your family will depend on taste — yours and theirs. You don't have to serve poached fish and celery when everyone would rather be eating Mexican or Italian meals. The most important thing is to plan a menu for the week and then base your grocery list on that menu.

Here are a few tips to keep in mind:

- ✔ **Plan for at least five family dinners a week.** Studies show that families who eat together tend to have fewer weight issues, perhaps because everyone is focused on the gathering and paying attention to what they're eating. Weekends can be a bit more relaxed, and you may find that instead of ordering pizza and wings out of necessity, you have some healthy leftovers to serve up at a moment's notice.

- ✔ **If your family has never been big on meals together and you have no idea what to feed them, start thinking about your main dishes.** Will you feed them meat, fish, eggs, vegetarian meals? Your favorite ethnic or family recipes can be modified to be less fattening and healthier, so don't count them out just because you've been preparing them with lard for the last 15 years. For more on modifying recipes, see Chapter 9.

- ✔ **How you prepare food is just as important as what you prepare.** Bear in mind that it's not enough to choose chicken over pizza with the works; *how* you prepare the chicken determines how healthy a choice it is. We discuss food preparation more in Chapter 9, but know that frying even the healthiest foods negates their good qualities. So although your kids may love fried zucchini at every meal . . . it's really no better for them than French fries.

Although getting the weekly menu up and rolling takes some effort (particularly if you've been shopping by the seat of your pants for decades), in the long run, you're likely to find that it simplifies your life. No more scrambling for dinner ideas night after night, and you'll free up some time every day that's otherwise spent waiting in line at the market. Plus, posting the menu somewhere in the kitchen not only reminds you of what you need to defrost for that evening's meal, but it also lets everyone in the house know what they'll be eating for the week. This information can be particularly good for family members who don't accept change easily. (Conversely, waiting until dinnertime to spring a healthy surprise on these same folks can backfire in a big way.)

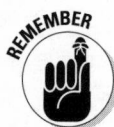

To a large degree, an obese child's success or failure with a weight-loss program depends on his parents' attitudes and efforts. Changing your own views on food can be difficult, especially if *you* don't particularly want or need to lose weight. But if you're worried about your child's size, you just can't stock the pantry with healthy foods for your obese child and junk food for the rest of the family. Most children don't have the willpower to walk away from their favorite treats, no matter *what* their size or weight. For this reason, it's very important to keep high-fat, sugary foods out of the house.

Don't forget the produce

No more breezing right on through the produce section on your way to the bakery! Make sure your weekly menu includes a vegetable dish for each dinner. If your kids have a favorite, great; if they've never eaten veggies in their lives, start off with something safe before branching off into Brussels sprouts territory. Most kids will eat a couple of the following choices:

- Corn (canned, frozen, or on the cob)
- Carrots (boiled or raw with plain yogurt or low-fat dressing for dipping)
- Cucumber slices (it may help to peel the cuke — the skin can taste bitter)
- Celery sticks (another option that's often best served peeled)

Slow and steady wins the race; you don't have to convince them in one day that all vegetables are as delicious as potato chips (although one day they may come to decide this for themselves).

Introduce one vegetable at a time, go easy on the butter and salt (and don't even think about hiding those veggies under Hollandaise sauce, which is basically just liquid fat), and set a good example for the kids by eating your own veggies. Although veggies are healthiest *au naturel,* a fat-free salad dressing may be just the thing to convince a reluctant vegetable eater that these goodies from the garden are actually edible and don't taste so bad after all.

Take it easy on the bread and pasta

When it comes to bread and pasta, try to include as many whole-grain choices as you can. They're filled with fiber, minerals, and vitamins — all elements that refined flour products (such as white bread and regular pasta) just don't offer (at least not naturally).

Feeding the early birds and packing a power lunch

Your grocery list isn't limited to dinnertime entrées and side dishes; you still have to think about healthy breakfast and lunch options.

Breakfast is a tricky, sometimes volatile meal, especially if you have kids who aren't morning people. You'd do almost anything to get them off to school without any major emotional meltdowns, and if that means serving doughnuts and a fruit drink at the breakfast table, then so be it. You figure that they have a long day ahead of them and need their energy, which the ton or so of sugar contained in this unhealthy meal should provide.

All right, so you're not offering up an officially calibrated ton of sugar, but you can do much better. For one thing, sugar contains empty calories, which means that although the body takes the calories contained in sugar and either uses them or stores them, no actual nutrients are absorbed along with those calories. Sugar has no protein, no vitamins, no minerals . . . not much except fat-building potential.

A hiker or runner may need (and easily convert) sugar calories into energy, but the average child has enough natural energy (and then some) to make it through the day without a sugar boost.

Rather than sugar-laden breakfast treats, consider these alternatives:

- ✔ **Low-sugar, high-fiber cereals,** with fruit added if they really need something sweet in their bowls
- ✔ **Eggs,** which are packed with protein (something kids need for healthy growth)
- ✔ **Whole-wheat toast with low-sugar jelly** to deliver fiber a-plenty and some vitamins as well
- ✔ **Oatmeal** that isn't supersweetened

Even though your child gets on the bus and out of your hair, you still have to do your best to monitor her meals. If you happen to live in a school district that takes healthy meals seriously, you can feel good about sending your child off to school with lunch money. (Chapter 12 talks about checking out school lunch programs.) More typically, though, kids attend schools that pay a lot of lip service to balanced meals but don't follow through in the cafeteria. If fried foods, heavily buttered veggies, and ice cream treats are the rule at your child's school, consider loading up on the following lunch staples to pack in her lunchbox:

- ✔ Whole-wheat bread
- ✔ Tuna fish packed in water (and prepared with light mayo)
- ✔ Pita pockets or tortillas to fill with veggies and/or cheese
- ✔ Fresh fruit

Your goal is to eventually convince your child that a banana or applesauce is a treat all by itself. But if she just isn't buying this and insists on some sort of dessert, try these alternatives:

- ✔ Graham crackers
- ✔ Animal crackers
- ✔ Fig bar cookies
- ✔ Low-fat yogurt

Fight the temptation to buy the lighter, low-fat versions of your child's favorite treats. She may accept the low-fat cookies initially, but in several weeks, she may have a craving for a cookie with all the bells and whistles (that is, sugar and fat). She's more likely to fall back into old habits if her tastes haven't truly changed and she's just been tricking her taste buds for a while.

Attacking snacks

When your child comes home from school, he's starving, of course. He's put in some tough hours learning, and he needs something to tide him over until dinner. Snack time is no time to let your good intentions slide! Forget the brownies and offer the following instead:

- Cut-up fruits and vegetables (the less work kids have to do to make these foods ready-to-eat, the more likely they are to eat them)
- Dried fruits
- Low-fat yogurt
- Air-popped popcorn
- Pretzels
- Cereal-based snack mixes
- Fig bar cookies, animal crackers, or graham crackers
- Low-sugar cereals

You don't want to starve your kid, but you also can't let all heck break loose at snack time. If he sits down to eat an entire bag of pretzels and follows that up with three containers of yogurt, that's just too much. Remember, he's accustomed to ingesting large portions, and he may not realize what a normal portion looks (and feels) like. If he's old enough, try to explain that he has to relearn the feeling of being full and also the feeling of true hunger. Smaller portions will be the norm from this point on.

The bottom line: Snacks are okay — in moderation.

Make sure snacks have their parameters; for example, your child may be allowed to fill a small bowl with pretzels, but draw the line at letting him take the entire bag to his room while he does his homework. That's not a snack; that's just excessive eating.

A sample shopping list

When it comes time to figure out what good food items should go on your weekly grocery list, plan ahead and think about keeping the pantry stocked in preparation for healthy last-minute meals, school lunches, quick breakfasts, and low-fat snacks. Your list should include staples like:

✔ **Skim or 1 percent milk:** Soy milk is another low-fat option that some kids just love. Other dairy products should be at least part skim. Margarine is much lower in fat than butter, and cheese made with skim milk is lower in fat than regular cheese.

✔ **Whole-grain breads:** Whole-grain pitas and wraps fall under this category along with whole-grain pastas.

✔ **Vegetables:** Fresh veggies are preferable, but canned or frozen are better for long-term planning and storage. Just make sure that butter and/or cheese aren't added to your veggie choices.

✔ **Fruit:** Load up on fresh fruits (berries, apples, bananas, oranges, kiwi — whatever your kids will eat!) whenever you can, but avoid fruits that are canned or frozen in heavy syrups. For convenience, natural applesauce (without added sugar) is usually a pretty safe bet, as are raisins, prunes, and other dried fruits. And low-sugar jellies are great toppers for whole-grain toast in the morning.

✔ **Low-fat meats:** Chicken and turkey breast have lower fat contents than beef and dark meats (like poultry legs). On nights when convenience and quickness are priorities, try an already-roasted chicken (usually found in or near the deli section) rather than a fried bird. (Chapter 9 contains more information on choosing the healthiest meats.)

✔ **Soy products:** If you're thinking about cutting meat out of your diet altogether, give soy a chance. You can purchase it in blocks or cubes (as in tofu) to add to meatless dishes, or you can buy soy foods, like soy hot dogs.

✔ **Low-fat snacks:** Stock up on pretzels, graham crackers, popcorn kernels (for air popping), rice cakes, low-fat yogurt, ice pops made with real fruit (and no sugar added), granola bars, gingersnaps, and vanilla wafers.

✔ **Spices:** Salt and pepper, of course, are staples, but other spices add flavor to recipes without adding fat. Experiment with different tastes, or purchase spices for specific recipes.

Basically, your shopping list should contain mostly low-fat, low-sugar choices. A small treat here or there obviously isn't going to cause weight gain, but remember, you're trying to change tastes and cravings in your family. It's dangerous to bring home a box of donuts and expect an overweight child to stop at eating just one, especially if he's used to eating three or four in one sitting. And don't expect treats to just sit around uneaten — when you bring unhealthy foods into the house, they *will* get eaten.

What to leave off your list

Maybe you want to come at healthy grocery shopping from the other direction. The following kinds of things shouldn't make the cut when you prepare your weekly list:

- **Whole-milk diary products:** Butter, sour cream, cream cheese, cheese curds, blocks of cheese . . . they're all filled with fat. Look for their low-fat counterparts. You'll be surprised at how quickly your family gets used to the new taste.

- **High-sugar cereals:** Sugar is nothing but empty calories. Look for low-sugar cereals or choose plain oatmeal and let the kids stir in some fresh peaches, bananas, or raisins.

- **Pastries:** They're high in fat and sugar, which makes them no good. Leave the donuts in the bakery and the frozen breakfast pastries on ice.

- **High-fat meats:** Even the low-fat versions of bacon, hot dogs, burgers, sausages, and cold cuts are high in sodium, which contributes to the development of heart disease. You're better off cutting items like these off the grocery list for good.

- **Convenience foods:** Items like TV dinners, pot pies, and frozen pizzas contain high amounts of fat and sodium to prolong their shelf lives and improve their taste. They're also usually fairly expensive, so pass them by.

- **Sugary juices and soda:** These beverages are grouped together here because both have high sugar contents. Your child gets very few nutrients from sugared juices and *no* nutrients from soda. For the most part, these drinks contain empty calories.

- **Fake sweeteners:** The jury is still out on the long-term safety of some sugar substitutes, and anyway, you don't want to replace a real sugar addiction with a fake one.

- **High-fat snacks:** TV dinners and frozen pizzas have no place in a healthy home, and chips, microwave popcorn, cookies, cupcakes, and ice cream should also be replaced with low-fat snacks (see "Attacking snacks" earlier in this chapter).

- **High-fat condiments:** Replace regular mayo with a lighter version; ditto for salad dressings and sauces. Skip the sour cream and use plain low-fat yogurt instead.

Ideally, high-fat and sugary treats should be the exception to the healthy-eating rule in your household. We're not advocating complete self-flagellation and a lifelong sacrifice of desserts and such. Realistically speaking, everyone enjoys a treat now and then — but the fact that you *don't* eat them every single day is what makes them *treats*! Your child will probably be surprised at how much more enjoyable treats are when she gets them just every now and then; and you'll probably be surprised when you realize that the family doesn't miss having cake every night. With your support and determination to stick to your guns, your family can and will get to the point at which healthy shopping — and healthy eating — is just the order of the day and not something that requires a lot of thought. We know that to many parents, this sounds like a bunch of hooey. It isn't. This lifestyle isn't impossible, but an obese child needs at least one strong authority figure to implement and enforce it.

Getting the Kids Involved in the Planning

Kids are more apt to learn the finer points of choosing the best foods if they're involved in making decisions about the food that enters the house. You may have a hard time accepting your child's input if you like to be in control of everything in the household and especially when you first begin this weight-loss process. However, the sooner you let your child throw her opinions into the mix of meal planning and grocery shopping, the sooner you'll know if your words are having any effect on her. Sure, it's usually easier to take matters into your own hands and just do the cooking and the shopping yourself, but children have to know the difference between healthy and unhealthy foods if they're to have long-term weight-loss success.

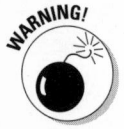

Some of the foods that you try when you're implementing a healthier diet for the family will be trial and error. Don't let a flop in the kitchen discourage you from continuing on with your new healthy eating plan. It takes time for the palate to adjust to these different foods. And in any event, there may be some foods that your family just doesn't like. Don't lose heart; just keep trying.

Deciding on the menu for the week

At some point, many moms get tired of hearing that there's nothing to eat and that the family doesn't really like what's being served for dinner. The simple solution is to get the kids involved in what goes on in the kitchen. Let them help you plan the menu for the week. Hand over the grocery list and allow them to add their own healthy choices.

There are a couple of benefits of getting kids involved in menu planning:

✔ **You allow them some freedom within the new eating plan.** You don't simply demand that they eat certain fruits and vegetables; rather, you lead them in the right direction and then allow them to choose *which* fruits and vegetables they'd like to try. Instead of being a dictator, you're instituting a plan for the kids, by the kids.

✔ **You educate them to make better choices.** When your son lists microwave popcorn as a treat he'd like to have for the week, take the opportunity to discuss why air-popped popcorn is better for his health. (In case you don't know why: Air-popped is lower in fat and calories; microwave popcorn is usually smothered in oil and a butterlike substance.) You want to have these conversations without being preachy or overbearing. Your job is simply to inform.

If you have to guide your child away from his first choices for the menu, be prepared to face some whining — at least initially — along the lines of, "Who cares if it's high in fat? I like it! I won't eat anything else!" Your response should be to take the grocery list back into your own hands. Your child can refuse to eat the healthy foods you bring home; that's his choice. If he's hungry enough, he'll have to try them. And after he tries them, he'll find that they're not nearly as bad as he expected them to be (even if he won't admit it). When he's ready, let him have another chance to put his two cents in on the grocery list.

What you're trying to do for a child who's reluctant to change his eating habits is just open a door in his mind. All he has to do is realize that there's another way to eat — a healthy way, a way that doesn't cause him to gain weight and feel unwell — and he'll be on his way to accepting the changes to his diet.

Helping out in the kitchen

Part of reeducating kids about food is letting them help prepare meals. When your child hangs around the kitchen while you're preparing meals, it's easy for you to say things like, "Baking this chicken is so much easier than breading it and frying it, and it's healthier for us, too." Sharing information in this casual manner goes over much better than throwing a nugget of information out there while you're driving to school. Other topics of conversation during meal prep may include:

✔ **Nutritional high points of certain foods:** Berries, for example, are high in antioxidants and thought to protect against certain types of cancers. Lycopene is an element found in high levels in tomatoes and is also believed to play a part in fighting off cancer.

✔ **Nutritional low points of particular foods:** There's some confusing information out there about some food groups. For example, kids need calcium, but they don't need it from whole milk. Your explanation of why you cut out unhealthy foods is imperative to your child learning to make good choices for himself.

✔ **Healthy substitutions:** You may mention to your child that you're substituting applesauce for vegetable oil in a cake recipe because it's lower in fat and better for everyone's health. (The recipes in Appendix A show you how favorite recipes can also be low fat when you use the right ingredients.)

Healthy Shopping on a Budget

You may be thinking that the advice in this chapter is fine and well for people who don't have to mentally tally up their grocery bill as they place items in the cart. Perhaps the reason your family eats unhealthy foods is because you can't afford to buy fresh produce and low-fat meats.

Some parents avoid the healthy-food route because they think that it costs more to purchase separate ingredients than simply to buy the prepackaged version of the meal. There's more to the story. The most expensive part of overhauling your refrigerator or pantry is the initial stock-up. (Spices, in particular, can be costly.) But after you make the switch from junk food to healthy food, as long as you continue to monitor the weekly specials at your grocery store, your food bill should settle out somewhere close to what you used to spend on convenience foods. You may not end up *saving* money when you switch to low-fat meals, but you won't go broke, either.

Avoiding the high-priced traps

Convenience foods are expensive, and we're not just talking about high-fat convenience foods like frozen pizzas and sandwich pockets. The price of healthy convenience foods, like baby carrots (you know, the cute little carrots that you don't have to wash, peel, or cut), can lead consumers to believe that it's impossible to feed a family healthy foods and still make ends meet. And as more and more grocery stores reinvent themselves into meccas of gourmet food, you see more and more healthy, convenient, and expensive offerings that only bolster this myth.

If you're choosing a snack for the kids, for example, a 99¢ bag of cheese curls is cheaper than a $2.99 bag of baby carrots. But the bag of baby carrots is more expensive than the big bag of whole carrots that need washing, peeling, and cutting but taste the same. If you consider the cost per unit, those big carrots come pretty darn close to the cheese curls, and they're obviously healthier.

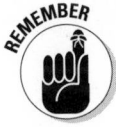

Keep in mind that healthy, fiber-filled foods tend to fill the stomach more than high-sugar and low-fiber snacks and foods. Your child may be able to consume half a bag of cheese curls without feeling satisfied, but a large apple and a piece of whole-grain toast will fill her stomach and tide her over until dinnertime. These are healthy snack choices, and of course, she also gets nutrients from the apple and toast that the cheese curls just can't offer.

As soon as you walk through the doors of almost any grocery store, you find yourself in the produce department, which nowadays often includes a refrigerated case of peeled and cubed fruits, expensive organic juices, and out-of-season fruits. These items are pricey, and that's why they're in the prettiest spot in the produce department. Take a look behind you and you'll see that almost everything else is laid out in plain bins. There are bargains to be found in the produce aisle if you know where to look and what to avoid.

Suppose you're thinking about tossing a nice salad to add to the family dinner. You head over to the bags of precut, prewashed lettuce and are shocked to find that one package costs almost $5. That's an insane amount of money to spend on lettuce, right? Head down the aisle a ways and you'll find an entire head of iceberg lettuce (generally the least expensive lettuce) for a fraction of the price. Sure, *you* have to wash and tear the leaves, but you get a lot more use out of an entire head of lettuce than you get from that bag of salad.

If you've been loading up your freezer with precooked or ready-to-cook foods, you may be surprised to find that your grocery bill *doesn't* skyrocket when you switch to raw materials, so to speak. When you purchase convenience foods, you're really paying for someone else to take most of the work out of preparing those meals or snacks. Conversely, when you purchase separate ingredients with which to prepare your meals, you not only save money, but you also have complete control over what goes into the dishes you make for the family. For example, when you serve up a frozen pizza, you have no idea about the quality or freshness of the ingredients. But if you make a pizza from scratch, you do.

Having a plan = saving money

Eating healthfully requires a plan, and shopping for healthy foods without going broke requires even more planning. You're right in thinking that people who have money to burn have an easier time buying the foods that they need — but you could say the same thing about anything in life. The lack of a bottomless bank account shouldn't prevent you from buying healthy foods; it only means that you need to do some extra research and planning before you head to the grocery store.

What kind of planning, you ask?

- ✓ **Get your Sunday paper.** It contains coupons and sale fliers from the grocery stores in your area and is worth every penny of the $2 you spend at the newsstand.

- ✓ **Know what's on sale for the upcoming week *before* you make your menu and shopping list.**

- ✓ **Clip coupons for extra savings, but only clip the ones for foods you would normally buy.**

- ✓ **Make a shopping list for the entire week.** The bill may seem high at first, but if your current shopping habits include popping into the store every day to buy essentials for only the next 24 hours, you'll probably end up spending more.

- ✓ **If you see a sale item that you know you want to keep around, such as whole-wheat bread or chicken breasts, stock up while the price is low.**

- ✓ **Check the unit or per pound prices on items that you use frequently.** Buying items in large quantities is usually less expensive.

- ✓ **Try the store brands.** They're usually just as good as the national brands and are often cheaper — which adds up to big savings when you're totaling up a basket full of groceries. In many cases, you can actually save more by purchasing the store brands than by clipping coupons for the national brands (which often require that you buy three or four units of an item in order to save a quarter).

- ✓ **Resist the temptation to stock up on high-fat convenience foods, even if they're on sale.**

Shopping wisely is much cheaper than eating out or swinging through the fast-food drive-thru. Consider this: You can take your family of four out to dinner at a sit-down family restaurant three times and spend $100. Or you can take that same $100 and stock your fridge and pantry for the week with just about everything you need for breakfast, lunch, dinner, and snacks — *if* you plan ahead and look for specials.

Putting food in the deep freeze

One of the best ways to get the most bang for your buck at the grocery store is to purchase items that are on special, plan several meals around those items, and then freeze the extras. That way, you're always preparing your healthy meals at the absolute lowest cost. For example, boneless, skinless chicken breasts are a healthy, versatile, easy-to-prepare item, but they tend to be fairly pricey. When you see them on sale, stock up for the coming weeks so that you don't spend twice as much on your meal next week as you did this week.

If you don't necessarily want to prepare meals ahead of time, at least stock up on the sale-item ingredients and plan to store or freeze them until you're ready to cook.

Prepare your menu, prepare your list, and then prepare to prepare more than you normally would in the kitchen. If you hate to cook, it may seem to you that merely planning healthy meals is bad enough; asking you to cook even *more* food is nothing short of pure torture. But that's where you may be a little shortsighted. If you're in the kitchen and cooking *anyway,* doubling or tripling the recipe and freezing the extra portions is nothing — in fact, it *saves time* in the future. Do the work once, and reap the benefits for several meals. (This idea is sounding better and better, isn't it?)

To put your freezing plan into action, you need to:

- ✔ **Prepare your list and menu.** You know the drill (see "Making a List and Checking It Twice: What to Shop For and Why" earlier in this chapter for a refresher).

- ✔ **Clear room in your freezer.** Toss the junk food (ice cream, onion rings, and the like) once and for all.

- ✔ **Invest in good freezerware.** You can go with trial and error here, but the more expensive freezer bags usually provide better protection for meats and veggies. Ditto for the better-quality plastic containers.

- ✔ **Know how to freeze.** Casseroles and soups are better off in glass or plastic containers; uncooked meat and raw veggies are best protected in freezer bags. (For more tips, see the bulleted list later in this section.)

Although family meals are important, we know that every family also has its wild and crazy evenings when it's darn near impossible to get everyone in the same room for five minutes, much less an entire meal. So you may also want to consider freezing individual portions of meals for nights when you know that your teenager will be fending for herself while you and your husband work late. She can fix a nutritious meal without having to do anything except pop it into the microwave.

Freezing individual portions also allows you to send a healthy home-cooked meal to school with your child. Defrost it the night before, heat it in the microwave in the morning, pack it in a thermos or insulated container, and stick it in her lunchbox.

Here are a few things you need to know about properly freezing and defrosting foods:

- ✔ **Meats have a "use or freeze by" label on their packaging.** Adhere to this advice. If you find chicken in your fridge that's a week past this date, throw it out.

- ✔ **Don't stick steaming hot food in the freezer, but don't let food sit out for more 30 minutes before freezing it.** It may start to grow bacteria.

- ✔ **Label everything that you freeze.** If you're using glass or plastic containers, write the name of the meal, the date, cooking instructions, and the number of portions on some masking tape and attach it to the container.

- ✔ **Remove as much air as possible from food storage bags before freezing.**

- ✔ **If you're using glass or plastic containers, leave at least 1½ inches of space between the food and the lid for expansion.**

- ✔ **Defrost safely.** Never defrost poultry and other meats at room temperature. Put them in the fridge instead. Roughly speaking, it takes about four hours per pound to defrost poultry and eight hours per pound of beef.

- ✔ **To defrost quickly, put frozen items in cold water.** Make sure that the frozen item is in a watertight wrap or container, and change the water every 30 minutes to guard against contamination.

- ✔ **Defrost in the microwave.** Use a low power setting to defrost frozen foods, and check the food intermittently to make sure the edges don't get overcooked. When you nail down the perfect defrost procedure for a particular dish, write it down and attach it to the container the next time you cook and freeze that meal.

With freezing and defrosting, you'll eventually figure out which meals freeze nicely and which don't. Melted cheese, for example, tends not to regain the right consistency after defrosting. For this reason, if you're freezing something like low-fat lasagna, freeze it *uncooked.*

Changing the Way You Look at the Grocery Store

When you head to the grocery store, you want to be able to walk in as an educated consumer and stick to your guns and your plan while you shop. Grocery stores almost always follow a standard setup, and they do so for one reason: To get you to stay longer and spend more money. So that you don't fall victim to this trickery, this section advises you on how best to handle all those aisles and options.

Which aisles to avoid

You've been going to the grocery store for . . . oh, about forever. You have your routine, and you're very attached to it. Or maybe you're taking the shopping duties over from your spouse and aren't all that familiar with where to find everything. Don't be intimidated; the key is knowing what you *don't* need.

If you and your child have created a menu of healthy meals for the week (see the section "Deciding on the menu for the week" earlier in this chapter), the majority of your ingredients are *not* in the center aisles of the grocery store. Some items, such as cereal, canned fruits and vegetables, and whole-grain pasta may be located in the middle of the store, but there are also entire aisles that you can pass by, like the candy aisle, the soda aisle, and the chips-and-microwave-popcorn aisle. If an item you need is next to an unhealthy food (if pretzels are on the shelf below the chips, for example), grab your list item and keep on walkin'.

The aisles in the middle of the store are there to keep you shopping. For example, many people stop and buy milk on their way home from work. You'd think putting the milk near the store entrance would be a pretty good idea — maybe next to a separate checkout line for milk buyers, even — but store owners would lose money if that were the case. When you're forced to walk through an entire warehouse-sized building, past cookies and candy and nacho chips, just to get your milk, chances are pretty good that you'll stop and grab a couple of extra things in addition to your must-have item. The same thing happens when you shop without a list or stray from the list (for shame!) — you end up buying more than you need. Ka-ching! Someone just made more money off of you.

Where to best spend your time and money

The freshest foods — and therefore, usually the healthiest options — are almost always located around the perimeter of the grocery store. These items include:

- **Dairy:** Low-fat milk, yogurt, and cheese
- **Produce:** Fresh fruits and veggies
- **Seafood:** Universally low in fat, as long as it isn't fried
- **Breads:** Whole grains are best
- **Meat and poultry:** Low-fat beef and white-meat poultry

Because your list should be heavy on these items, you should spend little time in the interior of the store. However, you may need to venture into the interior aisles to pick up:

- Canned fruits and veggies
- Legumes
- Cereal
- Whole-grain pasta and brown rice
- Frozen veggies
- Low-fat snacks like crackers and pretzels

And that's about it. Honestly. Sure, you may need to pick up mustard or a spice now and then, but you can plan a menu and prepare your meals with these basic foods. (Note that frozen pizza is nowhere to be seen on these lists.)

Reading Nutrition Labels

One of the most important things that you can do to help reorganize your family's diet is read and evaluate nutrition labels. As you probably know, nutrition labels appear on every food item you purchase. The only exception to this rule is sometimes produce, but chances are good that if you look hard enough, you just may find some nutrition facts posted near a bin of apples or potatoes.

In any event, reading the label is one thing; understanding what that label is trying to tell you is another thing. When you become adept at understanding nutrition labels, you can teach your child how to break down the label information himself, thus educating him in the finer points of nutrition.

Take a look at Figure 8-1, which presents a sample nutrition label from a healthy breakfast cereal. In the list that follows, we start at the beginning of the label and work our way down, focusing on what you need to know for weight-loss purposes.

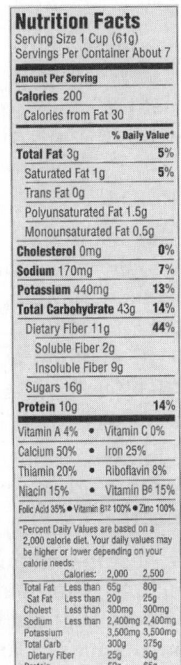

Figure 8-1:
A nutrition
label.

✔ **Serving size:** Tells you what portion size the rest of the label deals with — and it's usually not the entire box or bag of food. In this example, the serving size is 1 cup.

- **Servings per container:** Tells you how many servings are contained in the entire package.

- **Calories:** Refers to the number of calories contained in *one* serving. In this example, if your child eats 1 cup of dry cereal, he takes in 200 calories.

- **Calories from fat:** Tells you just that — in this example, of the 200 calories your child ingests, 30 come from fat. That's about a 7:1 ratio, which isn't too bad. Conversely, a hamburger patty may have about 250 calories, 150 of which come from fat. Over 50 percent of those calories came from fat — *that's* a high percentage.

- **Percentage of daily value readings:** Tell you how much of a particular nutrient the food item contains based on recommended daily allowances for a 2,000-calorie diet. In this example, the serving size provides 3 grams of total fat, or 5 percent of the daily recommended allowance of fat.

- **Total Fat:** Breaks down into subcategories, like saturated, *trans*, polyunsaturated, and monounsaturated fats. These fats are listed in descending order, from the worst type of fat — the types that are most likely to contribute to high cholesterol and heart disease — to the types that are less harmful to the heart.

- **Total Carbohydrates:** Tells you how much of the body's main source of energy the food contains. Debate has raged in the last few years over whether people who are trying to lose weight should cut carbohydrates out of their diet. The answer is no. Everyone needs carbohydrates — just in moderation. Children should get around 60 percent of their calories from carbs. Try to avoid *refined* carbs, like those found in white breads and white sugar. Whole grains, fruits, legumes, and vegetables contain carbohydrates in their natural forms and are best for the body.

  - **Dietary Fiber:** Listed under Total Carbohydrates. Foods high in fiber tend to be filling and also help to keep the bowels moving. The label in Figure 8-1 is from a high-fiber cereal.

  - **Sugars:** Listed under Total Carbohydrates. The location of the sugar count can be confusing because fruits, for example, may be high in sugar but are still a healthy choice because they're also packed with other nutrients (like fiber and vitamins). Candy and soda, on the other hand, contain high amounts of added sugar and no nutrients to speak of.

- **Vitamins and Minerals:** Tells you how much of these elements are contained in one serving of the food. When you see nice, high numbers here, you can feel confident about feeding the family something that's good for them.

It's not that hard to get used to reading and assessing food labels, but it may be time consuming on your first few trips to the grocery store. Here are a few things to keep in mind as you get started:

- ✔ **When you're initially trying to cut fat out of your child's diet, look for foods that are low in total fat but high in nutrients.** Children need vitamins and minerals for their bodies' essential functions. Remember, they're still growing and need plenty of energy to sustain them throughout the day. They just don't need a whole lot of fat.

- ✔ **Not all calories are the same, which is why the nutrition label contains a Calories from Fat measurement.** Instead of cutting total calories, it's sometimes just as helpful for weight loss to make sure that your child consumes foods that don't provide a lot of calories from fat and have a low percentage of saturated and *trans* fats. Saturated and *trans* fats are more likely to end up as artery-clogging junk. Polyunsaturated and monounsaturated fats, on the other hand, don't seem to contribute to clogged arteries in the way the other fats do.

- ✔ **Don't be misled by labels that claim a product is "Lite," "Fat-free," "Sugar-free."** Take the time to read the nutrition label in its entirety and evaluate the food based on its sugar, fat, vitamin, *and* caloric contents. A food can be fat free, for example, but still quite high in sugar and calories (and contain no nutrients to speak of).

As we discuss in Chapter 7, when an obese child is trying to lose weight, a good range for caloric intake is about 1,500 to 1,800 calories per day (but never lower than 1,500). When she gets into a healthy weight range for her age and height, she can gradually start adding 100 to 200 calories per day until she's able to maintain a healthy weight. Teach your child that her calories are like money — she only has so much to spend every day. Snacks should be lower in calories than meals, and she should try to shoot for as few fat calories as possible. This new way of thinking about food, combined with increased activity, will help her on the road to weight loss.

Chapter 9

Cookin' Up a Healthier Lifestyle

In This Chapter

▶ Laying down some new laws at the dinner table

▶ Adopting the healthiest cooking styles

▶ Avoiding unhealthy foods and preparations

▶ Getting kids involved in healthy food preparation

*N*o one can become an expert on healthy eating in the span of 24 hours. It takes time, a willingness to learn, and a certain amount of dedication to first educate yourself on the merits of a healthy lifestyle and then put the knowledge you've gathered into action.

Because food is one of those things that we all need for survival, some people scoff at the thought of exploring its complexities. "What is there to know?" they ask. "You eat it, it tastes good, and you're hungry again later in the day. Hand me a blue ribbon for being an authority on the subject." While we appreciate the content of this "lesson," there's far more to know about food than just when to eat it. In Chapter 8, we talk about how to navigate the grocery store and choose the healthiest options for your family. In this chapter, we help you do something with those choices by explaining how to prepare and serve food in the healthiest and most family-friendly ways possible. It's not enough to opt for fish over marbled beef, for example; you have to know how to keep your fish dish healthy throughout the preparation process.

Cooking healthier meals for your family can be stressful, particularly if you don't like to be in the kitchen in the first place. In order to ensure that your family gets the healthiest meals possible, though, you have to take the reins at the stove, so to speak. Your family may be reluctant to accept your new ideas, but they'll come around to your way of thinking as long as you show them that healthy cooking isn't a whim — it's the way things are going to be from now on.

Dealing with Different Palates

Some children are very set in their ways where food is concerned and are completely unwilling to stray from their favorites. Any kid can be stubborn and uncooperative when it comes to trying something new, which makes exposing your family to a healthy diet one tough task. And it certainly doesn't help if there's also an adult in the house who gags when steamed veggies appear on the dinner table.

Dealing with picky palates is no fun. In fact, hearing a whining chorus of, "I don't like this!" or "This looks too weird to eat!" may just send you right back into the drive-thru lane. This section offers tips on how to ease your family into low-fat meals and make your healthy cooking a smashing success.

Taking on picky eaters

No one really knows how picky eaters develop. Some people think that kids are just born with certain preferences, while others swear that parents allow their kids to challenge food choices and ultimately take charge of meals. We think that the truth lies somewhere in the middle of the two arguments. The good news is that you can do certain things to take back control of what your family eats — and make life easier for yourself. After all, you're the one doing the cooking!

Some studies suggest that from birth, some children are very sensitive to taste, including bitterness or sourness. This theory may explain why some people (adults included) just don't care for strong-tasting vegetables like peppers, broccoli, and Brussels sprouts, and certain fruits (grapefruit, in particular, can taste very bitter to some).

The best way to deal with picky eaters (both young and old) is to make it clear from the beginning that *one* meal is served each night. (For more on limiting the family menu options, see the section "Putting your foot down on separate meals" later in this chapter.) If the kids want to have some input on what they'll be eating, that's great. Let your kids help you plan the menu for the week (see Chapter 8). The more they start thinking about healthy foods for themselves, the faster they'll learn about good nutrition. Let each child plan a dinner, even if it's something that the other kids moan and groan about. Kids are more apt to try something that another kid has chosen, even if that child happens to be a pesky sibling.

Of course, just about everyone has one or two foods that they just don't like. We're not suggesting that you go out of your way to feed broccoli to a child who screams at the very sight of it. As long as she isn't screaming at the sight of every veggie, you have plenty of other options for healthy side dishes. And if she hates all veggies equally, chances are she's a *little* picky and you have some work ahead of you. Start by introducing her to tame veggies like corn, carrots, and beans before moving on to really exotic fare like beets and turnips.

If your children are teenagers and refuse to eat what you make, so be it. You can't always convince a stubborn 15-year-old to try a dish, and sometimes the coaxing can make matters worse. Teens are old enough to prepare healthy meals of their own, and if they get hungry enough — and if you only bring healthy foods home from the grocery store — they will.

Putting your foot down on separate meals

If you're new to the kitchen and chef duty, you may be wondering what you, as the person preparing your family's meals, are supposed to do when one kid only eats Mexican food, another one wants to try vegetarian meals, and your spouse just wants red meat. Do other parents really prepare separate meals for every picky eater in the family?

No! Although some parents get pulled into this type of appeasement, the person doing the cooking usually gets sick and tired of so many special requests. You don't want to spend the entire afternoon fixing what amounts to a restaurant-style menu of choices for the family. That's beyond the call of duty. And anyway, if your family has been subsisting on high-fat, high-calorie meals for as long as you can remember, part of the reason you're cooking now is to help them change their preferences towards healthier foods.

Your family can't possibly develop new tastes if they're allowed to successfully avoid all but one or two healthy meals per week. In other words, the more healthy foods you expose them to, the better their chances are of finding several meals that they really like — and then they can build on *those* tastes.

Obviously, if tears and tantrums accompany every meal, you're working on an entirely different level. When your son objects to something new you set before him, continue to be encouraging, and *don't* fix him a separate meal. Let him wrap up his dinner plate, put it in the fridge, and leave the table. When he gets hungry enough, he'll either try your healthy dinner, or he won't. Either way, he *will* survive.

Here's where parents tend to get bogged down in the meal department: We all want to do what's best for our kids, and we want them to be happy to boot. If one meal makes them unhappy, many of us are only too eager to fix something else that's sure to please them. In a household with a significantly overweight child, this eagerness to please the child may be the root of food problems. In the end, servitude doesn't do anyone any good — you're stuck playing the role of short-order cook, and your child discovers that he can get away with eating just one or two healthy meals every week. That's not your goal.

Cook one palatable meal for the entire family and be done with it. You'll be happier, and in the long run, you'll break your kids of their pickiest habits. You may never convince your son that red onions are tasty, but he'll end up eating a lot of healthy foods that he otherwise wouldn't have tried. (It's amazing what happens when you stop playing Cook. They eat what you make!) And as long as you're keeping the junk out of your house, you can be sure that your children aren't bingeing on candy after refusing to eat dinner.

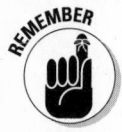

A healthier lifestyle means that you change the way you do everything in your home: the way you shop, the way you cook . . . and the way you serve dinner. Regardless of what you did in the past, dinner consists of one meal for everyone. Be firm on this rule. You're trying to teach your family about healthy options and making good choices out in the real world. When your child's at a friend's house, that mother or father won't prepare two separate meals — one for the family and one for your child. And when your child goes to school, he won't choose the tossed salad over the onion rings as a side dish if he's never had a salad in his life. You're the one who has to introduce your children to good foods so that when they leave home, they consider good foods valid options!

Encouraging everyone to try new things

Is it right to essentially force a child who hates salad to eat a bowl of crisp greens? Of course not. It's wrong to force-feed anyone anything. But getting your child (and other family members) to try something new doesn't mean you have to cram it into his mouth with a plunger. You can be much more subtle than that. Muster up a good supply of enthusiasm because you're going to play the middleman between your family and healthy food.

Get everyone involved

Arm yourself with some healthy recipes you'd like to try out (either from Appendix A of this book or from other cookbooks), and just do it. Not everyone will be head-over-heels excited about cutting the fat out of their diets, but in due time, they'll come around. Just remember that choosy eaters sometimes need someone to get them on the right track before they can jump in and participate.

Experimenting with a whole new way of cooking is exciting. You're constantly looking for new recipes, you're bringing different foods home, and you're approaching cooking from a whole new direction. Let your family see your excitement. Encourage them to give you ideas, and listen to what they say. Your goal is not just to cut the fat from your family's meals but also to teach them how to take care of themselves and how to make good choices where food is concerned.

If you get positive input from your children on the weekly menu from the very beginning, that's great. If they're acting as though this healthy menu-planning thing is complete torture and suggesting things like fried chicken and bacon cheeseburgers for your healthy meals, then you just have to take control and plan the menu yourself. When they're ready, they'll suggest appropriate foods.

Another way to get the kids involved at mealtime is to let them set the table however they see fit. Encourage them to make place cards, fold napkins into unique shapes, or set up a picnic-style dinner (in the family room or out in the yard). If they feel they're playing a part in bringing everyone to the table, they'll be more likely to join in on the actual dining.

Ease into it with small changes

If your kids aren't happy about the changes you make in the kitchen, take it slowly. In other words, don't try to switch them from eating fast food almost every night to a completely vegan diet in a week's time. Instead, start out with some healthy meat options (like grilled chicken breasts or turkey burgers) or a healthy pizza in order to make the transition from high-fat foods to healthy meals easier.

After you win them over with some normal-sounding (albeit healthy) meals, you can use parental logic on them: "You loved the pizza I made last night. The chicken I made tonight is just as good, but you'll never know until you try it!" If this argument convinces them, you're good to go. If it doesn't, you may want to try out a rule that many parents enforce at the dinner table: Everyone has to try one bite of the meal in order to give it a fair shot. As long as you're not serving something extremely spicy or exotic, this "try it and see" rule may work wonders for opening up a stubborn mind. If your son has never had any problem eating French fries, for example, there's no reason he can't at least try a baked potato. If you can just get that first bite into his mouth without him dissolving into tears or a major meltdown, he may discover he actually likes it . . . and the rest of your meals may go much more smoothly.

Part of the reason you want your family to try as many foods as possible is so that they know that healthy eating isn't boring. You're not asking them to eat a bowl of plain lettuce every night or give up every food that they love. Healthy eating just means that the food is prepared differently.

For example, suppose your preteen daughter has been hooked on chicken nuggets ever since she was a toddler. Instead of telling her that she has to give up her favorite food immediately and for the rest of time, find a way to help her broaden her horizons — slowly, at first. Serve grilled chicken sandwiches for dinner one night (with low-fat condiments, of course, like low-fat mayo or mustard); add some carrot sticks and low-fat dressing as an alternative to French fries. You haven't taken her into some land of completely alien food; you've just taken what she likes and restructured it so that it's healthy. She may complain that it's not fried, and that's where your encouragement will make all the difference. By saying, "No, it's not, but it actually tastes very good," you're being encouraging; responding with "Too bad. You're not eating fried food anymore," won't improve her attitude about accepting the changes to her diet.

Prepping and Cooking the Healthy Way

Maybe you're a pro in the kitchen and whip up gourmet dishes so good that the neighbors appear at your door when they catch a whiff of your cooking. But if you've been using fat as one of your main ingredients, it's time to explore a healthier way to prepare tasty meals for your family. On the flip side, if you've successfully avoided cooking lessons up to this point, it's time to become skilled in preparing low-fat food in your own kitchen.

When you're trying to help your child lose weight, cooking your own meals is unavoidable. Even though many sit-down restaurants provide healthy menu options and some fast-food places are starting to look out for their customers' health, eating out every night is very expensive. And besides, it limits your family's options and taste experiences to what's offered on menus. When you open yourself up to healthy cooking, you find that you can prepare almost any meal in a healthy way.

In this section, we talk about the basics of setting up a healthy cooking environment and ways you can go about cutting the fat from your cooking.

The fresher, the better

When you're cooking healthy, choose your ingredients wisely by reading nutrition labels (for more on deciphering nutrition labels, flip back to Chapter 8) and cook from scratch as much as possible. When you're planning your meals for the week, steer clear of any foods with a high fat content, which include convenience foods such as frozen TV dinners, frozen pizzas, or prepackaged meals of any sort (see Chapter 8 for more on convenience foods). These foods are usually very high in fat and sodium, both of which add to the flavor of the meals but also contribute to weight gain and the development of high blood pressure. Cooking from scratch lets you rest assured that what you're feeding your family doesn't have any hidden fat.

Now, you may be thinking, "If I'm not *serving* a TV dinner, I obviously won't be using it to *make* dinner." True enough. But convenience foods extend beyond entire meals to include frozen or flaked mashed potatoes, canned soups, and macaroni and cheese if it's partially prepared.

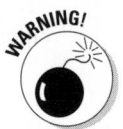

Frozen vegetables are an acceptable option for a side dish — but *not* if they're smothered in cheese. And because overcooking vegetables lessens their nutrient-packed punch, buying fresh rather than canned is best, although canned is better than nothing (and also better than fried, obviously).

Even though some healthier convenience foods are available these days, convenience foods still tend to be more expensive in the long run than preparing your own meals at home, and they don't really provide you (and more important, your child) with the hands-on learning she needs concerning healthy cooking. At some point, your child will have to choose a meal that doesn't come in a can or box with a low-fat label on it. She has a better chance of choosing well if she's been in the kitchen watching you actively cut the fat from your family's meals.

We're not suggesting that you till your backyard and turn it into an organic garden to supply your kitchen (although if you're interested in that sort of thing, go for it). Instead, try to break recipes down into their most natural components. When you're preparing a casserole, for example, don't use canned meat, which is almost always high in sodium. Try to use fresh vegetables whenever possible because they have more vitamins than canned veggies. In other words, if you're cooking a healthy meal, you may as well make it as healthy as you possibly can.

Preparing veggies

Veggies make a great snack or side dish for any dinner. Your family probably likes them slathered in butter or — gulp — fried, but you know that those preparations just don't fly with limiting fat intake. So what's the best way to serve up veggies that aren't objectionable? Here are a few tips:

- **Choose vegetables that are acceptable to everyone.** We all have foods that we just don't like, and some people are very sensitive to the bitter-tasting chemical contained in some vegetables. If everyone moans over spinach, pick something else. Beans, carrots, corn, and peas agree with most kids' taste buds, so give them a try.

- **Go raw.** Raw veggies are excellent because they're full of nutrients and easy to serve. Carrot or celery sticks served as a side dish with a low-fat or yogurt-based dressing may just satisfy everyone at the dinner table.

- **Resist the urge to cut veggies into teeny-tiny pieces before you cook them.** While it takes less time to cook chopped veggies, leaving them in large pieces helps to keep their nutrients intact.

- **Leave the peels on whenever possible; they're packed with nutrients.** Leave the skins on potatoes when you mash them, and serve snap peas in their shells.

- **Steaming veggies in a double boiler or microwave basket is the best way to preserve their nutrients.**

- **If you boil vegetables, use just enough water to cover the veggies, and boil just until they become tender.** Overcooking causes vegetables to lose vitamins and minerals.

After you start working with vegetables on a regular basis, you'll know what your family will eat without complaining — and hopefully that complaint list will be on the short side. If they continue to balk at eating anything green, leafy, or grown in a garden, just look for new ways to prepare those veggies. For example:

- Toss veggies into soups.

- Add lettuce, cucumber slices, avocado, and/or tomato to sandwiches.

- Slice up some potatoes, brush them with olive oil, and bake in the oven for about 20 minutes at 350 degrees. *Healthy* fries!

- Skewer veggies, brush them with some olive oil, and grill them.

- Stir-fry veggies and serve them over brown rice.

- Experiment with different herbs to give steamed veggies a whole new twist.

Vegetables have endless possibilities, and the more comfortable you become in the kitchen and the more familiar you become with herbs and different cooking methods, the more creative you can be. (And the better the possibility that your kids will come running to the dinner table rather than hide behind the sofa when you call them.)

Getting fruity-licious

Fruits make great snacks, anytime, anywhere. Thanks to modern technology and transportation, you can find almost any fruit at any time of the year, although out-of-season fruits tend to be expensive. Still, the luxury of eating fresh red raspberries in the middle of January makes them worth every penny!

As with vegetables, many of the nutrients that fruits offer are in their skins, so offering your child an *unpeeled* apple or pear is best.

Children are often more willing to accept fruits than vegetables in their diets because although fruits aren't candy, they do contain some natural sugars and hardly ever have a bitter taste. So, finally, there's something that may work in your favor — Mother Nature created a sweet snack for kids with a sweet tooth!

Although raw fruits are considered healthiest, canned or dried fruits sometimes travel better, particularly in lunchboxes. (Smashed bananas and apples bruised beyond recognition may result in a child's refusal to eat the brown fruit — and can you blame him, really?) When you need fruit that travels well, keep the following things in mind:

- ✔ Purchase small plastic containers to protect fruit on its journey.

- ✔ Fruit juice counts as a serving of fruit and comes in handy portable boxes and pouches. Read the labels, though, and make sure your child's getting real, 100 percent juice. Most so-called fruit juices contain very little evidence of actual fruit (or nutrition).

- ✔ Raisins, banana or apple chips, and dried cherries, blueberries, papaya, and mango are all very sweet and completely uncrushable.

- ✔ Make sure that applesauce and other canned fruits aren't packed in (or contain) high-fructose corn syrup. Fruits packed in their own juices are best.

One way to expose your child to a whole grove of fruits at once is to make a fresh fruit salad. Fruits tend to blend together well, so toss in whatever you can find in the produce section, including grapes, apples, oranges, mango, strawberries, bananas, kiwi, and pears. If the mixture seems too dry, add a little 100 percent fruit juice to the mix, and serve it up for a snack or as dessert.

And speaking of desserts, fruits baked into pies don't count as a healthy choice unless you've personally cut the fat from the pie crust and haven't added any sugar.

Ahoy! Eating from the deep blue sea

If the thought of eating fish makes your family crinkle their noses, or if the only way your family would ever consider eating fish is if it were deep-fried, the time has come to reevaluate those feelings about our friends with fins.

As for health benefits, fish has a lot going for it:

- ✔ Most fish is very low in fat.

- ✔ It's packed with *omega-3 fatty acids,* which have been shown to have wide-reaching and significant health benefits, mostly in the reduction of heart disease.

- ✔ Researchers have found evidence that eating fish may help prevent asthma, improve the health of the brain and eyes, possibly reduce the risk of certain cancers, improve the health of diabetics, and alleviate symptoms of depression.

You may have heard media reports about fish being associated with high levels of mercury in the bloodstream, which in turn can cause neurological problems. So are we crazy for advising you to feed fish to your family? No. Almost every variety of fish has traces of mercury, but only certain kinds tend to have very high levels. The FDA recommends avoiding shark (at the table *and* in the water), king mackerel, and tilefish, which all tend to have high levels of mercury. According to the FDA, shrimp, canned light tuna, pollock, salmon, and catfish tend to have low levels of mercury.

Frying fish (or anything else, for that matter) isn't the way to go when you're trying to improve your family's health and help your child lose weight. Instead, you can broil, bake, poach, steam, or grill fish, depending on the variety and the thickness of the cut. When you purchase fresh fish, ask the fishmonger for cooking recommendations.

Marinate or sprinkle fish with herbs before cooking it, and serve it with a slice of lemon, which really does add flavor and cut the fishy taste. If your child can't do without a condiment, give her some ketchup instead of tartar sauce, which is high in fat.

Shellfish such as lobster, shrimp, and scallops are also low fat and contain the good omega-3 fatty oils. Not long ago, doctors advised that shellfish be eaten only sparingly because it was thought to be high in cholesterol. Turns out it's lower in cholesterol than was previously believed, so go ahead and serve your family a lobster or clam bake! (Just skip the drawn butter.)

The lowdown on meat: What's healthy and what's not

As we explain in Chapter 8, there are healthy ways to include meat in your family's diet. In fact, healthy cooking should include meat because meat provides protein, something a growing child needs. Forget everything you know about meat, and read the following sections to find out how to choose the right cuts and prepare them in healthy ways.

Fowl's anything but foul

Chicken breasts and turkey breasts are both healthy meat choices that are easy to prepare, even for kitchen novices. To seal in the juices, bake or grill chicken breasts. A turkey breast requires no more preparation than defrosting it, unwrapping it, and following the cooking instructions on the wrapper. (Heck, it may even include a handy pop-up timer!) If you've never cooked a turkey breast and believe you're just not capable of doing so without ruining it, you're wrong. (You can thank the experts at the turkey factory for making the process *incredibly* easy.)

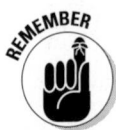

Before serving them, be sure to remove the skin from chicken and turkey. The skin holds the juices in during cooking, but it's also very high in fat and turns a healthy meal into a not-so-healthy one. Needless to say, frying poultry also detracts significantly from its health benefits.

When your family gets used to the taste of baked or grilled poultry *sans* the skin, something really interesting is waiting for you at the grocery store: ground chicken and turkey, which you can substitute for ground beef in any recipe. Think turkey burgers, spaghetti sauce with ground chicken, and turkey meatballs. If you don't reveal the switch to your family right away, they may not even notice the difference in taste. These meat products look almost identical to ground beef both before and after cooking, so if you're worried that your youngster will think that you're mean for serving up Chicken Little tacos, keep that information to yourself for the time being.

When you're choosing a package of ground turkey or ground chicken at the grocery store, read the label carefully to make sure that you're purchasing ground *breast* meat! Ground dark meat (from the legs and thighs) isn't all that healthy; you'd be better off buying lean ground beef.

Some safety concerns you should consider when working with poultry include:

- ✔ When you bring poultry home and stick it in the fridge, make sure to use it or freeze it within 48 hours.

- ✔ Defrost frozen poultry in the fridge to keep bacteria growth at bay.

- ✔ Poultry contains salmonella, bacteria that can cause severe gastrointestinal illness. To protect yourself and your family from contamination, wash your hands after touching raw poultry or its packaging, keep raw poultry and its juices away from other foods in the fridge, and use a separate cutting board and knife when preparing poultry.

- ✔ Cook breasts to an internal temperature of 170 degrees and whole birds to 180 degrees before pulling them out of the oven. Ground poultry shouldn't appear pink when it's fully cooked.

With so many ways to serve it, poultry can become a staple of your family's diet. You can cook whole birds or whole breasts, cut up breasts, or use ground poultry. Because breast portions are low in fat and high in protein, you have no reason not to add poultry to salads, soups, sandwiches, casseroles, stir-fry, pizzas, tacos, and more!

Lean and not mean (to your health)

Walk through the meat department of your grocery store and you'll realize just how many different cuts of meat there are. Some are much better for you than others, and getting it all straight may seem like an overwhelming task. Never fear! Here are some simple guidelines to follow when looking for the leanest meats:

- ✔ **Pay attention to the labels.** Meats that have a USDA Prime label tend to have a higher fat content than meats labeled USDA Choice or USDA Select. Pass those Prime labels right by.

  Ground beef labels give you fat content information, usually in the form of "75/25," "85/15," or "90/10." The second number indicates the percentage of fat in the meat, so choose ground meat that's 15 percent fat or less.

- ✔ **Don't choose meat that has a marbled (white, streaky) appearance.** That's fat you're looking at.

✔ **Sirloin, round, chuck, and tenderloin are lean cuts of beef.**

✔ **To get really lean ground beef, ask the butcher to grind up some sirloin.** Also ask him to remove the fat from the edges before he grinds it.

✔ **Lean pork cuts include tenderloin and loin chops — *not* bacon or pork sausage.**

After you go to all the trouble to buy lean mean, you want to keep it lean on its way to your table. In order to keep lean meat lean, bake it, broil it, or grill it, but *don't fry it!* When preparing meat for cooking, get yourself a sharp knife and cut off any excess fat around the edges. After browning ground beef, drain the fat off by placing the meat in a colander. To get even more fat out (or off), rinse the meat in the colander with hot water before using it in a sauce or casserole.

Meat requires the same safety precautions as poultry: Use it or freeze it within 48 hours of purchase, defrost it in the fridge, and avoid contaminating other foods or surfaces with the juices. Beef may contain *E. coli,* a bacteria that can produce serious illness in children, so make sure any beef you serve to your kids is cooked to 155 degrees (there should be no pink left). This high temperature kills any E. coli that may be present. Undercooked pork, meanwhile, may contain a parasite which can cause an illness called trichinosis, so make sure you cook pork products to at least 144 degrees before serving.

Knowing What to Avoid

Giving up certain recipes can be difficult because they mean so much to us. They're more than food — they're comfort, a way to pass the time, and a big part of who we are. The good news is that many, many recipes can be modified to be low in fat and all-around healthier.

Modifying your eating habits begins with understanding why certain foods contribute to poor health. This section explains what makes some foods and cooking choices far less healthy than other options.

Pass the fried whatever

It's possible to deep-fry just about any food, and by gum, it seems as though people are out to prove that point these days. Take a look at this list of foods that are regularly dipped in boiling fat and served to kids and their families:

- ✔ Chicken
- ✔ Vegetables
- ✔ Cheese
- ✔ Dough
- ✔ Meat
- ✔ Fish

Here's the amazing thing about this list: Everything on it can be 100 percent healthy if it isn't fried!

Frying foods usually involves oils that contain trans fats, which are among the worst offenders when it comes to clogging arteries and contributing to heart disease. (For more on the kinds of fat, see Chapter 7.) Imagine taking a lovely little eggplant, full of vitamins and yearning to do your child some good, and dipping it in egg and bread crumbs (nothing too offensive yet). Then . . . you toss it in a hot pan of oil and watch its fat content jump through the roof!

Some foods don't have a shot at being a healthy choice in the first place, so frying them just makes them even worse. At county fairs, for example, the big thing these days is frying up cookies. Now, no one is fooling anyone here — cookies aren't a healthy snack even before they hit the oil. But the thing that sometimes trips people up — kids, in particular — is thinking that because a fried food *started out* healthy, it must retain some good qualities even after it's been soaked in hot fat. Needless to say, this isn't true. A fried "healthy" food (like a vegetable or lean meat) is no longer a healthy choice. Even if the food in question manages to hold onto some of its nutrients, the amount of fat it gains in the frying process pretty much negates the lingering nutrients. In other words, the bad qualities of fried food completely overshadow any trace of goodness that may remain after the frying process.

In the end, we can say without reservation that fried food is just not a healthy option, especially not for a child who is already overweight. We know that fried foods taste good. We also understand that when a child loves his fried foods, he truly *craves* them. But you have so many other options for cooking tasty, healthy meals that frying should go right out your kitchen window.

Curb the bad carbs

You're probably somewhat familiar with the debate over carbohydrates: Do they cause people to gain weight, and should we all do away with carbs in our diets? *Carbohydrates* are natural sugars, and the fact is that humans' primary source of energy comes from carbohydrates, so it's especially important for a child to eat enough carbs. The *type* of carbohydrate a person consumes, however, is what determines the effect on weight gain.

The following foods contain carbohydrates:

- ✔ Fruits
- ✔ Vegetables
- ✔ Whole grains
- ✔ Bread (and breadlike products, like crackers and cereals)
- ✔ Pasta

Carbohydrates fall into two vastly different groups:

- ✔ **Low glycemic index:** The carbohydrates you find in most fruits, veggies, and whole grains (including whole-grain bread products) have what's called a *low glycemic index,* which means that the body easily uses the natural sugars found in these foods for energy. For the most part, these foods are in a fairly natural, unrefined state, which means that all their vitamins, minerals, and fiber is intact, and this condition makes it easy for the body to use those elements for energy and essential functions.

No hope for "healthy" frying

When you see packaged fried chicken advertised as containing "all white meat" or "all breast meat," don't be lured into buying it for your kids, thinking that it's a somewhat healthy option. After all, it's fried, which means it's high in fat and not a healthy choice. Period. Nothing else matters — not where the meat came from or how lean the cut was before it fell into the deep fryer.

If you're looking for a healthy way to fry your family's favorite foods, you're not likely to find one. The chemical processes that take place between hot oil and food have led scientists to theorize that in addition to adding loads of fat to the diet, fried foods may also cause a cancer risk. And changing your frying method to use different oils only changes the risks, it doesn't eliminate them.

Different oils containing different types of fat (saturated, polyunsaturated, monounsaturated, and trans fats) have been tested to see if any can produce a healthy fried food. The end result of these tests is basically this: The chemical composition of each type of fat and the way it reacts with food results in different health risks, like cancer and cardiovascular disease.

✔ **High glycemic index:** Foods that contain white sugar and/or white flour (like white bread, pasta, cookies, crackers, and doughnuts) have a *high glycemic index*. These foods have high levels of *refined* carbohydrates (meaning that the natural grain has been stripped away), which cause the body's blood sugar levels to jump higher. If that blood sugar isn't used fairly quickly, it's stored as fat.

Like we said, everyone needs carbohydrates for energy, but when you serve up bread and flour products, make sure they're in as natural a state as possible. Stick with good carbohydrates by following these guidelines:

✔ **Buy whole-grain foods, like whole-grain bread and brown rice.** Whole grains provide vitamins, minerals, and fiber.

✔ **Use whole-wheat flour, and avoid using white sugar as much as possible.**

✔ **Avoid white-flour breads and pastas.** If you compare a white-bread label to a whole-wheat bread label, you can see that the vitamin and mineral content of the white bread pales in comparison. (No pun intended).

Cheese: Friend or foe?

Cheese contains calcium, which kids need for growing bones, so can it really be that bad? If whole-milk cheese is a part of your child's daily diet, she's probably gaining weight unless she's extremely active. Low-fat dairy is an excellent alternative and is readily available in stores these days.

Steer clear of cheese sauce, which is very high in fat. Cheese sauce is an even more unhealthy choice when it's poured on top of a refined carbohydrate (like pasta) or a fried food (like tortilla chips). If your kids have a hankering for some cheese to top their broccoli, melt a sprinkling of low-fat shredded cheese on top of the veggies in the microwave.

When preparing pizza at home, use low-fat mozzarella for the topping and your kids will never know the difference.

Mom, I'm Starving!

No matter what age group you're dealing with, when kids are looking for something to eat, seize the opportunity to teach them about making healthy choices, first by making sure that your kitchen is loaded with healthy, edible foods, and then by making suggestions for a healthy breakfast, lunch, or snack.

Getting help in the kitchen

You probably already know that cooking at home takes more time and energy than ordering out or even using convenience foods on a regular basis. To ease your kitchen burden, take advantage of opportunities to let your child help with the cooking. Don't be shy about giving him duties at mealtime. Requiring his help in the kitchen:

✔ Makes your life a little easier, which may, in turn, allow you to maintain your enthusiasm surrounding your new, healthy recipes (as opposed to feeling as though you've taken on *so* much work and no one appreciates it).

✔ Encourages conversation between you and your child about the upcoming meal. Working on the meal together is a great time for you to drop little pearls of wisdom concerning making healthy choices.

✔ Encourages conversation about the day and what's happening in your lives, and fosters a sense of support, which is just what your child needs right now. If he can talk to you about his math test while he washes the lettuce, he also may be willing to talk about his hopes for weight loss.

But what kinds of kitchen jobs should you give to children? Isn't it dangerous to hand a kid a knife and a hunk of meat? Sure, *that's* dangerous. Ultimately, the tasks you give your kid really depend on the age of the child. Younger kids can do easy tasks, like washing vegetables and tearing lettuce for a salad, setting healthy condiments out on the table, and setting the table with plates and silverware. Older kids can take on more responsibility, within reason. You may not want your 10-year-old using a food processor, but you can have him chop veggies for stir-fry with a small, plastic, dome-covered chopper. You can also show your preteen how to work the stove while you teach him what kind of safety measures are involved in using lit burners and hot pots and pans.

If you have a budding chef on your hands who wants to add herbs and spices to every meal, let him go at it. The two of you may come up with something your family will love.

Giving lessons in portion sizes

Before you let your child loose in the kitchen, even a kitchen that contains nothing but healthy foods, you have to explain portion sizes, or how much food he should be eating at a single sitting. Some experts say that a handful of whatever a kid's eating is an appropriate serving size. We think a better, more helpful-in-the-long-term method is to teach kids how to read food labels and then apply the label information.

What the heck are we talking about, you ask? Here's an example: Suppose your child wants some cereal after he comes home from school. That's fine; you've purchased whole-grain oat rings, which provide lots of vitamins and minerals. The serving size on the label is 1 cup. Hand him a measuring cup and let him pour 1 cup of cereal into it and then into a bowl he regularly eats out of. Do the same thing with the milk — find the serving size, and then let him measure it out and pour it into the bowl. If he wants a banana in the cereal, no problem. Again, it provides essential nutrients — but one banana is enough.

Now, let him look at the bowl in front of him. That's a normal serving size of cereal, milk, and fruit. Overweight children and adults are often so used to eating larger-than-average food portions that they don't realize how much or how little they *should* be eating to adapt to a healthier lifestyle. Encourage your child to measure out portion sizes until he's able to easily estimate the amount of food in an appropriate serving size. (Even better, some serving sizes are listed in quantities, like "12 pretzels" or "10 crackers.") Measuring may seem like a lot of trouble to go through every time he has a snack, but it won't take long before he realizes what one serving of pretzels looks like.

Encouraging self-sufficiency

Giving kids certain responsibilities (like feeding themselves from time to time) encourages good decision making and, in turn, bolsters their confidence because they know that they really can take care of themselves — and others, if need be. The biggest bonus of teaching your child about making healthy food decisions is that she learns skills she needs in the real world. When she slides her tray past the choices in the school cafeteria, she knows which foods are better for her, healthwise, and she chooses the plain turkey sandwich on whole-wheat bread over the suspicious-looking macaroni and cheese.

Take things slowly at first. When you begin to bring healthy foods home, talk about them as you put them away. Explain why you've chosen whole-grain flour over white flour, for example, and why you've switched from whole milk to 1 percent or skim. Of course, there's a fine line between explaining and lecturing (especially as far as kids are concerned), so do your best to keep the tone light and friendly, and don't get pulled into any kind of debate or argument over why you won't bring home donuts or cupcakes.

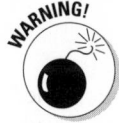

Although you need to teach your child about the healthy choices the family is going to be making from now on, take care not to overwhelm her with too much information all at once. Obviously, an older child can understand more complex information than a toddler can, but even an adolescent has her limits on how much she wants to hear from her parents. When she seems like she's had enough of the conversation, continue it at a later time.

After you talk with your child about healthier options and why you won't bring certain foods into the house anymore, she's ready to start preparing her own snacks and meals. Watch from a distance, and resist the urge to criticize her preferences. (Just because you would never dream of dipping pretzels in plain yogurt doesn't mean that she shouldn't.) Make sure she's paying attention to serving sizes, but give her guidance without making decisions for her. Encourage the transition from learning what's best for her health to putting what she's learned into action.

Promoting creativity

Experimenting with healthy foods is something to play up in your household. So many times, people — not just kids, but adults, too — hear the words "healthy foods" and immediately conjure up an image of dry toast, cottage cheese, and a leaf of lettuce . . . at every meal. You know that this isn't the case; plenty of foods are legitimately great tasting *and* healthy, so no one has to feel as though they're surviving on something that tastes like cardboard.

As long as you make sure that you're bringing healthy foods into the house, you can feel comfortable letting your kids make their own choices at snack time and whenever they may be left to feed themselves. Your daughter seems to like low-sugar jam on a toasted pita pocket? Great! She wants to pack a low-fat cheese stick and graham crackers for a snack at school? Wonderful! She's stirring low-fat granola into her yogurt for an added kick? Terrific! These are all healthy snacks, and whether anyone else will find her preferences appetizing is beside the point. She's experimenting with new tastes and textures, she's making good choices, and she's learning that healthy does *not* equal boring. That's the lesson you want her to remember.

When kids are ready to start preparing actual meals on their own, you may see an added burst of creativity. Herbs, spices, and low-fat condiments can all make or break a meal, so encourage your child to try out these new tastes and combinations. She may discover a new way to fix a meal she already enjoys, which will give her more reason to continue experimenting with healthy foods — there's just so much to discover!

Chapter 10

Move It and Lose It: Getting Physical

*E*ating the right kinds of foods in the right amounts, as we discuss in Chapter 7, is essential to leading a healthy lifestyle. However, a truly healthy lifestyle isn't possible without some form of regular physical activity.

Although it *is* possible to be heavy, active, and healthy, most overweight people aren't physically active. And the less physically active a person is, the more weight he's likely to gain, making it even harder for him to become physically active even if he wants to. In Chapter 3, we talk about the orthopedic pains and strains and the breathing problems that obese kids sometimes deal with on a daily basis. If your child doesn't feel well physically, he can easily make a legitimate argument against engaging in physical activity by saying, "I can't go outside and play. I can't breathe when I move, and it hurts my legs to walk very far." Unlike a child who's unwilling to break away from the TV simply because he doesn't *want* to, an obese kid often has genuine health issues that discourage him from becoming more active.

But these are the exact reasons that it's so important for him to do something. The more time he spends being inactive, the more likely it is that he'll never believe he's capable of turning his physical state around. We're not suggesting that a significantly overweight child turn over a new leaf by running around the block a couple of times. When someone is obese, *any* increase in his amount of daily physical activity is an improvement. The goal is to increase activity little by little. The more your child moves, the better he's going to feel — both physically and emotionally. You may encounter some bumps in the road, but throughout this chapter we talk about ways to handle them and to continue encouraging your child's progress.

In this chapter, you find out about the best ways to introduce children to physical activity (which aren't necessarily the same methods we'd offer for adults). The name of the game is to keep it fun and interesting so that it doesn't seem like *work!* (Come to think of it, this *is* the same kind of advice we'd give to grown-ups!)

If your child isn't obese but you fear he's headed in that direction, it's important to start adding physical activity into his daily routine. As with all adverse physical conditions, preventing obesity is better than treating its myriad side effects, so discovering how to incorporate exercise into your youngster's life now will have long-lasting positive effects.

I've Fallen Onto the Couch and I Won't Get Up: Battling Laziness

Obesity doesn't just happen on its own — not in kids and not in adults. Most cases of obesity are caused by unhealthy diets and lack of exercise. We talk about establishing a healthy diet in Chapters 7, 8, and 9. This section addresses the bad habits associated with a sedentary lifestyle. The combination of eating low-fat, low-sugar foods and adding physical activity to your child's day packs a one-two punch against obesity.

Doctors often say that some people are *predisposed* to weight gain, but that doesn't mean that someone whose entire family is overweight will absolutely, positively become obese; it means that a person who comes from an overweight family has to be especially vigilant in his or her efforts to prevent obesity. And if that person happens to be a child, a predisposition means that his or her parents have to take a very proactive approach to keeping their kid healthy.

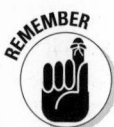

The U.S. Department of Agriculture (USDA) recommends that *everyone* engage in at least 30 minutes of moderate activity each day for good health, but *any* improvement in your child's level of physical activity is for the best, no matter how small it may seem at first. Minor victories are *still* victories!

Living the sedentary life

Many times, when a doctor or nutritionist is calculating how many calories a person needs each day, they ask the person about his or her level of activity: Is it active, moderately active, or sedentary? What do these terms mean where kids are concerned?

- ✔ **Active:** Playing hard for sustained periods of time. For example, a kid who's outside playing football for hours on end is considered active.

- ✔ **Moderately active:** Thirty minutes of physical activity every day in addition to the everyday tasks of life (such as physical chores like raking or mowing the lawn, walking to a friend's house, and so on).

- ✔ **Sedentary:** Sitting in one spot, watching TV or playing video games. Movement of any kind is extremely limited.

Most obese children fall into the sedentary category, which starts a vicious cycle. The less active a child is, the more likely he is to become overweight. As he becomes more overweight, he may be less able to easily engage in physical activity, plus any health issues that arise from being overweight (like asthma or aching joints) make it less likely that he'll participate in some sort of regular exercise. As time goes on, the situation worsens until the child feels as though there's just no way that he can get up and get moving.

Things may be made even worse by the child's embarrassment over his weight and lack of participation in activities. For example, a school-age overweight child who's never been one to play outdoors with the other neighborhood kids isn't likely to be eager to start when his weight reaches a crisis point. He may fear that the others will make fun of his weight or his lack of coordination, and if these fears become reality, he'll be discouraged from pursuing physical activity in the future as well.

The best way to introduce your child to a lifetime of physical activity is to start out slowly and to keep expectations to a minimum. Exercise helps burn off body fat, but it doesn't happen in one day or even in a week. Losing weight, like gaining weight, takes time. (The difference, of course, is that it's a heck of a lot easier to put on extra pounds than it is to take them off.)

In the beginning, don't concentrate on how long it will take before your child starts seeing the results of physical efforts. Instead, think of physical activity as a way to improve the health of your entire family, and encourage everyone to do the same. Throughout this chapter, we give you tips for including exercise as a regular part of your family's lifestyle — *that's* your primary goal. The weight will come off with regular activity and a healthy diet, but you can't force it and you can't make it happen any faster than Mother Nature intends.

Gaining weight, losing health in America

Turn on the news any day of the week and you'll probably hear about how Americans are more overweight than they've ever been in the past. Sixty percent of adults in the United States are heavier than their ideal weight, and obese kids make up about 10 percent of the population. These percentages have skyrocketed in the past ten years, so what's going on here?

The typical, modern American lifestyle includes a lot of sitting around — in cars, in offices, at home — and munching on high-fat and/or high-sugar convenience foods and junk foods. It's really no wonder that, on the whole, Americans are heavier than they were several generations ago, when people moved more and ate healthier out of necessity. What's most unsettling is

that the obese children of today are the obese parents of tomorrow, and research has indicated that heavy parents are more likely to have heavy children, at least in part because of the poor lifestyle habits they model for their kids. Are Americans destined to become heavier and heavier?

No. You already know the ways to turn this problem around: a healthy diet and more physical activity. Although not every child (or adult) will become stick thin by incorporating these elements into their lives, they *will* become healthier, and years down the road, they'll pass good habits on to their own kids, which is a starting point for turning around the health of the entire country.

Sneaking activity into your family's day

The younger the kid, the less engrained her unhealthy habits are and the easier it is to convince her that moving her body is fun, fun, fun! Plus, you're in complete control of her day, so when you tell your 5-year-old that it's time for the two of you to walk the dog, that should be the end of the discussion. Get the leash, grab the dog, grab the kid, and head out the door.

If you're encountering resistance with even starting to incorporate physical activity into your family's lifestyle, other ways to get everyone moving without them really realizing it include:

- **Taking the kids on little errands:** Safety is always your first concern, of course, so you may have to accompany young children on walks to borrow eggs from a neighbor down the street or to the corner market for fresh vegetables.

- **Giving the kids work to do:** Hand the kids shovels after a snowstorm and tell them to clear the driveway instead of hiring someone to plow. Let them rake, mow, and haul yard debris. Or if you don't have a yard for them to work in, give everyone a list of indoor chores. Dusting, mopping, vacuuming, and even washing windows gets them up and moving and accustomed to some light physical activity.

- ✔ **Trolling for the *farthest* parking spots:** When you head to the mall, grocery store, or anywhere else, choose a parking spot that's a good distance from the door. The relatively short walk is a good way to ease your child into a physical activity.

- ✔ **Creating a fun zone in your house:** If your kids don't have any room to let loose inside, they may be less apt to give up their seats on the couch. Turn a corner of the basement or a spare bedroom into a well-padded place where they're free to dance, jump, or roll to their hearts' content.

An older child is more likely to know what you're up to when you park far, far away from the entrance to the store. She may want to debate the physical activity issue with you and, in fact, may argue with you until she's worn herself out. What do you do with this kid? Drag her outside? Force her to have fun in the yard? With an older child, you have to take a step back, think about the reasons she's opposed to activity, and find out what's going to work best for her. She may be holding back because of:

- ✔ **Physical pain:** Her knees, hips, lower back, ankles, and legs may ache when she engages in physical activity.

- ✔ **Difficulty keeping up:** Whether she has asthma or she simply becomes winded easily, not being able to breathe can be a real deterrent to any form of exercise.

- ✔ **Embarrassment over her lack of coordination:** If she's concerned about being able to move easily or about what others will say to her concerning her weight, she may protest against any efforts you make toward her physical fitness.

Even something as seemingly innocuous as walking a long distance from the car to the store can seem like torture to a child who's sensitive about her weight, so do everything in your power not to make it an issue. All the changes you make are for the health of the entire family, and that's the card you need to play with a child who's reluctant to jump on the Active Train. Simply tell her, "Honey, we're parking here because *I* need the exercise." Even if you don't need to lose weight, approaching exercise from this angle is a really effective way to set a good example for your child.

Aside from making small changes like walking to school or to the store rather than driving, the best way to get a reluctant older child moving is to find some sort of sport that she can tolerate physically and that she enjoys. We talk more about this option in the section "Organized sports" later in this chapter.

Exercise Is Not a Form of Torture

Physical activity is essential to a healthy lifestyle, and not because it can make your child skinny. In addition to burning off calories, exercise provides the following benefits:

- ✔ It helps to lower cholesterol and improve heart health.
- ✔ It can help lower blood pressure.
- ✔ Activity aids the proper development of bones and muscles in children.
- ✔ Exercise releases endorphins into the bloodstream that help to lift one's mood.

Exercise jump-starts a healthy cycle of feeling good both physically and mentally. Although it may be difficult at first, the more your child moves, the more she'll be able to do. She'll feel those endorphins kicking in, which will give her a sense of well-being during and after an activity. In addition, as she continues to exercise, her self-esteem and physical feeling of wellness will both improve.

And then there's the fat-burning benefit that exercise offers, as well. Simply put, an obese child can't lose a significant amount of weight *without* exercising — at least not in a way that would be considered healthy. Starvation isn't an advisable means of losing weight for anyone, let alone a child or teen who's still growing and developing. Although an undernourished body will eventually look to fat reserves for the calories it needs, eating a low-fat diet and burning those calories off through exercise is a *much* healthier way to achieve a weight-loss goal. Finding one or more activities that your child can stick with in the long term is also a way to ensure that her health improves no matter what the number on the scale reads.

Getting the whole family involved

An overweight child usually comes from a family for which weight is an issue. His parents are overweight, and his siblings probably are, too. Although obesity is sometimes linked with a genetic predisposition, it's often caused or exacerbated by unhealthy lifestyle choices. When choices like overeating high-fat foods and watching TV around the clock are the norm inside a home, everyone usually suffers the adverse effects in the form of weight gain.

Our point here is that most families for which obesity is a concern aren't dealing with only one overweight member of the clan, so no one feels singled out when a plan for leading a healthy lifestyle is put into effect. That's not to say everyone is happy about the changes in the household, but the alterations in diet and activity level should be enforced across the board. What's good for the kids is good for the adults, and vice versa.

Taking that idea one step farther, what's good for an overweight member of the family is just as good for a member of the family who doesn't have a weight problem. Unhealthy choices are unhealthy regardless of how they affect weight. High-fat foods contribute mightily to the development of cardiovascular disease (namely clogged arteries), and recent studies have shown that this type of damage can start in childhood! Pairing a low-fat diet with regular exercise helps counteract this damage, so cutting out the fat and getting those bodies moving is in everyone's best interest!

Start with fun and easy activities

Some low-impact, low-key activities that are great for your family's initial foray into becoming more active include:

- ✔ **Walks:** Find a park with a decent trail, and explore!

- ✔ **Swimming:** Because of the buoyancy water provides, swimming is a great activity for overweight kids or adults who suffer from aching joints.

- ✔ **Bike rides:** Biking is an activity that you can adapt to everyone's individual athletic abilities. Take it slowly at first — no need to break any records!

- ✔ **Toys that encourage activity:** Invest in a basketball hoop, rollerblades, a skateboard ramp, a badminton net . . . anything that gets the family out the door and doing something.

The more active the entire family becomes, the more apt each member will be to find his or her own favorite modes of exercise.

Avoid the "E" word

"Now wait a minute," you're saying. "My family hasn't participated in physical activity in years. What are you suggesting we do, break out the Jane Fonda tapes?" Well, if your family happens to find these tapes entertaining and inspiring, then sure — dust off the VCR and give it a whirl! But realize that *exercise* is sometimes a loaded word, fraught with all sorts of (negative) expectations and likely to meet with resistance. And the fact is, kids don't "exercise" in the same way that adults do.

For some people (including kids), exercise can conjure up images (or actual memories) of becoming breathless, sweating profusely, and generally feeling completely helpless. Physical education class can be a nightmare for overweight and obese kids (see the "Evaluating Your Child's Physical Education Class" section later in this chapter); unfortunately, these bad experiences are often linked to exercise, souring kids on the whole idea of getting physical. If they've been in situations in which they couldn't keep up and were teased by other kids or even put down by a teacher for their lack of stamina, sometimes there's no winning kids back to the idea that exercise is a good thing.

Ultimately, you may want to avoid using the term *exercise.* Call it "getting out of the house." Or call the activity by its name, as in "Let's go for a walk," "Hey, we're headed out for a little hike this afternoon," or "Why don't we jump in the pool for a swim?" The most important thing, at least initially, is to make the family realize that they can be active without feeling as though they're going to drop and without feeling as though they've failed at something (those gym class memories again). If you can get this message through, they'll end up feeling as though participating in activity can be fun!

Encouraging your kids to move it (and lose it)

As we say in the introduction to this chapter, kids usually don't exercise the way that adults do. Adults are eager to quantify everything about physical activity: what they did, when they did it, how long they did it for, and how many calories (and even how many *fat* calories) they burned in the process.

Children, of course, just want to do something that's fun. Your obese 8-year-old isn't going to keep checking her watch to see how many more minutes she has to walk before she can feel good about herself and her weight-loss efforts today. She'll feel good about herself as long as she does something that she enjoys. The goal is to work 30 minutes of activity into most days, but if your child isn't expected to keep track, then how do we expect this whole physical activity thing to work? Does it run on some sort of honor system or what?

The initial goal isn't exercising for a specific amount of time; it's teaching your child that physical activity is enjoyable. When she's confident that she can participate in activities, it's up to you to encourage her to find one that she likes well enough so that she'll do it on her own. You won't have to sneak around with a stopwatch because active kids like to *be* active. Here are two points to ponder:

 ✔ Most kids really enjoy and are encouraged by group participation in physical activity.

> ✔ When they aren't playing in organized, scheduled activities (like soccer games), most kids play in short spurts — ten minutes or so at a time. It's okay, then, for your child to run around in the yard for relatively short increments of time, as long as she does it several times a day.

Although teens are usually in the age group that's big on keeping journals, some younger children may also benefit from keeping logs of their activities, just to have a visual concept of how things are going. Appendix B provides an exercise log that they can use.

Organized sports

Participating in sports can really give overweight kids the boost they need, both physically and emotionally. Feeling a sense of accomplishment — that realization that, "Oh my gosh, I really *can* do this!" — is something that these kids really need in order to continue on the healthy-living track.

Let your child decide what kind of sport she'd most enjoy. Don't push her into ballet lessons when she'd much rather be somersaulting in a gymnastics class. Also, if she's not an athletic child and wants to try out a sport that she's never played before, make sure you sign her up for a noncompetitive teaching league, at least for her first time out. (This is good advice for any kid, regardless of his or her weight.) Jumping into a league with mini-pro players (kids who were either born with a gift for athleticism or who have been playing the sport practically since infancy) may leave her feeling like a deer in the headlights, like an outsider, and like this whole physical activity thing stinks just as badly as she feared it would.

Competitive sports leagues are all about the competition, naturally. Inexperienced or weaker players often sit on the bench and end up feeling ashamed of their lack of prowess on the playing field. Teaching leagues, by contrast, are all about learning the basics of the sport and giving everyone equal time and opportunity to play. As a result, these leagues are much better starting points for *any* child who isn't well versed in a particular sport.

Your child probably won't be confined to choosing between gymnastics and soccer. Kids' sports are big these days, so when your child is ready, look for all sorts of opportunities to sign her up for something she'd enjoy. Some activities to research in your area include:

✔ Hockey

✔ Speed skating

✔ Figure skating

✔ Skiing

- ✔ Snowboarding
- ✔ Baseball
- ✔ Softball
- ✔ Lacrosse
- ✔ Horseback riding
- ✔ Basketball
- ✔ Football
- ✔ Dancing
- ✔ Rowing
- ✔ Swimming
- ✔ Martial arts
- ✔ Tennis
- ✔ Skateboarding

Many sports leagues are coed (at least until adolescence, when the difference in size and strength between the average boy and girl becomes more of a safety issue), and a child can choose between team activities and being a team of one (in activities like skiing, running, or horseback riding).

Activities for youngsters

The youngest children usually offer the least resistance to including physical activity in their regular routines. It truly *is* fun for them to chase and be chased, and preschoolers don't yet feel self-conscious about their weight — they're more interested in playing, either with other kids or with Mom or Dad.

If you have an overweight youngster, start improving her physical fitness by cutting *way* down on her TV time. She doesn't need eight hours of educational programming each day. When she does watch TV, choose shows that have some sort of physical component to them. Many kids' shows these days ask the kids to get up and dance along with the characters, for example. From a health standpoint, these interactive programs are the least objectionable form of TV (even though kids jumping on the couch tend to grate on parents' nerves!).

When you want to get her moving outdoors, think back to your own childhood. Kids love a good game of chase, hide-and-seek, or tag. A friendly game of kickball is a blast for little ones, and walking the dog around the block is nothing short of an adventure! Here are some other ideas for getting little ones outside and having some physical fun:

✔ Visit local playgrounds and encourage her to run and climb to her heart's content.

✔ Take her on scavenger hunts in the yard or park. Hunt for pine cones, rocks, and pretty leaves.

✔ Sign her up for a kid-friendly gymnastics class or a learn-to-swim group.

✔ If you're a stay-at-home parent, look for play groups in your area. Keeping her busy is easier if she has other kids to run around with!

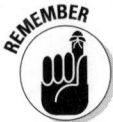

Although little ones thrive on routine, some young kids always seem to be switching gears. The name of the game here is being open minded and flexible. She doesn't need to follow a strict exercise regimen as long as she's doing *something* that involves moving her body!

Weight resistance training: Added activity for adolescents

In addition to aerobic activities, which are an effective way to burn calories, adolescents may become interested in weight training, which is also a good way to fight a weight problem. Muscle tissue burns calories even when it's at rest, so an activity that adds muscle to the body is good for anyone.

If your child is interested in weight training, make sure he's doing it safely! Don't stand by and watch him try to lift a 300-pound barbell when he's never lifted anything heavier than a laundry basket in his entire life! Take your child to meet with a professional trainer, or do some research together to lessen the possibility of mild or severe injury.

A weight machine is safe for a teenager to use as long as he's not straining to lift the weight. Before you buy him that bench press that he's got his eye on, though, remember that bench-pressing should only be done with a *spotter* — someone who can lift the weight off your teen's chest if he's unable to do it himself. If you know you're not capable of this feat of strength (and no one else in the house is, either), *don't* bring the bench press into your home.

Remind your child that weight training is a gradual process and that results often take several months to become visible. Trying to do too much too soon can result in an injury that will hamper his future progress and maybe turn him off the whole idea forever.

Keeping boredom at bay

Ever heard the phrase "Familiarity breeds contempt"? Repetition of any activity — whether it's physical activity, school, chores, or playing with the same friend for days on end — can lead to boredom. Although some kids find one or two activities that they love and will stick with from now until the end of time, most kids need to shake things up a bit in order to stay interested in physical activity.

Parents, meanwhile, are easily frustrated by children who seem to be darting from one activity to the next, never quite settling into anything permanently. If your child begins Tae Kwon Do lessons, for example, and complains about having to go to his classes midway through the three-month session, should you let him quit? What about the wasted time and money?

Here's a good rule of thumb for your child (and not just for sticking with physical activity, but for making his way through life): When he makes a decision, he has to see it through to the end. You want to give him the power to choose the activities he wants to try, after all, and you don't want to force him into doing something he truly hates. Fine. But before you hand over a check to a sports league, gym, or dojo, explain that after he's signed up, he has to honor his commitment to this activity until the class or season is completely finished.

 Even if your child ends up disliking the activity he's chosen, seeing something through to the end provides a valuable life lesson: Don't quit in the middle of anything because you're bored with it. If he actually ends up liking the activity after some hesitation, that's an even *better* life lesson: Give everything a fair shot because you just never know how things will turn out.

Staying with an activity even when it's more difficult and/or less interesting than he expected it to be also speaks volumes about his efforts towards improving his health. If the kid quits enough activities in his life, he'll never feel as though he's capable of finishing anything. But if he learns to stick with things, he's going to feel far more confident in his abilities to try just about anything.

 Kids often get bored or discouraged with activity when they don't see immediate results in their weight or when they hit a weight-loss *plateau* (a standstill). Encourage your child to continue his efforts but switch to another type of exercise. Sometimes changing activities is just the thing to jump-start weight loss.

Taking weight and health into consideration

Everything about adapting to a healthier lifestyle takes effort and time. We don't expect an obese child to show immediate results, compliance, or even an eager attitude when it comes to physical activity. Obviously, a school-age child who's never been active in her lifetime may have to work up to the *idea* of becoming physically fit. And we know it's difficult for a child with legitimate health issues to begin an exercise regimen of any sort.

On the other hand, we also know that introducing physical activity into a child's routine is well worth the effort in the long run. Engaging in any sort of physical activity is better than doing nothing at all, but we aren't advocating tossing your obese child into a sports league at this very moment. The basic start-up plan involves turning off the TV, putting the video games away, and taking part in some sort of low-impact activity, like walking or doing yard work. That's enough for this initial stage. As your child's stamina increases, encourage and help her to do more.

Slow and steady wins the race! Every little bit of activity helps, but trying to do too much too soon can definitely hinder her progress and make her feel as though she's faltering.

The benefits of helping your child achieve a certain level of physical fitness are twofold: Not only do you see her health improve, but you also may notice an improvement in her self-esteem. The better she feels physically and emotionally, the more likely she is to continue on with a healthy lifestyle and not fall back into her old habits. All these elements of healthy living work together; if one falls out of place, you can expect that the others will, too.

Snowed In or Rained Out?

In the sunny, warm areas of this country, physical fitness is often a way of life. Families walk, bike, and skateboard year-round. They wonder how people survive in the colder climates, where physical fitness is often a seasonal thing: In the spring and summer, everyone looks and feels fit, but come winter, it's time to hunker down in the house and hibernate.

If you live in an area where it's cold literally half the year, you have to know how to adjust and find a way to keep physically active even when it's below freezing outside. Shutting down for months on end just isn't physically or mentally good for anyone. Committing to a healthier lifestyle includes finding a way to keep the family active from January through December and then doing it again, year after year.

Studies have shown that people who live in northern, cold climates are often negatively affected by the lack of sunlight in the winter months. They may develop a condition called Seasonal Affective Disorder (SAD), which is like the winter blahs but worse. Exercise has been shown to alleviate symptoms of depression in people who suffer from SAD.

Finding fun indoor activities

You may feel as though the only options for activity available in the winter months are skiing, snowboarding, and sports of that nature; and because your entire family hates the cold, you're pretty much out of luck. Not true! You live in an era in which the surgeon general is worried sick about the epidemic of obesity, and, as a result, more and more communities offer year-round indoor activities in the interest of maintaining physical fitness throughout the winter months.

For you nonskiers, here are some ideas for finding indoor activities when it's cold, rainy, snowy, or all three for months on end:

- **Look for a community gym in your area.** Private gyms are often expensive and may not allow young children. Gyms run by municipalities, in contrast, tend to be much more family oriented, with activities for every age group.

- **Check out after-school activities.** After-school programs are often a great place to find the teaching leagues we talk about earlier in this chapter (see the section "Organized sports" earlier in the chapter).

- **Research indoor athletic arenas in your area.** Because some areas are snowy from October to April, you may be able to find indoor pools, indoor horseback riding rings, or even a sports dome offering soccer, lacrosse, baseball, softball, or golf during the coldest months.

- **Think about investing in home equipment.** Obviously, you aren't going to put a preschooler on a treadmill, but if you have a teenager who's trying to lose some weight, a treadmill in your home may be a terrific way for her to maintain her fitness routine when it's too cold and icy to walk outside. Before you make any big purchases, however, make sure that your teen is interested in exercising at home and able to test out the equipment (so that you don't spend a lot of money on something that eventually turns into a clothes hanger).

- **Let them dance.** Although cutting back on video games is wise, if your kids want to play Dance Dance Revolution, let them! The game's really popular with kids, and it gets them working up a sweat!

Keeping the little ones busy

If you have small children, get creative and make a safe play area indoors where they can run and climb without getting into too much trouble! A small indoor climbing gym may be just the thing to keep your preschooler busy, or maybe she'd prefer a tricycle to ride in the basement.

 Take a good look at your home and think about the safest options (taking things like stairs and sharp countertops into consideration). Pad hard surfaces with foam rubber, old towels, or pillows; remove rickety furniture that your child may be tempted to climb on; and use old furniture cushions to create soft landing pads for crazy jumps. In addition to wearing herself out, your child will come to think of certain times of the day as times to be physically busy. (Although that may wear *you* out, it's actually one of the best things you could hope for in terms of her health!)

Resisting the tube

Before you dismiss indoor activity ideas in favor of letting the kids have a little extra TV time during the cold months (after all, those gray winter days can be *mighty* long without some form of electronic entertainment to help pass the time), realize that limiting TV time is one of the essential components in a healthy lifestyle. Studies have shown that without any other intervention (like actually becoming more active), cutting back on TV time cuts a child's percentage of being overweight significantly! And we know for a fact that sitting around staring at a screen does *nothing* to help kids lose weight, so stick to those TV-viewing limits, even when it's 3 degrees outside.

 If your child has a TV in his room, get it out! Not only does that type of access lead to time spent not being active, but it can also lead to a dependence on TV at bedtime. Many kids stay up late watching their shows or movies, fall asleep with the TV on, and don't get a full night's rest — making it harder for them to be active the following day.

Playing It Safe Outdoors

In this chapter, we talk a lot about taking the family out of the house and into the great unknown (which may be nowhere more exotic than your local playground). Although physical activity is your goal here, safety is your very first priority, no matter where you're headed or what kind of activity you have planned. Accidents are the leading cause of injury and death to children in this country, so please take the time to make sure that you've addressed every possibility whenever you take your child out of the house.

A little prep work goes a long way

Part of being safe is packing the appropriate gear when you're off on a family outing. For example, if your family is heading out on a hike, you need to dress them for the changing climate as you head up the mountain, and you need to pack food and water, a map, sunscreen, bug repellent, and bandages. Packing up the bikes for a long ride? Same deal: Fortifications, appropriate clothing, bandages, sunscreen, bug repellent, a map if you're headed off-trail, and repair gear for use in the event of a flat tire.

Your motto should be, "Be prepared for any event that's in the realm of possibility." It's possible, for example, that your child could sustain a scrape while on a bike ride, so you should have some bandages handy; it's much less likely, however, that she's going to need to use the headlight on her bike in the middle of the afternoon, so you can leave the extra batteries at home. Get creative with your thinking, but stay on *this* side of the sane parenting line.

Common sense is usually your best instinct as long as it's not coupled with a "That will never happen to my family" attitude. Here are some very basic safety tips that you should enforce every single time your children engage in a particular activity:

- Cyclists always wear helmets.

- Skateboarders also always wear helmets. Elbow and knee pads and wrist guards are also advisable for kids.

- Swimming is only allowed when an adult is present. Nonswimmers wear floatation devices when they're near a pool or body of water.

- Use the buddy system when riding bikes or walking in the neighborhood, and never talk to strangers. Of course, an adult should always accompany young children.

- Hikers always carry a map of the area they're visiting, dress for the elements, and let a third party know where they're headed.

- Walkers walk facing traffic; cyclists ride with traffic.

- Children don't ride bikes or walk from house to house after dark. Teens and adults who are out at night wear reflective clothing.

- Kids need to inform a parent of where they're headed (to a friend's, over to the playground, and so on) before they leave the house.

The great thing about your child becoming more active and confident is that he'll probably be busier — and that's exactly when your safety antennae have to go up and stay up. These are nonnegotiable rules. Things that may be negotiable are the time your son needs to come home from a friend's house or whether he's allowed to bring a friend home for supper. When it comes to your child's safety, make no concessions. Expect the rules to be followed, and enforce them to the very best of your ability.

Evaluating Your Child's Physical Education Class

If you pay fairly high school taxes, you probably assume that your child is getting plenty of bang for your buck in his gym class at school, right? Well, that depends on where you live and how your community feels about physical activity. In some areas of the country, physical education classes are disappearing, while in others, schools are installing state-of-the-art gyms in an effort to catch kids' interest in exercise — and maintain it.

No matter how your school fares, there's no doubt that, if done correctly, physical education class can produce lifelong benefits, such as:

- ✔ Learning about working as part of a team
- ✔ Learning the old adage, "You win some, you lose some"
- ✔ Learning fitness skills that carry over into adulthood

A good physical education program emphasizes these lessons in an attempt to enhance a child's overall learning experience. In other words, gym class shouldn't be about taking a break from the school day; the lessons learned there should carry over into the classroom and back home, also.

What to look for

If you're unsure about how your child's gym class compares to the physical education classes offered by other schools, go in and observe the class in progress. While you're watching, ask yourself these questions:

- ✔ Are all the kids participating, or are only the most athletic kids having fun?
- ✔ Is the class actually learning something of value, or are they playing a game of elimination (and humiliation) like dodge ball?

✔ Is what they're learning in any way relevant to a healthy lifestyle? In other words, are they learning about a sport or game that they could actually play outside of the confines of gym class?

The problem with a gym class that emphasizes games of extreme competition and/or elimination is that the most athletic kids end up playing, and everyone else ends up sitting around, waiting for gym class to be over. The game's great for the athletes, of course, but it's a big waste of time for the other kids. Gym class activities should be fun and fair for everyone. After all, the athletic kids play their sports after school anyway. The kids who are most likely to be turned off by these types of classes take home the lesson that physical activity is boring, humiliating, and something to be avoided.

How to take action and improve phys ed class

The number of gym classes available to high school students, in particular, is dwindling because of the amount of schoolwork and other classes (such as computer, foreign language, and college-level courses) that kids are expected to complete these days. High schoolers may be required to take only one year of physical education in order to graduate, which obviously doesn't send the message that physical fitness is important! Of course, academics are extremely important, but teaching adolescents about the long-term benefits of a healthy lifestyle is also vital.

So what can you do if your child's school has a less-than-adequate physical education program? Take your concerns to the administration. If the school district simply doesn't have the money to provide high-tech equipment (like a rock-climbing wall or a weight room), think about becoming active in fundraising for this purpose. Physical fitness is such a timely issue that you're likely to find a lot of support from other parents and businesses who are more than eager to jump on the "Helping Kids to Become More Fit" bandwagon (or whatever label you happen to choose for your efforts).

If, on the other hand, your main objection is to the types of "sports" the kids are playing, then make that clear. A teacher who has a degree in physical education can (and should) do much better by his or her students than forcing them to participate in activities that end up with half the class sitting on the sidelines. In this day and age, kids should be learning about ways to keep themselves healthy, and they also should be exposed to activities that they may actually want to take up in real life, like swimming, badminton, tennis, and golf — *not* dodge ball!

Part III

Managing, Troubleshooting, and Keeping the Weight Off

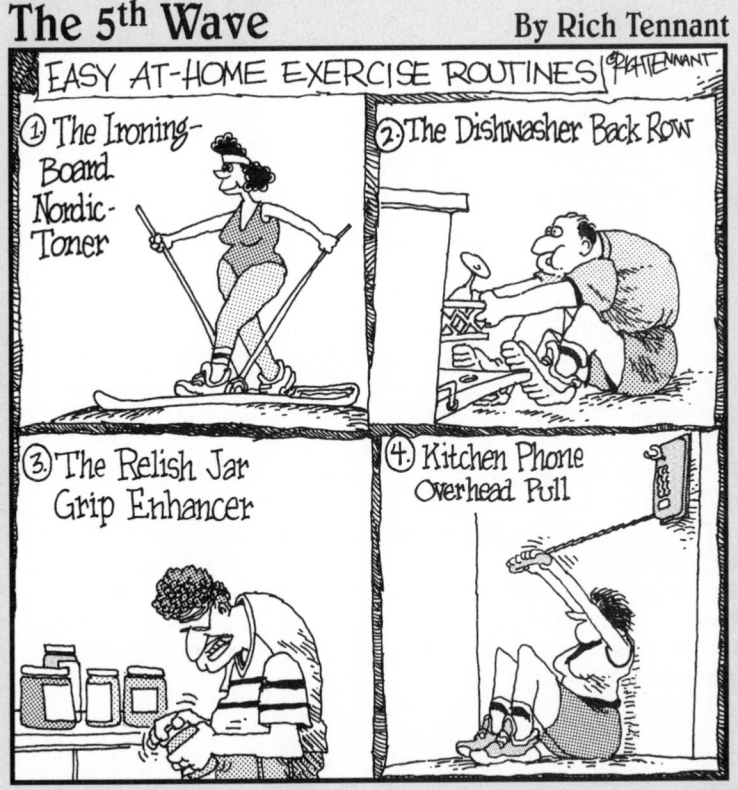

In this part . . .

One of the hardest parts of weight loss is the maintenance of a healthy lifestyle. It's just so easy to slip back into old habits, especially in times of stress or boredom. In this part, we offer tips for helping your child stick to the new way of doing things and encouraging her continued success. We also talk about how to find outside help if you feel as though you've done all you can for your child and have seen less-than-encouraging results or suspect that she may have an eating disorder.

Chapter 11

Supporting Your Child's Weight Loss

*W*hen you see your child succeeding in his or her weight loss venture, you may be tempted to breathe a sigh of relief and think that you're out of the proverbial woods. You can feel good about the direction your child is headed in, but it's important for the entire family to stay tuned in to the issue of obesity. Healthier habits should be a lifetime goal, not things that you come back to only now and then to lose a few pounds.

Studies show that obese children (especially preteen and younger) who don't have full parental involvement and support are more likely to fail in their attempts to lose weight and/or keep that weight off long term. An 8-year-old can't do the weekly grocery shopping, after all. He has very little control over the rules of the house and what kind of food comes into it. If a child is eager to lose weight but faces snack cakes and chocolate cookies every time he opens the pantry, he's at a disadvantage and has to work even harder. However, if the child is clamoring for snack cakes but there aren't any in sight, he just has to learn to live without them.

Parents play vital roles in children's weight loss — not just in jump-starting the process but also in teaching them that weight loss isn't a short-term goal. It involves choices that we make about what goes in our mouths every single day. Your attitudes about food and physical activity are contagious, so make sure that you send the right messages to ensure that your child stays on the right track toward weight loss and a healthy lifestyle. In this chapter, we talk about how you can help your child by setting a good example with your actions *and* your attitude toward this healthier-living venture.

Setting Realistic Goals for Your Child

You'd never do anything to purposefully hurt or discourage your child, but expecting too much too soon in the way of weight loss can backfire. We're sure you've seen stories on television talk shows about people losing 100, 200, or 300 pounds over the course of a year, so you may expect your child's weight loss to come about relatively easily. After all, if you're changing the family's diet and exercise plans, the weight should just melt away, right?

No. It took a long time for your child to become obese, which means that he needs adequate time to take the weight off. Experts recommend a loss of ½ pound per week for children and 1 pound a week for adults (older adolescents fall into the latter category). Did you read that correctly? *Eight ounces a week?* Although that may seem like a pitifully small expectation, your child is far more likely to keep weight off when it comes off slowly.

Don't expect too much too soon

Quick weight loss is often attributed to water loss and/or the effects of what amounts to malnutrition (see the sidebar "Beware fad diets"). You can't cut your child down to 700 calories a day and expect her to be able to function normally. Sure, she loses weight that way, but you take two big risks:

- ✔ She's hungry all the time, which means that, eventually, she has to give into that hunger and eat whatever she can get her hands on.
- ✔ She may become ill, suffering from dizziness and exhaustion, experiencing heart palpitations, and having difficulty concentrating.

Your goal is to teach your child to make healthy choices about food and exercise that eventually become second nature to her. You just can't accomplish that overnight, no matter how badly you want to. So take things slowly, and cheer her on every time the scale shows that she's lost a fraction of a pound. She's moving in the right direction, and she'll get to the finish line when she gets there.

Beware fad diets

Part of being a good role model for your child is making the healthiest choices where food is concerned. If you're always jumping on the latest fad diet bandwagon, stop. These diets show very poor results as far as long-term weight loss goes and even worse results where nutrition is concerned. (You really can't expect to eat nothing but cabbage for a month and have your body thank you for it.) More important, don't encourage your child to embrace fad dieting as a means of controlling *her* weight!

These diets are designed for adults, not growing children whose daily nutritional needs are very different and far more complex. You also don't want to send the message that there's a quick fix for her weight problem. Conquering obesity once and for all requires long-term planning and permanent changes. She's more likely to learn how to keep the weight off if she's well versed in good nutrition and healthy foods (not just cabbage).

Cutting your child's caloric intake by just 250 calories per day is enough to produce weight loss of ½ pound per week and significant long-term results. To give you an idea of how much food you actually have to cut from your child's diet, here's a list of some food items that contain approximately 250 calories each:

- ✔ A full-size candy bar
- ✔ A 16-ounce can of sugar-sweetened soda
- ✔ Two 8-ounce glasses of sugar-sweetened juice
- ✔ A small bag of chips
- ✔ Three average-sized chocolate chip cookies
- ✔ Six chicken nuggets
- ✔ Three to four fried (small) mozzarella cheese sticks
- ✔ A small serving of French fries
- ✔ One regular plain fast-food burger

These are fairly average snacks, so you can see that it doesn't take much to start the weight-loss process. (Increasing daily activity is the other factor in this equation and something we talk about in the section "Getting Everyone Moving" later in this chapter.) By eliminating sugar-sweetened drinks from your child's diet, for example, you subtract more calories than you probably realize. Do the math: The number of cans of soda your child drinks per day × 250. If you're shocked at the final tally, you should be more resolved than ever to get the food issue under control in your home.

When you eliminate one hidden source of calories, be sure not to replace it with another. For example, at dinnertime, don't replace soda with whole milk, which is loaded with calories *and* fat. Skim milk is a much better choice; not only is it low in calories, but it also contains calcium, which is an essential nutrient for bone strength.

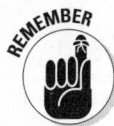

It may be easier than you think to make small changes in your family's diet. Don't close your eyes to the obvious: Take an honest look at some of the hidden calories your child ingests each day and eliminate some of them. Paying attention to nutrition labels is a vital part of removing hidden calories from your child's diet; you can find out more about these labels in Chapter 8.

The beauty of helping a younger child through the process of losing weight is that you're the one controlling the purse strings. Learning to say no to some of your child's requests (or demands, depending on the child) is part of supporting her weight loss. "No, we aren't having chicken nuggets for dinner," or "No, we aren't buying soda anymore," are just two phrases you can work into your parent-in-control routine. And don't waste time feeling guilty, even when she cries that she simply can't live without French fries. You don't do her any favors by allowing her to continue ingesting foods loaded with fat and sodium. Remember, everything you do is intended to help her, even though she doesn't see it that way — or at least not yet.

Accept that setbacks happen

Don't expect perfection from your child. We can't say it more simply than that. Either from personal experience or from watching friends or family members struggle with their own weight issues, you know that losing weight and sticking to a new diet and exercise regime can be tough for an adult. Because kids are more adaptable and far less set in their ways than adults, you may think that settling into new eating and exercising habits is easier for them, but that's not always the case.

Some kids accept change better than others. For kids who have come to depend on food as a comfort measure or who have been settling down to watch after-school cartoons with a bag of chips for as long as they can recall, understanding that certain behaviors are no longer acceptable is a real challenge. Some days will be fine; other days, you may find yourself at odds with your son when you spot what looks suspiciously like chocolate cake crumbs clinging to his chin.

Don't flip out if your child has ice cream or cookies at a friend's house. An *occasional* slip-up shouldn't affect his long-term weight-loss goal. If he's doing well otherwise, let an isolated incident go without lecturing him about it.

What should you do when your child is losing weight at a steady clip and then starts putting pounds back on? Take a minute to realize that your child is struggling in some way. The pounds are obviously not reappearing by themselves; he's either consuming more calories or not getting enough activity, or both. Get his opinion on how things are going. Ask where he thinks he's having difficulty; maybe he just needs to find some activity he enjoys more than what he's doing now, or perhaps a friend offers him snacks when they play after school, and he doesn't know how to say no without hurting his pal's feelings.

Try to rule out the most obvious problems (which are, of course, a high-fat diet and lack of exercise) before you start investigating other possible causes of weight gain (see the sidebar "Keeping thyroid concerns in check"). Remind him that you're in this together and you'll help any way you can. Ultimately, especially in the case of an adolescent, he has to do the work. You can't always shield him from his generous (but misguided) friends, and you can't exercise for him. You *can* continue to encourage him without nagging him about the weight, which is dangerous territory, especially where teenagers are concerned. Weight issues are such emotionally laden topics that harping on slip-ups can make things much, much worse; he may tune you out completely and do the exact opposite of what you suggest.

The worst thing you can do when your kid is regaining weight is to make a setback seem like the end of the world. Your child is *trying*. Even though you're frustrated and anxious about what may happen to him if he doesn't get with the program, remind yourself that you're the adult in this scenario and therefore need to keep cool.

Keeping thyroid concerns in check

Among parents of overweight kids, thyroid function is sometimes a source of major concern, especially when it seems that a child is having trouble losing weight despite his efforts. The *thyroid* controls the body's metabolism, so if your child's thyroid is somewhat sluggish and not doing its job, then it makes perfect sense for your child to be overweight. Correct the thyroid problem and the weight issue will fall right into line, right?

Sure . . . except more often than not, overweight children do *not* have thyroid problems. Testing the thyroid of an obese child is standard procedure for pediatricians, but usually the findings reflect that the thyroid just can't keep up with the child's caloric intake. Parents looking to the thyroid as a way to achieve a quick fix for their child's weight problem are sometimes disappointed to hear that the problem is more complicated. Reduced calorie intake and increased activity levels are usually the most effective cures for what ails an overweight or obese kid.

To deal with your child's weight-loss setback calmly and rationally, acknowledge these facts:

- ✔ Your child isn't putting on weight to make you mad.

- ✔ Your child is *just a child,* with a child's viewpoint. Even if he's an adolescent, he may not realize the seriousness of his weight problem and, by extension, how serious backsliding can be.

- ✔ Backsliding is correctable if you catch it early and don't make matters worse by punishing him or belittling him for it.

Your best bet is to nip a backslide in the bud, so to speak. Brainstorm new activities. Correct any errant eating habits. Offer helpful bits of advice. In the case where a friend is supplying snacks, the solution may be as simple as teaching your child to say, "I don't want to spoil my appetite for dinner," or, "I'm really not hungry, but thanks anyway."

Don't say things like, "When you're ready to lose weight, let me know!" or, "I can't help you if you're not going to do what I tell you!" Continue with business as usual, stick to your low-fat cooking and plans for more family activities, and assure your child that you aren't angry with him.

Laying a guilt trip on a backsliding child or otherwise turning the situation into one in which *he's* hurting *you* only serves to further damage his self-esteem. This kind of reaction on your part also may drive a wedge in your relationship with your child to the point where he stops trying to lose the weight or decides he'd rather go it alone than deal with you at weigh-in time. Either way, the weight becomes an issue that separates the two of you, which leads to incredibly painful emotional wounds — for you and for him.

Remind your child how great you think he is right now and that you love him just the way he is. Make it clear to him that you don't want him to lose weight so that he'll be better looking or more popular but so that he'll feel better physically and emotionally. In other words, the weight loss should be all about your child, not about your ideals of how he should look or what his classmates want him to look like. Let your child know that you support him in every phase of his weight loss (good and bad) and that you'll see him through to his goal.

Being Consistent and Supportive

Supporting your child through the long process of losing weight requires consistency, a skill that comes naturally to some parents and not so naturally to others. Even if you know that you've been less than consistent in your parenting up to this point (for example, you tell the kids they can't have a friend over but then give in when they cry about it; or you tell them they can't have another bowl of ice cream but relent when they beg and beg), it's not too late to set a firm resolve now. Obviously, helping your child lose weight means saying no to some of her less-than-healthy food requests, but it's important to remember that "no" means absolutely nothing to your child if she knows that you'll give in if she just keeps asking.

Chances are you've heard the timeworn advice: "Kids love rules. They need limits." Well, we don't know that kids love being told what to do, but they do need someone older and wiser to set limits for them. Most children can't institute and follow through on major lifestyle changes without at least one parent helping them out, cheering them on, and leading by example. However, even with an amazing support system, some kids are still reluctant (to say the least) to stick with the changes associated with weight loss. Your consistently positive attitude about a healthier way of life provides a stable environment in which weight loss is more likely to occur. Remind yourself that you really do know what's best for your child, at least when it comes to conquering her weight problem.

Making a permanent lifestyle change

This weight-loss project isn't a temporary solution; it's a lifestyle makeover. Don't talk to your child as though all he has to do is lose the weight and then he can go back to eating snack cakes for breakfast and nacho cheese on crackers for lunch. Make sure he knows that the days of sitting around eating junk are over — for the entire family.

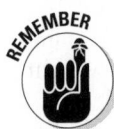

Weekends, holidays, and birthdays aren't free passes to take a break from this healthy new lifestyle. Healthful eating and exercise are regular parts of your family's life from this point on — this plan doesn't have an expiration date. If you hear your child saying things like, "I can't wait until we can have fried chicken every Saturday night again!," or, "The first thing I'm going to do when I lose all my weight is order a pizza all for myself!," gently remind him that those habits got your family into this situation to begin with and that you're all able to make better choices now. You don't want to instill panic in him, where all he can think is, "I can never, ever have fried food again. What is my mother doing to me????" The goal is to kill his craving for that kind of food, and that takes time. Hopefully, by the time he reaches his goal, your child won't still be dreaming of hitting all the fast-food places in town in one night.

Any kind of permanent lifestyle change is heady stuff for a kid, so it may help your child to keep a weight-loss journal where he can keep track of how he feels and how things are progressing. Writing down his feelings about certain foods may help him sort them out and actually minimize his cravings. (If he's really expressive in his writing, for example, he may come to the conclusion that although he loves fast food, it was harming him physically and emotionally — and that realization may be enough to make him turn his back on it for good.)

A journal also can be a real blessing for an older kid who needs to be able to look back on how far he's come over the course of a long weight-loss journey. It may be just the thing to keep him going when he's midway to his goal and feels like he'll never get there. He can easily remind himself of his continuing achievement and be proud of the fact that he's already done half the work.

Setting a good example

Working on a weight-loss program with your child is not the time to fall back on the "Do as I say, not as I do" defense, especially if you're struggling with your own weight issues. You can't expect a child to tackle her obesity problem on her own; she's much more likely to succeed if she's following your lead. For example, she's more likely to resist changes to her diet if she's eating steamed veggies and grilled chicken at dinnertime while everyone else enjoys pizza.

Increasing your child's activity level is another sticking point: You may have the best of intentions when you tell her to go for a bike ride, but you're undermining yourself when you get in your car to drive three houses down to visit your neighbor. You're full of knowledge about how to help her lose the weight; now show her that following through isn't impossible. Even if *you* don't need to lose any weight, get on your bike and go for a ride with her, or take her for a long walk in the park. If you've never been an active person and she sees that you're making a real effort to get out and move your body, your actions will impress her more than anything you could ever say.

Setting a good example involves making changes throughout the household. Convincing other members of the family to jump on this healthy lifestyle ride can be difficult if only one child has a significant weight problem. Your thin kids may present a very reasonable-sounding case, telling you that whatever they've been eating hasn't hurt them, so there's no reason for their treats to be curtailed (or for them to move their fannies off the couch). You know better now, though. Tell them that scarfing down saturated fats and leading a sedentary lifestyle isn't good for anyone, no matter how old they are or how skinny they may be. Be the leader and take charge of your entire family's well-being.

When setting a good example, do it in such a manner that your child takes notice, but don't constantly call attention to your actions. A child quickly learns to ignore preaching about healthy foods and exercise, so live by example, give your child relevant information (such as what you'll be having for dinner or where the family will be hiking this weekend), and leave it at that.

When your child realizes that the entire family is doing things differently now, she's more likely to accept healthful foods and activity as a natural part of life as opposed to something she alone is being forced to do. You can see the difference in the mindset: If it's a family affair, she's just following along with everyone else's healthy choices; otherwise, she's completely on her own, and, as a result, she may be scared and resentful of being the odd one out and less than eager to comply with the program.

Sticking with it when the going gets rough

Parents of severely overweight kids are sometimes faced with a kid who loses interest in the weight-loss program or who finds it hard to accept the changes that are expected of him. These reactions are to be expected. Like any major life change, adapting to a healthy lifestyle can be tough and, at times, dull. Don't be afraid to shake things up when you notice your child's interest waning. Explore new, healthy recipes, for example, or introduce the family to a fun new activity, like checking out your park's bike trails or joining a family swim program. Expose your family to the possibilities life has to offer in the way of interesting food and enjoyable activities — things that they may have been missing out on when they were parked in front of the TV for the last few years. (For more ideas on how to keep your family's attention focused on healthy living, see Chapter 13.)

When your child is in a rough patch, resist the urge to throw your hands up in the air and say, "Well, if you aren't interested, we'll come back to this when you are." You're trying to be consistent, right? Teaching your family to make healthy choices is undoubtedly the right thing, so don't give up on them when they start grumbling about whole grains and vegetables. You're breaking them down, but your goal is to build them back up, stronger and more confident of themselves than they were before.

Are your kids bored with the healthy choices routine? Let them pick their own activities every once in a while. If they want to skip the family excursion next weekend and instead play a game of soccer with their friends, let them. They're finding independent, kid-friendly activities, and they aren't angling for TV time (and you can't ask for anything better in the way of progress). Finding their own preferred activities is a huge step in embracing a healthy lifestyle.

Refusing to give treats for tears (or make other common mistakes)

Following your plan has been easy, you say. You're an organized person, so all you had to do was create a healthy menu and an activity chart, and everything just worked itself out. Except for that time your daughter cut her finger and you had to give her a brownie before she would stop crying. Oh, and there's that time she fell and needed some ice cream to make her feel better. And what about that time she ran right into the wall? A couple of cookies helped to soothe those bumps, but . . . wow, is it possible that this weight-loss program is making her clumsy? She sure seems accident prone all of the sudden.

More likely, she's too smart for her own good. If she knows the only way to get a treat is to come to you howling in pain, guess what? She can come up with all sorts of ingenious ways to feign injuries (at least let's hope she's faking them).

Obviously, you want to make sure she isn't really hurt. But even if she legitimately skins her knee, a piece of candy can't heal that wound. What does an injured child truly need? Some medical attention if the injury is significant, and some TLC from Mom or Dad (or Grandma, Grandpa, or Aunt Sue . . . whoever happens to be in charge).

Aside from the fact that she may be lying to you in order to score some sugary treat, you don't want your child to equate food with anything other than hunger and nourishment. Like everybody else, she's going to face hard times sooner or later in life. Using food as a comforting tool is one of the worst habits she can develop because it creates a vicious cycle of depression linked to being overweight (which is caused by overeating . . . which leads to being overweight . . . which leads to depression . . . which leads to more overeating to comfort herself).

Other food messages to avoid include:

- ✔ **"Eat your peas and you can have ice cream."** Meals don't have to end on a sugar-high note! Promises like this one reinforce the importance of a super-sweet dessert rather than underscore the importance of eating a balanced meal. Peas become a punishment your child has to endure rather than a building block for a healthy body.

- ✔ **"Let's have a clean-your-plate club."** Even if you're attempting to get your kids to eat their veggies, let them decide when they've had enough. Part of controlling one's weight is recognizing the feeling of fullness, something your kids are likely to ignore if they're competing against one another for "first-one-done" status.

> ✔ **"You can't leave the table until you've finished your dinner."** Your child needs to be able to recognize his own inner physical feeling of being satiated. Preparing a healthy meal is great; forcing him to finish every morsel of it when he's no longer hungry cancels out your best efforts and confuses your child. (Should he eat when his stomach is rumbling or when you tell him to? How will he know when he's full if he depends on you to tell him when he's through?)

Just about every parent has used one of these lines at one time or another, usually in an attempt to get kids to eat the healthy foods on their plates. Knowing that these tricks can backfire in a huge way should be enough to put them to rest for good in your own home. Focus on the good foods, but don't force 'em down.

Setting Mealtime Ground Rules

It can be difficult or darn near impossible for a child to lose weight and/or keep it off if the rules of the house don't support this venture. Skipping meals and eating in front of the TV sabotage healthy-eating efforts. On the flip side, getting everyone involved in preparing and gathering for a meal focuses attention not only the meal itself, but on the family unit. This meeting of the minds is an important step in the weight-loss process.

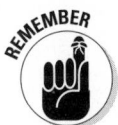 Successful weight loss is most likely to occur in households with lots of parental involvement and support. Rounding up the troops at mealtime allows plenty of time for chitchat about the day while simultaneously allowing you to set a good example with your own eating habits.

Establishing family dinner nights

For years, experts in various areas of child development have lamented the loss of the family dinner table, arguing that:

- ✔ Young children in particular thrive on the routine that regular dinners provide.

- ✔ Sitting down together on a regular basis gives everyone in the family a chance to talk about the day.

- ✔ Family dinners give parents the chance to model good eating habits for their kids.

- ✔ Family dinners set the precedent for kids to prepare balanced meals for themselves when they're off on their own, in college and beyond.

We know that finding time to eat together (let alone cook an entire meal) is hard when you and/or your partner work and your kids' schedules are jam-packed with friends, music lessons, and sports. But you need to do whatever it takes to gather your family for dinner together at least three to four times a week. Your obese child needs this kind of consistency and modeling in order to learn long-term healthy eating habits; your other kids benefit from the togetherness, too.

Rounding up the family for dinner several times a week may sound like an impossible task when one kid has soccer, another has band practice, and you regularly take conference calls during the dinner hour. Think about moving dinner time to a later — or earlier — hour when everyone is able to sit down and connect for 20 minutes or so.

Some parents are overwhelmed just thinking about plunking an entire home-cooked meal on the table, especially if they haven't done this before. If you're in this camp, start by concentrating on your main dish, and don't fret over how to prepare veggies and other healthy side dishes — yet. You can always offer the kids raw carrot sticks with a low-fat dressing for dipping or purchase salad and add a tomato or cucumber to the mix before serving it up. When you get into a groove preparing dinners on a regular basis, you can expand your repertoire to include more-involved vegetable dishes. Check out Chapter 8 for useful advice about planning family meals and Appendix A for recipes to try.

Obese children (and adults) often eat large portions of whatever food strikes their fancy throughout the day. Planned mealtimes give the day structure as far as food as concerned so that the whole family eventually understands that they shouldn't eat plates of food that amount to an entire meal unless it's an *actual* mealtime.

If your child is still hungry after he finishes his main course, steer him away from a complete second helping by offering more of the vegetable side dish. After all, veggie dishes are full of fiber, low in fat, and a great way to fill up a stomach without adding a lot of calories into the mix. Fresh fruit is another great choice for dessert for these same reasons.

Sticking around for breakfast

Adolescents, even those who have grown up in households with healthy eating habits, routinely scoff at balanced meals. They delight in eating junk and rebelling against their parents' best intentions at mealtimes — especially breakfast.

Teenagers are apt to skip breakfast, either as a way to lose weight or because sitting down to a bowl of healthy grains when you're in high school just isn't cool. You can't force a piece of whole-wheat toast down your child's throat, but you can mention to him how important breakfast is and that kids who skip breakfast tend to drag through the morning and overeat at lunch. The most you can do is provide the meal and set a good example. Make sure you prepare yourself for the day by taking the time for breakfast before you head out the door; otherwise, your words fall on deaf ears.

Interestingly, studies have shown that kids are more likely to eat healthy meals if parents are simply *present* for those meals. You don't have to hold your teenager's hand and help him operate the microwave so that he can have his oatmeal in the morning. Rather, like the family dinner concept (see the preceding section), your presence makes the morning seem like more of a family mealtime, even if the morning is all hustle and bustle in your home (as it is in most homes with school-age kids). Of course, taking the time to prepare a healthy breakfast for yourself makes the morning something of a follow-the-leader event: You take the time to eat breakfast so your child will, too.

Turning off the TV

No TV (or computers, books, or anything else distracting) during meals can be a tough rule to enforce, especially if your household includes TV junkies of the adult variety (that is, you and your partner). Sure, catching the news at dinnertime is a great way to kill two birds with one stone (and to hear the full report about that poor little bird being assaulted with some sort of rock). But think about what a distraction TV is: You know how hard it is to concentrate on a show and talk on the phone at the same time, or how difficult it can be to read a book when the kids have their cartoons blaring. The TV seems to command all your energy and attention, and *you* have a fully formed adult brain. Just imagine what it does to your kids!

Here's what we know about TV and its negative effect on weight-loss programs and healthy lifestyles:

- ✔ TV is chock-full of commercials that encourage kids to eat unhealthy foods.
- ✔ No one burns a significant amount of calories while watching the tube.
- ✔ Kids who watch a significant amount of TV (as in four or more hours a day) are more likely to have difficulty making social connections with their peers and other people.

Imagine what goes on in your child's head when the TV is on. Her full focus is on the show, right? So give her a plate of food and guess what happens: She ingests the entire thing quickly, without ever speaking a word to anyone else, and she probably doesn't realize how much she ate or that she ate anything at all.

The entire point of having a family meal is to pull everyone together and make the meal meaningful. It's a time to model good eating habits and to discuss — in context! — the benefits of certain types of foods. Sitting everyone down at the table and turning the TV on goes against everything that you're attempting to accomplish.

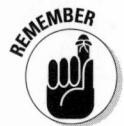

Pediatricians recommend no more than two hours of television a day for kids, and this time limit actually includes video and computer game usage. So if you're looking for a good way to cut TV out of your kids' day, banning it from mealtimes is an excellent place to start.

Having everyone pitch in

If you've never sat down to a family meal (not even when you were growing up), you may feel funny about suddenly using the kitchen table for something other than organizing the laundry and doing homework. And your family may roll their eyes when you tell them how nice it's going to be to eat dinner together every night.

The best way to get your family used to the idea of family mealtimes and comfortable with it as a normal part of everyone's day is to get them involved in the mealtime event. Here are a few recommendations:

- ✔ **Let the kids help.** Need to make a salad? Your 7-year-old can do it for you. Let him tear the salad, and consider purchasing a hand-held chopper (where the blades are all contained in a domelike device) so that he can manage most of the veggie cutting, too. Involving kids in meal preparations makes them feel more a part of it and cuts down on your workload.

- ✔ **Have your kids set the table for dinner.** Forks on the left, knives on the right, napkins at each place or in a big basket in the middle of the table, if you prefer. Everyone needs a glass, and the serving dishes need serving spoons. Tell the kids what the meal is and let them decide what kind of (low-fat) condiments to put out. If you have some particularly crafty and/or eager kids, ask them to make place cards or fold the napkins into creative shapes!

✔ **Let imperfect manners slide — at first.** Good behavior can be a very difficult part of learning to eat as a family. Be firm with basic rules (no throwing food, no whining, no dancing on the chair) but hold off on more stringent expectations (no elbows on the table) until your kids are more comfortable with the structure and routine of family mealtime.

✔ **Encourage conversation.** If your family doesn't sit down together on a regular basis, you may need to plan what to say to each other until casual conversation becomes a natural part of the process. Some families go around the table and share the best thing that happened to each person that day. It's a good way to get everyone talking.

Don't rush the meal; let everyone talk to their hearts' content, even if that means they take a break from eating their healthy dinner. Unlike TV viewing, computer use, and reading, conversation isn't a distraction from the meal and actually enhances the experience of coming together as a family. And if everyone ends up talking more and eating less, that's another benefit of friendly chitchat during dinnertime.

Family dinners should eventually evolve into a relaxed part of the day and hopefully something everyone looks forward to.

Getting Everyone Moving

Getting the family out of the house and doing something active together on a regular basis may seem silly if you've never done it before in your entire life. However, your obese preschooler isn't going to slim down all by herself (and an obese school-age or adolescent child is going to need some help and encouragement to get started, also). Like family mealtime (see the "Setting Mealtime Ground Rules" section earlier in the chapter), family outings serve a dual purpose: You bring the family together while teaching your kids that activity isn't harmful — in fact, it's a necessary part of life!

Here's the deal with family activities: Obese kids tend not to be very active. As they get older, even if they want to participate in sports or other activities with kids their own age, they're often too self-conscious about their lack of coordination and their weight to join in spontaneously (such as at recess). And because they're forced to participate in physical education classes at school, where they probably fall far behind their classmates skillwise, obese kids may equate physical activity with pure torture.

Boys in particular learn to socialize with each other through sports. Even though today's girls are more involved in sports than past generations, they still tend to solidify their relationships off the playing field. Regardless, although it's certainly possible for a child to go through life without playing football, soccer, lacrosse, baseball, or any other sport, it's heartbreaking to see a kid who so badly wants to play sitting on the sidelines and feeling out of the social loop because of it.

So if you find yourself debating the merit of family activities, remember that you want to give your children the basic skills to be able to keep up with their peers when they need to (in gym class), which will hopefully lead to a desire and enough confidence to join in on unorganized play (like recess or a neighborhood game of kickball).

If your older kids grumble about having to give up time with their friends for family outings, invite the friends along. The purpose of the outings is to make activity fun; a friend actually may be very helpful in helping you reach that goal, especially if it's a child who really loves to be outdoors doing *anything*.

Most obese kids have at least one parent who is also significantly overweight, so it's probably safe to say that activity hasn't ranked high on the family's list of priorities. Where do you begin if your family can best be described as totally inactive? Start off small. Don't attempt to conquer Mount Kilimanjaro (or your local equivalent) on your first foray out of the house. Do something that everyone will enjoy so that when it comes time for the next outing, you aren't faced with tantrums and complaints about how bored everyone was last time. Also consider taking turns choosing what you're going to do so that, at the very least, everyone is happy on a rotating basis.

Here are some tips and ideas for getting your family up and moving:

- ✔ **Walk.** Walking is one of the best exercises for all age groups and activity levels. Have the kids leash up the dog (he needs exercise, too!) and explore your local park or nature trail.

- ✔ **Dust that bike off.** Biking is a low-impact exercise that's perfect for families looking for a fun way to increase their activity levels. (Be sure to set a good example by wearing a helmet!)

- ✔ **Keep it fresh.** You'll undoubtedly find that the family enjoys some outings more than others, but you don't want your favorites to become stale. Explore new places and activities on a regular basis.

- ✔ **Ban TV, computer, and video games on outing days.** If your kids are griping about going on a walk in the woods, they may stop if they know that they're not missing out on TV time.

- ✔ **Bring along healthy snacks and water.** Pack a backpack with enough sustenance to get the family through your walk, hike, or bike ride.

- ✔ **Be patient.** You may be gung-ho to ride your bike five miles and chat the day away, but your kids may not take to these outings as quickly. Take your cue from them, and be encouraging but not overbearing. Eventually, they'll come around.

When you're feeling more confident in your ability to get the family out of the house and doing something physical, you can start getting more creative with your activities. Take the family ice skating, go for a hike up that mountain, or join your local YMCA and sign up for a family-swim program. And when the children are ready, let them choose more independent activities, like a Sunday afternoon of flag football with the neighborhood kids. You'll know you've done well by them when they're confident enough to go off and play with their peers. In the interest of keeping alive your message that this is an *active* family, find your own preferred method of exercise and continue to plan family outings at least once a month.

Sometimes going on a family outing just isn't possible because so much needs to be done around the house. The solution: Introduce your kids to chores. Older kids can push the mower, younger children can help rake leaves, and kids of all ages can help shovel snow. Work together, and show them that hard work never killed anyone (well, no one *their* age, anyway).

Keeping Up with Your End of the Weight-Loss Bargain

After you get the family off on the right foot and things seem to be going fairly well in the weight-loss department, you may be tempted to rest on your laurels, but you can't. Losing weight and living a healthy lifestyle is a lifelong quest. It doesn't have to be painful or dull, but it does take a certain amount of vigilance, especially on the part of the person who's planning the meals, doing the grocery shopping, encouraging activity, and setting the good example. (That would be you.)

Must you stand guard in the kitchen for the rest of time, making sure that no one sneaks an unhealthy snack? Should you get a bullhorn to announce morning exercise time? Only if your family responds well to these tactics. Keeping yourself interested and engaged in the weight-loss process is a much smarter way to lead the family toward a permanently healthy lifestyle.

Realizing you're the key to your child's success

We can't say it enough: Children who are successful at weight loss have support at home. This isn't a temporary project that you can toss to your child for completion in a few weeks' time. He needs you to be involved from the beginning and to stay involved.

Think about how easy it is to slip back into bad habits. We aren't dependent on these habits for survival (even though it may not feel that way when we're longing for another drag on a smoke, for example). Imagine that food is your bad habit — that's what your child is faced with. He can't just ignore his temptation completely because he has to eat every day for the rest of his life, and that means that he has to choose well every single day. He may slip up now and again, and that's where you come in, cheering him on in the right direction, reminding him that one cookie doesn't spell disaster, and making sure that he's doing what's best for himself. That's a parent's job, after all.

You may wonder when an older child, for example, is able to conquer his bad habit all by himself. When you see that losing weight and eating healthy foods aren't just chores to him but things he's eagerly accepted, and when you can see how happy he is to have shed his old skin, chances are he's almost there.

Keeping abreast of the newest info

These days, staying connected and up-to-date on matters of interest is so easy. The Internet is filled with information on obese children, weight loss, exercise programs, nutrition — just about everything you need to maintain a healthy lifestyle and infuse it with new ideas every now and then. The USDA's updated food pyramid site (www.mypyramid.gov/kids), for example, is entertaining, educational, and something that kids can navigate all by themselves. Parents can check out the American Obesity Association's Web site at www.obesity.org/subs/childhood for statistics, causes, and the latest research information on childhood obesity.

Alternatively, if you're just itching to talk to other parents of obese children, ask your pediatrician or nutritionist about local support groups. (Because childhood obesity is a growing problem in the United States, parent support groups are more prevalent than they were years ago.) If you're lucky enough to find such a group, don't shy away from attending a meeting and participating in discussions. You're likely to hear different points of view on everything from cooking to exercise (and dozens of other topics). You may be inspired to try something new that will work well for your own family.

Chapter 12

When You Can't Be There: Conquering Tempting Scenarios

*Y*ou can set down all the rules you want, but if your child doesn't have to follow through on them when he leaves the house, you're just wasting your time. Because you're probably like most parents and aren't with your child 24 hours a day, take some time to consider where and how your child spends his time away from home: Is he in a day-care setting where he can snack all day long (or are the snacks he's given less than ideal)? Do your parents stuff your children with sweets every time they visit? Are your child's friends undermining your best intentions by providing him with chips and soda every day after school?

And what about what happens *in* school? You may assume that your child is getting a healthy lunch every day, but very few school districts provide meals that are low in fat and high in vitamins and minerals. Snacks at school are another area where fat and empty calories sneak their way into your child's mouth.

If you've followed the advice in Chapter 8, you've taken control of your own pantry and refrigerator. But your child's faced with plenty of other opportunities to break your healthy-food rules each day. Although many of these opportunities are out of his control, particularly if he's a younger child, this chapter takes you through some of these situations and shows you how to teach your child to make good food choices.

Advising Caregivers of the New Rules

You know it's not easy to revamp the food and exercise rules in your own home. It took a lot of effort and determination to even begin that major project, but now that the plan is underway and your family's moving toward a healthier lifestyle, you can see that the work was well worth it.

Now how do you convince your mother and your babysitter of the same thing? If you're lucky, your child's caregivers care as much about what's best for your child as you do, and, more important, they agree that your child needs to start losing weight now.

If you're not so lucky and are, in fact, in a more typical situation, you may find yourself butting heads with your mother-in-law and pulling your hair when you tell her for the umpteenth time that a healthy snack for your child doesn't consist of Tootsie Rolls dipped in peanut butter with a tall glass of sugar-sweetened juice to wash it all down. So how do you handle caregivers who don't follow your family's new program?

Feeding issues at day care

First of all, let us explain what we mean by *day care:* It's the place you drop your child off when you go to work. Obviously, we advocate selecting a licensed day-care center for safety reasons: The center undergoes at least minimal inspections, and workers are supposed to be screened for criminal backgrounds. In reality, we realize that a lot of day-care situations out there aren't regulated by anyone, like neighborhood sitters and unlicensed day-care centers. For the sake of this discussion, however, we lump all these caregivers together. (For information on choosing good day care, check out *Choosing Childcare For Dummies,* which is published by Wiley.)

Suppose your child comes home from day care bouncing off the walls. Is she just imitating what she sees other kids doing, or is she burning off the sugar fuel in her tank?

Identifying feeding problems at day care

One of the many benefits of losing weight is an increased energy level, and obviously your daughter's desire to act as a pinball in the family room shows that she has plenty of vim and vigor. But if she's not eating healthy snacks and meals at day care, you'll notice it in the following ways:

✔ **She may still strongly crave sweets and fatty foods.** Cutting these unhealthy foods out of your family's diet should eventually change their palates. That's not to say that your child won't crave chocolate every now and then, but the occasional craving shouldn't feel like a *need* to your child if she's really off the fats and sweets.

✔ **She's not losing weight.** If you've cut out all the junk at home and you're taking walks after dinner and she's not losing, something's up. She's probably getting extra calories somewhere else.

✔ **Her energy level isn't picking up.** Sugar may act as rocket fuel to your child, or it may make her drowsy and crabby. Healthy foods usually provide healthy side effects — that is, more energy and a better overall physical feeling.

✔ **She balks at your healthy snacks.** If your child's getting her treats when you're not with her, she won't commit to this new plan you've come up with. To her, those carrot sticks you're offering are just a nuisance; she knows she'll get her chips tomorrow at day care.

The fact of the matter is that you can't be sure what your child is eating at day care unless you go in and check it out for yourself. But don't rely on someone else's word (or on the word of your 4-year-old). *Show up* at snack time and take a look at what the kids are eating. Yes, we know it can be very hard to negotiate time out of the office and that a story about checking out your child's snack may not fly with your boss; however, you have to acknowledge that everything you're trying to do for her is probably going to fail unless you *completely* remove the fats and sweets from her diet. Just take a minute and think of everything you've done to ensure healthier eating and more activity at home. It seems like a big waste if she can effectively take a break from this lifestyle every day, doesn't it?

If your day-care provider is licensed, she should be participating in the USDA Food Program, which provides caregivers with detailed instructions on feeding young kids and also cuts checks each month to reimburse caregivers for feeding children healthy meals and snacks. Ask your day-care provider if she participates in this program.

Getting on track at day care

At this point, you know what healthy snacks are and what they aren't. So let's say you pop into your child's day care and find her noshing on chicken nuggets and French fries while sipping whole milk (only the most outlandish day care in the world would give kids soda, but a high fat content in their lunches may be par for the course). She's as happy as a clam, looking forward to those home-baked cookies on the counter for dessert. Meanwhile, your hair is standing on end. You'd never allow this type of food!

Can you really hope to correct your chosen day care's errant feedings? Probably not. After all, the reason many day-care centers provide meals like nuggets and fries is they're cheap and easy and kids love 'em. The low cost of the meals and their nonexistent preparation methods, in turn, keep the cost of the day-care center down. And that's the Achilles heel of working parents everywhere — finding decent day care that you can afford. If your child is otherwise safe in this place, should you make a big deal about the food?

Yeah, you should. Your child will not be safe from physical harm if she doesn't start to lose her excess weight — or, at the very, very least, stop putting it on — right away. And you can't expect either change to happen in a place where she's being fed the very foods that spell certain failure for her new, healthier eating program.

So if you can't insist that the center improve its mealtime standards, what can you do? You have two choices:

- ✔ **Talk with the director about your child's nutritional needs and even offer to pack healthy meals for your child to have at snack and mealtimes.**

- ✔ **Start looking for another day care.** We suggest that you try a licensed provider who's required to follow certain dietary guidelines. If your child is in unlicensed day care, you can't force the care providers to feed your child healthy foods. Licensed providers are getting money from the USDA, and they have to prove that they're feeding kids according to the pyramid guidelines. It comes down to looking out for the best interest of the child, and if that means switching sitters, then that's what it takes.

The second option, looking to change your day-care arrangement, is better, for this reason: Imagine you're a preschooler, you're in a familiar environment, and suddenly you're eating differently from all your friends. You aren't allowed to have the cookies or even the same lunch as everyone else. How well does *that* go over with you?

Some day-care centers are equipped to deal with specific dietary requests; others aren't. In other words, your child's day care may accommodate your low-fat, pack-it-yourself menu, or it may just feed your kid whatever she wants when she starts whining and crying about it. There are different levels of care, and although some day-care providers may truly love your child, others may just go for the quick, keep-the-kid-quiet fix.

You may be tempted to look at this situation and say, "Hey, I'm the customer. I'm the one paying the bills, this is what I want for my child, and the sitter or center should cooperate." But you also know how compliant your child is likely to be when she's not able to eat the same things as her friends. If you think the change will be nothing more than a tiny blip on her daily radar and your sitter will follow your wishes, then give the new system a try. If you just know it's going to be a fight — between your child and the sitter and between the sitter and you — then difficult as it may be, you probably need to look for new day care.

Being proactive about activity

In addition to food, another concern with day care is activity. Although most young kids are naturally active, especially when put in a room with other children, you want to make sure that your child isn't allowed to opt out of physical activity. If her group is going for a walk and she refuses, does her "teacher" allow her to stay behind and play with clay with another group? Does her sitter allow her to sit in the corner of the yard rather than play tag with other children? Again, the level of care — and tolerance for an uncooperative child — varies from center to center and from sitter to sitter, so check it out for yourself.

If you suspect that your child isn't getting enough activity, talk with your child's day-care provider. Express your concern; explain that your child needs to get in on the action for her health. Get the sitter's take on the situation; after all, she's the one who hears your child's reasons for not playing. If your child is shy, for example, she may benefit from having a play date with a day-care pal at your home, where she and her friend can connect and strengthen their bond one-on-one (a bond that's likely to carry over into the play yard at day care). If your child complains that she gets too hot or too cold playing outside at day care, send a water bottle along or an extra pair of socks. Try to get to the root cause of her unwillingness to play and then correct it.

Breaking the news to cookie-pushing grandmas

Dealing with your day care or sitter is nothing compared to dealing with your own parents or — heaven help you — your in-laws. These people love your child just the way he is; they want to know why you can't just accept him instead of trying to reshape him.

Addressing sensitive issues with care

If the relatives in question are also obese or very overweight, you may find that it's especially hard to ward off comments and questions that force you to defend your parenting decision. In this case, your best intentions toward your child can be perceived as a blanket judgment on anyone who's heavy. But don't buy into this attempt at a guilt trip, no matter how skilled the other party may be at laying on the criticism.

If you feel that you're under attack, remind yourself why you took the reins of your child's eating and exercise habits in the first place: Not because you're concerned with the way he looks, but because you're concerned for his overall well-being. Now that you've educated yourself about the long-term physical and emotional effects that obese children deal with, you can inform others about the dangers of childhood obesity as well.

Even though you're well within your rights as a parent to explain and defend (if necessary) your family's new, healthier lifestyle to relatives who are actively working against you, resist the urge to preach to others about how they should change their eating habits. You run the risk of turning others off the idea of losing weight altogether.

As you well know, food and weight are highly charged issues; a suggestion here and there (about ways to cut fat or a great new exercise program you're involved in) to your overweight sister or mother is probably all right, but continual chatter about losing weight and eating healthfully may only result in your family members tuning you out. We know that you're excited about turning your family's lifestyle around, and you want to open everyone's eyes to the possibilities that a healthy life offers! The best way to get your message across is by becoming a living example. When others see that you're reaping the benefits of a healthier lifestyle, they may be inspired to follow suit.

In any event, you've established a healthy program for your child, one that simply can't be disposed of when he's visiting overweight relatives. One sweet treat isn't going to undo all the work you've done; however, if he's at his grandmother's on a regular basis and you know that Gram serves your child nothing but fried foods and sugary snacks, it's up to you to put a stop to it. Feed your child before he goes to Gram's, or buy healthy snacks for your child to eat at Gram's house.

Take care not to offend an overweight relative. As bad as her eating habits may be, she may not know any better. Also, she's probably fairly set in her ways, especially where food is concerned. Keep in mind that you're not trying to overcome *her* weight issue; your focus is on your child's health.

Dealing with someone who blatantly breaks the rules

What's worse than trying to sensitively deal with an overweight relative who feeds your child junk food? A relative who doesn't have a weight problem, who thinks your obese child is adorable, and who sneaks your child unhealthy foods not because she doesn't know any better but as a means of winning your child's love.

In this situation, the gloves can come off. It's one thing for someone who isn't well informed on the issue of obesity to feed your child fatty or sugary foods; that's like the blind leading the blind. A relative who purposely undermines your authority and does something that's actually harmful to your child is an entirely different matter. That's like tossing gasoline on a fire to watch the pretty colors it makes. (In other words, it's a dumb thing to do, especially when your child's weight problem is the fire. Everyone knows that fire can spark out of control when conditions are right.)

Don't worry about offending someone who's deliberately working against all the bad habits you're trying to change in your child's life. Lay down the law as often as you need to. Just take care not to hash things out in front of your child, lest he feel like his weight issue is the cause of a family rift.

Families are funny. The roles we all play as children never really change, even when we're adults. So if your younger sister is the one who's slipping your child candy when your back is turned, let her know that her childish behavior is no longer acceptable and that you won't tolerate it, especially when it affects your child negatively. Mothers, in particular, sometimes have a hard time letting go of their authority and try to run the lives of as many generations as they can get their hands on. If your mom is the offending cookie-pusher, remind her that *you* are the boss where your child is concerned and what you say goes.

Of course, in the end, you may find yourself doing battle over what seems like a nonissue. After all, as the parent, you have the final say of what's best for your child. So why must your mother-in-law (or sister, or father, and so on) feed your child foods that she knows you don't approve of? The answers to that question likely depend on so many things, from how she feels about you to how she feels about her own weight, so don't try to psychoanalyze her justification. Focus on what's most important — the health of your child — and don't stand for any actions that will only confuse or harm him (and make your job more difficult in the end).

Leading the way

Because you've reevaluated your entire household's eating and exercise habits, perhaps the best way to deal with nonsupportive extended family is to invite them to your home for a healthy meal. Show them what you're doing; give them a taste of healthy food. Heck, if you can manage it, take them along on an activity-focused family outing (but be careful not to expect too much in the way of compliance, especially if they're not particularly active people).

Sometimes, the resistance you meet from family members stems from your individual history with losing weight in the past. If you've tried and failed to drop your own excess pounds several times, your family may not believe that you're serious about helping your child or that you'll succeed in this venture. However, what they don't know is that you're better informed this time around, and more important, you have a child who needs your help. There's no better motivation than that.

Resist the urge to preach to your parents or siblings about your goals and plans for your child (and for yourself). Allowing them to see how well your child takes to this program may be all the incentive they need to stop fighting you and to actually encourage your child along the way. At the very least, witnessing firsthand the effort that you and your child put into his weight loss should be enough to stop any deliberate sabotage.

Sticking With It Away from Home

When your family's away from the controlled environment of home, you may be tempted to take a break from monitoring everyone's food intake and activity levels, but remember: Obesity doesn't take a vacation — at least not for long! Letting things slide for a week on vacation, for example, is the first step toward diving headfirst right back into the problems you've worked so hard to leave behind. Maintaining the new program takes vigilance and dedication, even when you're away from your everyday environment.

After your family truly turns the corner toward accepting healthy foods and activity (as opposed to just following along with whatever you're doing), it's much easier to stick to healthier lifestyle routines. No one bugs you to eat at the Deep Fried Palace because, first of all, they know you'll say no, and second, they know how bad that food is for them. Until then, it's up to you to make sure that healthy habits are enforced on special occasions and when the family is out of town.

Don't take a vacation from your healthier lifestyle!

Ah . . . the sun, the sand, the ocean waves . . . you're taking a well-deserved break from the harsh world. Who's this coming your way now? Oh, it's the waiter with frosty drinks on his tray. And there's the all-you-can-eat buffet stocked with corn dogs, fried cheese sticks, and bottomless tubs of ice cream. Oh, what the heck? You're all on vacation — let everyone live a little!

Not so fast. Loosen the rules a bit, and you'll be sorry. Vacations are prime weight-gain occasions for several reasons:

- People are eager to let others serve them, and they take whatever's offered.
- Resorts and cruise ships are often all-inclusive trips, meaning you can eat until you burst (theoretically, of course).

✔ Vacationers are more likely to honestly forget what they've eaten because they're off their normal routines.

✔ For many people, vacations signal a time to lie on a chaise lounge and do very little (aside from downing those cool drinks). Activity is out; rest is in.

"Well, so what?" you say. "Vacations only come once or twice a year, and we want to enjoy ourselves!" While it's true that most families have limited time or opportunity to escape from the real world, vacation shouldn't be an excuse to gorge yourselves on unhealthy food. Imagine a travel agent selling you *that* package: "Set sail with Silver Wave Cruise Lines and stuff yourself with fattening foods! Eat till you're uncomfortably full! Go to bed at night wishing you hadn't piled your plate so high! Lounge by the pool and *feel* your waistline increasing day by day!" (Hmmm . . . if only there were more truth in advertising.)

We're not saying that your family should stay home for the rest of your lives to avoid any possibility of falling off the healthy bandwagon. We're only reminding you that vacations require extra vigilance on your part because it's so easy to overindulge and slip right back into bad habits that may continue after the family returns home. One little break could turn out to be a permanent vacation from a slimmer, healthier, happier future, and no one wants that.

Stay active

Don't think of vacation as a time to do absolutely nothing but rather as a time to broaden your horizons. If you're headed to the tropics, take the plunge and try scuba diving, or make sure the kids spend afternoons in the pool — playing and swimming, not hanging out at the swim-up bar drinking milkshakes. Walk on the beach, go sightseeing on foot, and take a guided tour up a volcano or mountain. All this activity will make everyone hungry, so plan ahead for healthy snacks. For example, fruit is readily available in warmer climes, and it's fresh and juicy, so don't miss the opportunity to share it with the family.

Expose your children to as many new things as you can when you're out of town. You'll keep everyone active, and who knows? You may open the door to some lifelong interests they wouldn't have otherwise discovered.

Avoid temptation

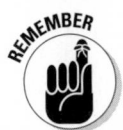

When it comes to mealtimes, skip the buffet! All-you-can-eat setups are just that — setups for weight gain. No one needs to pile a plate high and deep, time and time again, in one meal sitting. You don't need all that food to survive, and neither do your kids. Because your vacation activities are likely to leave everyone feeling famished, enjoy a piece of fruit or a salad before the main meal. Not only do these snacks help to fill the stomach, they're also healthier choices than buttered rolls or greasy appetizers.

Something else to outlaw on vacation: the dreaded hotel mini-bar. Don't even open it. Most of the time, these refrigerators are filled with candy, chips, and other snacks that the family doesn't need. In addition, they're outrageously expensive, so you're effectively paying exorbitant rates to make your family fat. By leaving the mini-bar sealed shut and only providing your family with healthy snacks, you eliminate a temptation that your kids may face every day. If unhealthy foods are kept out of reach, their decisions are already made for them. Skipping the mini-bar may be a good jump-start to healthy habits when you get back home.

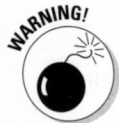

If the kids are crazy for room service, order the healthiest options. Look for low-fat meats such as grilled chicken breasts. A plate of fried chicken fingers doesn't cut it as a healthy meal, even if the kitchen swears that they only use white meat (which, unless it's processed and fried, as in this case, is lower in fat than dark meat). Fried is fried, and it's no good for the family.

In theory, vacations can be a great opportunity for weight loss as long as you don't base your entire trip around what the resort or cruise ship serves for breakfast, lunch, dinner, and snacks. If food has always been your focus when it comes to vacations, change it. Center your vacation on activities rather than food. Choose a particular cruise line because it sails to ports your family wants to get out and see — not because it serves the best drinks and has around-the-clock smorgasbords.

Making healthy choices when eating out

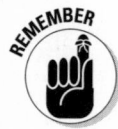

Meals should be about being together, reconnecting, sharing your views and experiences. Don't lose sight of that just because you're eating in a restaurant. Encourage conversation, and you'll find that everyone has plenty of food left over for a doggie bag — after all, you can't eat and chat at the same time (or at least you shouldn't — so here's your opportunity to teach table manners, too!).

You don't have to be halfway around the world on vacation to be faced with making healthy choices from a menu. Whether you're eating at your favorite restaurant or popping into the fast-food joint down the street, how can you be sure that you're choosing well?

The first thing to consider is portion size. Portions have gone haywire in this country in the last decade or so, and what you get at the typical restaurant is about twice as much food as you should have in front of you. Large portions are one reason why many families have a skewed idea of how much food they should be ingesting at one meal — they're used to servers bringing them large, loaded plates!

To combat portion problems, split an entrée with someone else in your party. Most likely, you'll find that neither of you goes home hungry (and the side benefit is that you spend less money). If your child is hankering for something on the menu that no one else wants to eat, ask for a to-go box as soon as the meals are served, and put half of her meal away for later. Although you could just tell her that she can only eat half of what's on her plate, removing half the food from her sight leaves her with a smaller portion and ensures that she won't be tempted to continue eating long after her stomach is filled.

When helping your child choose from a menu, take care to stay away from the following options:

- ✔ **Fried foods:** They're essentially soaked in hot fat, which, aside from exacerbating a weight problem, also clogs the arteries.

- ✔ **Cream soups and/or sauces:** These items are usually prepared with heavy creams and butter, making them loaded with fat.

- ✔ **Seared foods:** They're usually prepared with butter.

- ✔ **High-fat condiments:** Mayonnaise, tartar sauce, cheese sauce, salad dressings — they're all loaded with fat. Substitute lower-fat condiments such as mustard, ketchup, vinegar, and low-fat salad dressings.

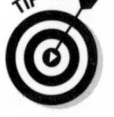

With salads, heavy-handed servers can effectively drown a bowl of goodness with several ladles of liquid fat. Instruct your child to order low-fat dressing (oil and vinegar or vinaigrettes are good choices, along with anything deemed "low-fat") and to ask for it on the side. Even low-fat condiments can become pitfalls if your child douses his food with them.

- ✔ **Sodas, milkshakes, and juices:** All three beverages are full of empty sugar calories, and shakes are also loaded with fat. Low-fat milk or water are better choices.

Going easy on the bread

You can probably remember a few instances of having loaded up on bread before your entrée arrived (and regretting it). The bread basket isn't exactly woven with evil (after all, one roll should actually decrease your child's hunger, making her less likely to consume an entire plate of food for dinner), but your child shouldn't have license to eat its entire contents. One lightly buttered roll (this means using one pat of butterlike spread — margarine is preferable to butter, and plain bread is even better) before dinner should be enough to keep her hunger pangs at bay, especially if you remind her to eat slowly. If her usual habit is to have three or four rolls while waiting for her meal, she saves several hundred calories by cutting back here.

Some families stick to a "no bread basket" rule in restaurants, passing up the rolls as soon as they're offered. This approach may be easier if your child is still young because you can bring healthy, predinner snacks (like animal crackers or cereal) along to tide her over until her meal makes its appearance. If you have a teenager who gets really hungry before dinner (and who would just die of embarrassment if you pulled some grapes out of your purse), stick with the one-roll rule or, even better, encourage her to order a predinner salad (with low-fat dressing, of course).

Turning to the light menu

Fortunately, many sit-down restaurants are coming around to a healthier way of thinking (and serving). Try the "light" section of the menu, making sure that what's listed there actually fits the bill. (Some places still put items like chicken fingers on their "light" menus, indicating that it's a smaller meal than anything offered on the regular menu.) Often, the light menu includes smaller portions of grilled foods and sandwiches that can easily be made to order. (Grilled chicken breast on whole wheat, hold the mayo and cheese? Sounds good!)

Light menus often include salads, too. Older kids, especially, may be interested in a bowl of lettuce topped with all sorts of food. Help your child choose carefully here. Just because there's salad somewhere beneath a pile of chili and cheese doesn't mean that it's a low-fat, low-calorie meal. When hidden from view by greasy (or fried) meat or encased in a fried tortilla shell, the salad is nothing more than a fibrous accompaniment to junk food. Look for a salad that's mostly vegetables (what a concept!); if meat's involved, it should be grilled.

If you're ordering your child a meal from the children's section of the menu, feel free to ask for healthy substitutions. Some restaurants offer kids a small salad or fruit in place of fries, for example.

Dealing with dessert

When dining out, your best approach is to adopt a "no dessert" policy. Remember, you're trying to change your child's palate so that she doesn't crave a syrupy-sweet ending to every meal. Many restaurants just don't offer healthy dessert options like plain, uncaramelized fruit or a plate of graham crackers. Desserts also are usually fairly expensive menu items, so if you must, use that defense to initially break the restaurant dessert habit ("Eight dollars is too much money for a piece of cake!"). Eventually, all you'll have to do is say "no" to the request for dessert, and your child will know why — and accept it.

If you absolutely can't get out of dessert (like if you're dining with your extended family, all the kids are having dessert, and you just know that denying your child a treat is going to backfire), split it between yourself and the child or between two kids. Dessert portions are usually far too large, anyway, especially for children.

Finding good fast-food options

In fast-food restaurants, healthy choices certainly don't overwhelm you. However, you can avoid choosing the worst things on the menu, which include anything fried, those heavy croissant sandwiches, and most breakfast sandwiches (they're often loaded with cheese and sausage). Triple-decker burgers are also out. Soda? Out. Milkshakes? Out.

So what's left that your child will actually eat? If your child eats grilled chicken or salad, those are usually the healthiest options on a fast-food menu. If not, a plain burger (no cheese, no mayo, no extra burger on top) is all right every now and then, and in place of fries, ask for fruit or salad. Choose low-fat milk or water rather than soda or a shake. Most of the time, kids are more interested in the toys that come with a child's meal than they are in the meal itself, so even if you can't substitute something healthy for the fries, let him have the toy, the burger, and the milk (and chuck the fries in the trash).

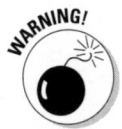

Don't negate the benefits of a healthy choice by adding mayo or cheese to a grilled chicken sandwich or heavy dressing to salad. Encourage your child to use low-fat condiments like mustard on sandwiches and low-fat salad dressing or vinegar on salads.

On Their Own: Preparing Children to Make Healthy Choices

When you think about it, controlling what your child eats at home and in a restaurant is relatively easy. (We said *relatively* — we know it's not truly easy.) When he leaves the house, you really have no control over what goes into his mouth — especially if he's older and more independent than a young child. (For the scoop on food-related issues with young kids and day-care settings, check out the "Advising Caregivers of the New Rules" section earlier in this chapter.)

Sleepovers, play dates, and junk food

What the heck can you do to prevent your overweight preteen or teenager from breaking all the rules when he's at a friend's house or even when he's at school? To start, he needs a solid foundation to stand on, and that comes from you. While you're helping him to lose weight, you also need to be educating him. Don't spare him the details: Tell him why he needs to drop his excess weight, and let him know that some serious health issues associated with being obese can be prevented if the two of you start working together.

Avoid using health issues as a scare tactic to threaten your child into a healthier lifestyle. That's just traumatic, for one thing, and it may only make him feel that there's something wrong with him; after all, "normal" teenagers aren't worried about heart disease.

Common sense tells us that teenagers love to rebel and take risks. They're immortal, in their own eyes. They truly believe that health risks don't affect them, so very few teenagers are likely to say to one another, "You know, I'm going to have some raisins instead of potato chips because I'm a little concerned about clogging my arteries. High cholesterol can start doing damage as early as childhood." (Yeah . . . we'd love to hear that conversation play out, too.) It's fair to say that plenty of teens don't adhere to healthy eating standards.

So, logically speaking, it's fair to assume that your preteen or teenager will come across some peer pressure when it comes to eating junk food. When he's at a sleepover, for example, he's bound to be faced with temptation. There's very little chance that his friends will also be snacking on carrot sticks and apples all night long. Educating your child in healthful eating is one thing; expecting him to educate others is quite another. Older kids just want to be like their friends, which is the problem. Your kid doesn't want to be the one opting out of the junk-food frenzy!

Fending off peer pressure

Banning your child from social situations isn't the answer to protecting him from temptation; the last thing an overweight child needs is encouragement to feel alone and different. Accompanying an older kid to parties and friends' homes to check out the cuisine is even worse (talk about being *different!*). Preparing him to ward off peer pressure is a much better approach. Consider the following suggestions of things you can do to help your kid before he visits the home of a junk-food junkie:

- ✔ **Have him eat at home before he leaves.** If he's not famished, he'll have an easier time passing up unhealthy snacks. A full stomach is also a good excuse for saying "No thanks" to a stack of cookies — he can simply tell the truth: "I'm not hungry; I just ate."

- ✔ **Give him his own fun (but healthy) snack to take along.** If your child is going to be at a friend's house for the entire day (or night), taking something to share is just polite. Even older kids get a kick out of animal crackers. (Don't believe us? Hand a couple of teenagers a box and watch them bite the heads off the lions and the toes off the bears and laugh about it.) If he arrives at his friend's place with a healthy snack, he'll know that there's something he can have when he gets hungry.

✔ **Remind him about portion control.** If he's going to a sleepover, for example, he'll probably have to eat a meal away from home. You can't exactly go over to the friend's house and cook a low-fat breakfast for the boys, so remind your child that he shouldn't load his plate up until the pancakes tower above him, *especially* if he's offered high-fat foods.

✔ **Discourage mindless snacking.** Video games, computer games, TV . . . these are the "activities" teens commonly enjoy. Remind your child that eating while lounging around is a bad habit and a bad idea for anyone trying to lose weight.

✔ **Tell him to take a football.** Or a couple of hockey sticks. Or rollerblades. Whenever possible, your child should try to be the one saying, "Let's go *do* something!", even when he's at a friend's house. Added bonus: Other parents *love* friends who drag their own kids away from the video games. If he gets everyone up and moving, your child is likely to be invited back.

When your child invites his friends over, should you let them have junk food in the interest of keeping his pals happy? No. Don't feel pressured to break with your own routine for anyone. Different parents have different rules; it's that simple. If your child is embarrassed, let him blame you for the lack of sugary, fatty treats in the house. It may be a lot easier for him to say, "My mom is on a health kick. She won't buy cupcakes anymore," than for him to say, "I need to lose weight, so we don't have any high-fat foods in the house."

Grading Your Child's School Lunch

Schools have all sorts of protective measures these days. Drug-Free Zones and Weapons-Free Zones surround the buildings where children spend most of their days, so why no Healthy-Eating Zones or Junk-Food-Free Areas? After all, consuming fatty foods is a major long-term health threat, especially in this country!

Take a look at your child's school lunch menu. You're bound to find chicken nuggets, cheeseburgers, hot dogs, French fries, macaroni and cheese, and pizza, among other things. You may as well be feeding your child at a fast-food restaurant every day. Find a few minutes to take a walk through your child's school's cafeteria. Are there vending machines in sight? What's in them? They probably aren't stocked with fruit and mineral water but rather with candy, chips, and soda.

The National School Lunch Program is responsible for feeding hundreds of thousands of schoolchildren around the country every day. The average parent may assume that the kids are being well taken care of in the cafeteria because schools that participate in the National School Lunch Program have to serve meals that adhere to specific dietary guidelines:

✔ No more than 30 percent of calories from fat

✔ Fewer that 10 percent saturated-fat calories

To find out if your child's school participates in this government program, simply call the school and ask. Schools that don't participate in the program are more likely to have even more unhealthy options (like fast food vendors right in the cafeteria) as a means of cutting costs.

However, many school lunches come processed and ready to be opened, warmed, and fed to the children. You can bet that these foods have fairly high levels of saturated fat to improve taste and shelf life. Most schools also only offer whole or 2 percent milk in their cafeterias. The bottom line regarding school lunches is this: Although the meals may adhere to government guidelines, they could be so much better if they included fresher, greener, truly low-fat options.

The real danger in the cafeteria lies in the a la carte items, like ice cream treats, chips, and soda. These empty-calorie foods do little except make children overweight. The treats, which are sold separately from the school lunches, are a major source of income for schools, which explains why they're within your child's reach.

To find out the nutritional breakdown of your child's school lunch, take the menu to a nutritionist. With a little time, she can evaluate the calorie count of each meal and snack.

Is it impossible to change the way your child's school feeds its pupils? Stranger things have happened, but your voice is more likely to be heard if you can gather up a group of concerned parents before bringing the issue before the school administration. Keep in mind that the National School Lunch Program provides low-cost or free breakfasts and lunches to students who otherwise may not have a morning or noontime meal, so your school district's reluctance to drop the program in favor of healthier (and more expensive) options may legitimately be out of concern for its less fortunate pupils.

Cafeterias go green

Some schools have adopted healthy, green cafeteria practices. Organic, naturally low-fat, high-fiber, pesticide-free foods make up the menus in these lunchrooms. In fact, some of these schools actually have gardens on the school grounds in which the produce for the school lunches is grown, picked, and sent straight into the kitchen. What a way to teach kids how easy it is to grow *and* eat healthy foods! As of this writing, most of these schools are located in the western United States, but the trend is growing.

So what can you do to help your child eat healthier at school? Let her choose one day a week to buy the school lunch, and make her a healthy lunch from home the other four days. (For tips on packing healthy lunches, check out Chapter 9.) Often, you have no control over how your child spends her lunch money. For all you know, your already overweight child could be purchasing an entire school lunch and four ice cream treats for dessert! When she chooses to buy lunch, send enough money with her to cover the cost of the meal — no extras.

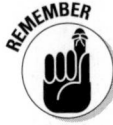

No matter how young your child is, encourage her (with a little guidance, especially for the youngest kids) to make her own healthy choices at meal-times, whether she's packing a lunch or purchasing one at school. If you pack her lunch in an effort to make low-fat eating as easy as possible for her, she's not really learning anything except that a nutritious meal magically appears in her lunchbox every day. Remember, your ultimate goal is for her to make healthy choices all by herself, and that's something she can learn to do best through hands-on experience.

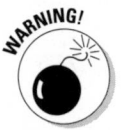

Don't send your child to school with loads of money! Granted, you can't do much to prevent your teenager from spending her own cash on soda at school, but you can keep money for treats out of the hands of a younger child. And no matter what your child's age, if the school has a prepaid lunch account system, don't put extra money in it! Often, you have no control over what that money buys.

Chapter 13

Dealing with a Child Who Hasn't Bought into the Program

The heartbreak of obesity and all its associated problems are enough to make a parent cry. But doing your best to improve your child's health when he seems to have no intention of following your lead can be incredibly frustrating and result in your abandonment of the whole thing. While it may be an understandable reaction, throwing in the towel is obviously bad news for your child's future.

Convincing a reluctant child to join the healthy parade that's marching through your home isn't just something you *should* do, it's something you *must* do. It's simply what's best for him. The alternative — his remaining obese, or worse, putting on more weight — is fraught with danger. As we say throughout this book, the best way to guide your child toward a permanently healthier lifestyle is to lead by example. So even if your child isn't jumping for joy at the thought of hitting the pool for some swimming or cycling around the block after dinner, his attitude doesn't let *you* off the hook.

In addition to being a coach, you're also a full-time cheerleader in this weight-loss game (although you aren't required to wear the skirt, wave the pompons, and smile incessantly). Obesity is certainly a cosmetic issue, but some of the most serious ramifications of carrying around excess weight can't be seen. Finding ways to remind your child of what's at stake — his health and his future — without getting sucked into argument after argument is essential to his success (and your sanity).

Shooting Down Arguments Before They Arise

Some children are naturally eager-to-please and ultracompliant (these kids usually don't even need to be told to do something; they just know what needs to be done and do it), while others must question every order they're given ("Why should I clean my room? It's just going to get dirty again" or, "Wash the dishes? Why can't we just use paper plates?!"). In some cases, personality styles are the result of how a child has been parented, but more often than not, kids are born with a certain temperament, and you can do very little to change it. If you have more than one kid and notice significant differences in each child's outlook on life, you know what we're talking about.

Even if you're fortunate enough to be dealing with a compliant child while establishing healthy guidelines in your home, you may still run into some problems with her adherence to a weight-loss routine. She wants to be healthy, but the process is long, slow, and sometimes arduous. In addition, your child has come to associate food with reward, and no matter how hard she works at this program or how much weight she loses, she knows a chocolate-covered, marshmallow-filled treat isn't waiting for her at the end.

Her desire to have sweet, salty, and/or fatty foods will hopefully wane over time (after all, one of the main goals of this whole program is to change her taste and overwhelming desire for goodies). But there's little you can do to speed up the weight-loss process, and that fact can be disheartening for even the most upbeat, enthusiastic child.

The ideal amount of weight loss for children is about 8 ounces a week, which means that you won't start to see a physical change in your child for a significant amount of time after you start a low-fat diet and exercise program. Although *you* may have the patience to wait for these lasting results, your child may become frustrated almost from the get-go when she's weaning herself off her favorite treats, increasing her activity, and seeing little in the way of results.

So how do you handle a child who isn't wholeheartedly onboard with the new healthy lifestyle? You don't want to set up a battle of the wills with a child of any age, of course. Remind yourself that you're the adult and she's the child. Then explore the following strategies for easing the transition, anticipating and preventing your child's resistance to the changes you're making, and getting your child back in the game.

Remove temptation from the house

The argument: "You let Jack and Emily and Dad eat all the cookies they want, so why can't I?"

Expecting your obese child to keep his hands out of a cookie jar filled with treats for you, your spouse, and your other kids is both unfair and unrealistic. By the time a child reaches an obese state, he's developed bad eating habits and insatiable cravings. Keeping unhealthy foods in the house is like leaving a pack of smokes in the nightstand of a person who's suffering from lung disease. Your child may legitimately yearn for his next candy or chip fix, and because he thinks the damage has already been done, he may figure there's no sense in not indulging himself.

Because he's already obese and feeling lousy physically, and because it may seem very unlikely to him that he could ever lose the weight, your child really can't see the harm in continuing down the same path. And because he may also be feeling isolated and depressed, food may be his sole source of comfort. You know that adopting a new, healthy lifestyle can change a lot of his negative feelings about himself and the future — but he's just a kid. He doesn't have an adult's perspective on life. All he knows is what's happening here and now, and as far as he's concerned, it ain't all that great.

Keep telling yourself and your child that the health risks and long-term implications of obesity are very serious and that your child still has a shot at a healthy, normal future if the two of you can work together now to lose the weight. This reassurance can be incredibly helpful when you're dealing with a child who doesn't necessarily appreciate what you're trying to do for him.

To keep your overweight child on track, your entire family has to be involved in a healthier lifestyle. You can't keep fruit pies and soda in the pantry for your average-weight daughter while you dole out skim milk and pretzels to your obese son. Even the most agreeable obese child will have a hard time accepting this arrangement, which in the end is only another reminder that he's *different* from everyone else. Clean out the pantry, clear out the fridge, and either toss or donate any food that's high in fat, high in sugar, or both. In particular, get rid of the following:

> ✔ **Juice:** Frozen cans of juice concentrate are nothing but water and sugar, for the most part, and sugar is just an empty-calorie food. Excessive amounts of sugar in the bloodstream of obese children is also thought to play a role in the development of type 2 diabetes (because the pancreas just can't keep its production of insulin high enough to meet demand).

✔ **Soda:** Each time your child drinks a soda, she's not getting any nutrients at all — just a bunch of sugar. Soda also rots the teeth; if a child has plaque on her teeth, the carbonation from the soda can cause a sort of chemical reaction with that plaque and eat away at the tooth's enamel. (Even diet sodas can cause this type of erosion.)

✔ **Whole milk:** Some dairy foods are fine, and for healthy bone development, calcium is a necessity in a child's diet. But skim milk has everything whole milk does — except a lot of extra fat. Pediatricians recommend keeping toddlers on whole milk or formula until the age of 2 (because they need the fat for brain development); after that age, however, you should replace whole milk with skim.

✔ **High-fat condiments:** Your child may be crazy about veggie wraps for lunch, but if she's covering her sliced carrots and tomatoes with high-fat salad dressing, she's adding unnecessary fat to her meal and sabotaging her own best intentions. In addition to regular salad dressings, eliminate regular mayo, dips, and high-fat sauces from your home. Grilled chicken smothered in a high-calorie honey-mustard sauce hardly counts as a truly healthy meal.

✔ **White bread:** Your child should get used to eating whole grains, which are full of vitamins, minerals, and fiber. White bread just can't hold up to the nutrients offered in a loaf of whole grain. The same holds true for pasta — whole-grain pastas are better, nutritionally speaking.

✔ **Sugared cereals:** Even the most innocuous-looking cereal (such as frosted wheat squares and frosted corn flakes) can be a sugar-laden choice. Whole grains are where it's at — plain oatmeal with fresh fruit is a very healthy *and* delicious breakfast.

✔ **The obvious treats:** Cookies, candy, chips . . . you know the drill. They're chock-full of sugar, fat, and salt — none of which your child needs.

✔ **And the not-so-obvious treats:** Replacing regular cookies and chips with low-fat alternatives may sound like a good option, but it's actually not the best idea. One problem with low-fat cookies and chips is that they taste too much like the real thing, so they aren't helpful at all in changing your child's craving for sweets and salty, high-fat snacks. You want your child to eventually choose healthier foods, like fruits, for snacks and desserts.

After you clean out your fridge and pantry and your child says, "There's nothing good to eat!," how do you respond? Offer up skim milk, fresh fruits and veggies, plain yogurt (and by "plain" we mean yogurt that doesn't come with cookie stir-ins), low-fat cheese, juice without added sugar, skim-milk cottage cheese, eggs, fish or chicken from last night's dinner, whole-grain cereals and breads, and low-fat, low-sugar treats like animal crackers and pretzels. Surely, your child can survive on these foods, right?

Absolutely. Even if she gives you a hard time, whining and complaining that there's nothing to eat, you can breathe a sigh of relief, for the moment. You've eliminated temptation at home, so she'll just have to eat whatever's on hand. (Chapter 8 offers plenty of additional ideas for healthy snacks to keep on hand.)

Set a good example

The argument: "You haven't changed the way you eat, and you watch TV all day long. Guess that means I can follow your lead, Mom [or Dad]."

Eating well and working exercise into *your* daily routine are two important things you can do to ensure your child's successful weight loss. In order to help your child lose weight, you have to know whether the foods you're offering her are at all palatable, and you can't know that unless you eat them, too! You can't convincingly sell her on the idea of a baked apple for dessert if you've just eaten a package of cookies hidden in your closet. (And lest you think that being forced to eat cookies *in a closet* is the extent of your sacrifice, it isn't. Check out the sidebar "Just say 'no' to a secret stash.") You have to join in the program; you have to *live* it — and live it in a credible manner.

You may find it difficult to adjust to healthier eating if you aren't overweight yourself. Remind yourself that eating high-fat and high-sugar foods can lead to major health issues like heart disease, even in thin people.

Eating together

Preparing a healthy dinner for the family tells your child that you're all in this together. Picking at the food on your own plate (without ever raising a forkful of salad or fish to your own lips) while you encourage her to eat her healthy meal sends an entirely different message: *She* needs to eat these foods, but you don't.

Just say "no" to a secret stash

Avoid the urge to keep your own stash of goodies around, reasoning that you aren't the one with the weight problem. Chances are, you'll slip up at some point: Your child will be able to smell chocolate on your breath, or she'll see you with a piece of candy — and what a betrayal that will feel like to her! Also, by keeping a hidden bag of candy in the house, you risk your child's discovery of these treats. Add her anger at your "cheating" to her frustration at being denied her own treats, and she may just sit down and consume the whole thing.

Refusing to change your own less-than-healthy eating habits almost guarantees that your child will fail to embrace the newest options on her plate. Remember, although an older child may seem mature enough to truly understand and appreciate the logic behind switching to a low-fat diet, watching the rest of the family indulge in a high-fat, high-sugar diet is a bitter pill for her to swallow. You can't continue to eat burgers and fries in front of her *and* convince her that eating unhealthy foods can lead to serious health problems in years to come.

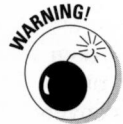

When you feed your child healthy foods while you continue to eat high-fat fare, you set up a serious credibility issue for yourself. When your child cries, "Hypocrite!" she has a point. No matter how skilled a debater you may be, you'll have a hard time counteracting her argument that if you're eating that food, then it can't be all that bad.

Moving together

Fitting exercise into an otherwise jam-packed day may be difficult, but you can't expect an obese child to get moving all by herself. Even if she's highly motivated at first, that excitement may fade over time, and that's where family support comes into play. Planned activities ensure that your child knows what she will be doing, where she'll be doing it, and with whom.

For a younger child, lead the way by taking her outside and playing with her. If you haven't played with a child since you were one, some activities to consider include:

- Tag
- Kickball
- Soccer
- Bike rides
- Foot races in the yard or driveway
- Walking the dog
- Walking to a friend's home

Fun stuff? You bet! All these activities get the two of you off and running without thinking about how hard you're working. Make sure that you allow your child as many water breaks as she needs, and concentrate on making outdoor play as enjoyable as possible so that when you call her outside after lunch every day, she won't kick up a fuss.

An obese teenager will probably refuse to play a game of tag with you in the yard (and who can blame her?). If she seems to lack direction in choosing an exercise she enjoys, suggest something the two of you can do together — at least initially. Embarking on this part of the program alone can be very scary for an overweight adolescent because she's naturally self-conscious and not in top physical form. Suggest low-impact exercises that are easy on the joints, like:

- ✔ Walking
- ✔ Swimming
- ✔ Biking

These activities are easy to do in pairs (just you and her) or with the rest of the family. They're also easy enough for beginners while leaving lots of room for gradual improvement. You and your teen may start out walking just one mile, for example, but as your stamina increases, you'll find yourselves covering twice the distance in the same amount of time.

Starting a fitness routine isn't easy. If your child tries an activity and comes away feeling as though it was a disaster, she won't be eager to try again. If you're not a regular partaker of exercise, let her know that you understand how she feels. Then give her some helpful suggestions, like walking in a park instead of on a busy road where she's more likely to feel as though people are watching her. And go with her. If she doesn't want to talk, let her wear her headphones.

Getting physical and showing your child that you're as committed to finding fun activities and getting fit as she is reassures her that she isn't in this all alone. Buddying up to walk or swim together is a great way for both of you to stick with a program because you know that you're going to hold one another to your exercise "dates."

Focus on other traits

The argument: "I'm sick and tired of talking about my weight!"

Adapting to a healthy lifestyle can be all consuming. Changing the way the family eats and exercises affects so many aspects of everyone's regular routine that, for a while, it may be all the family can talk about (for better or for worse).

Concurrent with the discussion of food and exercise, the topic of your child's weight may be front and center, and that's completely understandable when you're starting to make major changes. After time, though, you need to make sure that your child's weight isn't the only thing you ever discuss with him.

When your child begins his weight-loss program and is weighing in each week, you'll naturally talk about how well he's doing and areas in which he feels he may be struggling. Discussions about the grocery list or ideas for dinner over the course of the following week are a normal part of everyday life in almost every house. They're fair game — for now.

But you don't want to make your child's weight the center of attention after you get the healthy lifestyle ball rolling. He's more than an obese child; he has other traits aside from being overweight, so talk about those. This may be easier said than done if your child seems to have no interests outside of watching TV and snacking. Many overweight children aren't involved in *any* extracurricular activities, which is part of their weight problems. They need to fill their time with healthy habits, like music, art, or sports, instead of spending their afternoons in front of the tube. Encourage your child to *find* some other interests, either at school or in the neighborhood. He'll come to see himself differently when he's involved in multiple activities, and as a result, he'll be far less likely to fall back into his old habits.

In some homes, weight has been the central topic for so long that no one can think of anything else to talk about. If this is the situation in your house, it's time to find something to do — and then talk about that. Here are some ideas to get you talking about other topics:

- ✔ Play a game together — inside or outside.

- ✔ Go visiting to a friend's house.

- ✔ Ask your child about school, friends, his hobbies, or a good book he's reading.

- ✔ Talk about goals for his healthier future: Does your child want to learn to ski next winter? Is he looking forward to making an academic honor society?

The great thing about entering into a healthy lifestyle program together is that it gives your whole family the opportunity to get know each other all over again. Start by making sure that the conversations at the family dinner table focus on the day's events rather than your child's size and shape. (For more about family meals, turn to Chapter 11.)

Promote harmony at home

The argument: "You're too hard on me! You want me to be like my perfect skinny sister [or brother]!"

Being obese isn't easy in a culture obsessed with thinness and beauty, and it can be even more difficult to be extremely heavy in a *family* obsessed with weight and appearance. This book advocates getting the entire family involved in a healthier lifestyle, but concentrating on one child's weight problem while holding his thin sibling up as an example of ideal thinness is *not* conducive to a supportive weight-loss atmosphere. Comparing children is one of the most hurtful things a parent can do, even if it's not done with malice. The differences between a thin child and an obese one are stark enough, and no one needs to point them out.

Some parents compare their children to one another as a means of creating good-natured competition and lighting a fire under everyone to see who can do their best in any given situation. Grades, behavior, neatness . . . nothing seems to be off limits in these households. Some families may thrive in this type of competitive environment, but most often, siblings end up resenting one another for making their own lives difficult. Even the child who's hailed as the brain of the family may come to feel as though she's sick and tired of playing that role. In extreme cases, a child may shut down and decide that she's no longer going to be whoever it is that her parents and siblings think she is.

Your intentions for using one child as a model of the ideal body may be good, especially if there's no preexisting tension between the siblings. If your younger, obese child really looks up to her thinner sister, for example, then perhaps you figure that using the older child as an inspirational tool can only help matters. But the younger child already wants to be like her sister, so there's no need for you to push the matter any farther.

Each child needs to feel special and loved for who she is regardless of her weight. By pitting a heavy child against a thin one, either by saying "Your sister doesn't eat two sandwiches; and neither should you," or "Look how skinny your sister is; if she can do it, you can too," you create distance between your kids. And during this period of weight loss, your obese child needs all the support she can get. No matter what her relationship is with her siblings, she doesn't need to feel singled out and separated from them.

Pointing out another child's weight to your obese child may send the message that you want her to be just like her sibling in every way — and that's never going to happen. In fact, the heavy child may end up feeling disappointed (or feel as though she's disappointed you) when she drops the weight only to discover that she's exactly the same person she's always been, only lighter. (And if she doesn't lose the weight, that feeling of having disappointed you will be magnified.)

Comparing your children also harms your relationship with your overweight child. When she hears you praising another child's traits — and knocking her down in the process — she gets scared of disappointing you or angry at you for humiliating her. Or both. Either way, she's less likely to view you as a source of unconditional support, and that's what she really needs from you throughout this entire weight-loss process.

Even if you've used comparisons of the kids to some success in the past, *weight is off-limits!* The possibility of long-term emotional wounds is just too great and could prevent your child from *ever* feeling good about how she looks.

Reining In Those Sneaky Little Devils

Suppose you're a little surprised at how well your child has adapted to the changes in your household. He isn't at all upset about packing a salad for his lunch, and he readily accepts the no-more-soda rule. Maybe this weight-loss thing is going to be easier than you thought. Maybe you were worried for no reason. Things couldn't be going any better.

And then you find a candy bar wrapper in the washing machine and an empty soda can under his bed. After the initial shock of this active deception wears off, you feel your blood pressure rising. Haven't you told him time and time again how dangerous obesity is? Doesn't he understand that the whole family has made lifestyle changes in an attempt to help him overcome his weight issues? Doesn't he want to get healthy and feel better?!

Weight is an issue that's all wrapped up in other emotions: guilt, sadness, anger, and low self-esteem. You don't want to make matters worse, but you can't allow him to break with the program on a regular basis and, even worse, become a huge sneak. The danger of confronting him is that he'll try harder to make sure he doesn't get caught again. This section gives you some tips for talking with a child who's willing to go to great lengths to get his sugar fix. We talk about whether punishment is the best option and recommend alternative measures you may find useful in this situation.

Breaking with the program at school and friends' homes

When your kid leaves the house, you have to accept that he's at the helm of his own ship. You can't stalk him to make sure he's not down at the pizza place or peek through the windows of the school cafeteria to make sure he's eating a healthy, well-balanced meal.

School lunches aren't always the healthiest meals. Most schools offer treats in the lunch line, like cookies, cake, brownies, ice cream, and chocolate whole milk. Some schools even have fast-food vendors on campus selling their fat-laden wares to the innocents and making the obesity crisis in this country even worse. (Okay, we're stepping down off the soapbox now.)

In Chapter 12, we talk about ways to make sure your child gets a healthy meal at lunchtime. But what do you do when he's eating everything *but* the salad he packed in his lunch box this morning? Can you march into that cafeteria and spoon-feed him a low-fat, low-sugar diet? Should you make him wear a sign that says, "My mom won't let me buy snacks"? Of course not; humiliating your child doesn't do anything but make him feel as though he can't trust you.

To help ensure that your child has a healthy lunch:

- **Close your wallet.** If you're not handing out money for treats at school, your young child will be hard pressed to come up with the cash for a cookie or other treat.

- **Have your child pack his own lunch.** Provide him with plenty of healthy, tasty options for his lunchbox: low-fat turkey slices, whole-grain breads or pita pockets, fresh fruits and vegetables, and low-fat condiments like mustard, balsamic vinegar, salsa, hot sauce, or low-fat salad dressing.

- **Think beyond the sandwich.** Healthy soups, whole-grain pastas, low-fat stews, or last night's healthy leftovers are easily packed in an insulated container or thermos and pulled out at lunchtime.

- **If your child insists on buying lunch (many kids would rather die than brown-bag it), review the school's lunch menu with him.** Point out the healthiest choices; explain why the high-fat, high-sugar items aren't conducive to good health. Because they're often armed with their own money, older kids really need to have a firm grasp on the concept of what makes one food healthier than another. (Chapters 7, 8, and 9 are filled with information on healthy versus unhealthy food choices.)

When he's heading to a friend's house, reduce the chances that he'll sneak unhealthy snacks by doing any of the following:

- Feed him at home before he leaves.

- Give him a fun (but healthy) snack to take along and share.

- Tell him to take along a game, football, soccer ball, or something else that will get him and his friends active.

Sneaking snacks happens every once in a while, and it's not the end of the world. But *why*, you ask, would your child jeopardize his weight-loss progress? For the same reasons we all eat unhealthy foods at times: He may be truly hungry, and he may just be tempted beyond his ability to say no at this point in time. Don't forget that he's used to eating whatever's handy, and you can't expect a miraculous change in behavior overnight. Even the most motivated kids slip up now and then, and one misstep won't hinder the headway he's making.

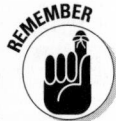

Even if he's going off to college in a few years, your child isn't a mini-adult. He doesn't have the ability to think long term like you do. While you're worried sick about the risks that obesity pose to his health, he's probably taking those threats much less seriously, especially if he's been lucky enough up to this point to avoid serious medical issues related to his weight.

Emphasizing choices

How do you deal with a child who has grabbed autonomy by the horns and is leading a double life (a healthy one at home and a not-so-healthy one elsewhere)? Drive home the concept of choices, explaining that the goal is to avoid making bad choices that can lead to lifelong ramifications. Explain this concept to your child in language that she can understand.

In Chapter 3, we talk about the serious long-term health risks associated with being obese. Even though you may have discussed these issues with your child (hopefully without scaring the living daylights out of her), she may not fully appreciate the seriousness of what lies ahead. Teenagers are notorious for thinking that nothing bad is ever going to happen to them.

You've got to get this newsflash through to her: Obesity is serious, the damage is happening now, and she doesn't have the luxury of time to decide whether or not to get with the program. If she waits too long, her health could be too far gone to do much about it. Tell her:

- She has a choice between a healthy future and one filled with fear over what will happen with her body.
- She has a choice to feel better or to suffer the pain (emotional and physical) associated with obesity.
- She has a choice to participate fully in life or to be sidelined by her weight.

She's the only one who can make these choices for herself, and they're dependent on her making the right decisions on a day-to-day basis. You can help her by educating her about which foods are healthy and which foods aren't, but you can't always be there to make the right choice for her.

You may be tempted to pack her lunch every day and prepare her snacks at home, and that's fine when you're first beginning a weight-loss program. Just make sure your child is at least nearby, watching and learning how to do these things for herself. After a couple of days of instruction, even a young child can prepare a healthy veggie wrap for herself or decide that she'd rather have fruit salad for lunch. An older child can and should pick up on the process very quickly.

Children learn about making good choices when they're allowed to think for themselves. If you have a child who's overwhelmed by decision making or who chooses unhealthy foods time and time again, narrow the choices down for her. Let her know what she *can* have instead of only telling her what isn't allowed. For example, if you're preparing the grocery list and your daughter asks for a fish-fry dinner next week, do the following:

1. **Definitely say no to that request and remind her that fried foods are high in fat and are something the entire family is no longer eating.**

2. **Let her choose from some healthier options, such as grilled chicken, fish, vegetarian dishes, or egg-white omelets.**

   For additional healthy food options, check out Chapter 9.

Resisting the urge to punish

You may be disappointed to hear that there's no punishment system for obese kids who break the rules (and hence, their mothers' hearts). Punishing and/or shaming a child for sneaking unhealthy foods will only make her better at hiding the evidence. Younger children are usually easier to get back on track simply because they have less freedom and opportunity to stray from your new rules regarding food. Teenagers, though, need to feel as though parents aren't completely in charge of their lives anymore. That's why they can be so cranky and even outright mean when you're just trying to help them. They want to do it themselves, and they don't want to have to say, even to themselves, "My mom helped me figure this out."

Although doling out serious punishment may seem like the right thing to do when you've had it up to your eyeballs with your teen's lack of cooperation, back off for a minute and cool down. Yelling at her, grounding her, and making her do the worst chores in the house for two weeks only feed the resentment she feels toward the situation. And yet, by completely ignoring the issue, you may send the message that you don't care, that it's all right for her to continue breaking her weight-loss rules, that you don't mind if she stops off for a submarine sandwich with the works on her way home from school.

Find some creative way to continue to educate her on the topic without making it seem as though you're truly punishing her. Let her prepare dinner for you a couple of nights a week. Take it one step farther and ask her to make the grocery list for next week. Give her the responsibility of taking care of her own health.

Keep in mind that true change takes time and that backsliding isn't the end of the world. Whatever her age, continue to support your child, and don't berate her for her shortcomings and mistakes. Before you know it, your child will be out the door and living her own life. And when she reaches that point, the decisions she makes will have to be her own. (Sorry, but you can't move into her dorm room and cook for her.) If you've done all you can to educate her on the dangers of remaining obese and how to care for herself, no matter what the outcome is, you'll know you did everything possible to help her control her weight problem and commit to a healthy lifestyle.

Chapter 14

Bringing In Outside Help

· ·

In This Chapter

▶ Evaluating the state of your child's weight-loss program

▶ Talking things out with doctors and support groups

▶ Moving on to more serious issues and treatments

· ·

*I*n theory, the (relatively) easy modifications to your family's lifestyle that we recommend throughout this book should help your and your child's goal to achieve better health. However, we know that some families have a really tough time adjusting their eating and exercise habits. When you've been doing something a certain way for years and years, figuring out and sticking to an entirely new system takes time and effort and can be exhausting, both mentally and physically.

You may reach a point when you've tried everything you can think of and still nothing seems to be helping your child. Or perhaps the weight is coming off slowly, but your child is still unhappy. Or maybe your child's dropping the weight extremely fast and you're concerned that your child has lost too much weight, that's she's developed an obsession with becoming too thin. When you hit the wall of frustration or worry, don't be afraid to seek help outside of your home. You want your child's emotional state to improve as a result of adapting a healthier lifestyle; a slimmer body is no consolation if her mindset is suffering.

Do We Need Professional Help?

It can be difficult for any parent to know what's "normal" for a child and what isn't. That's one big reason so many parents gather in formal playgroups or informal meetings at the playground — they want to touch base with other moms and dads to figure out if what their kids are doing and experiencing at any given stage of childhood is typical or slightly out of the ordinary.

If you're fortunate enough to have a network of friends who are also turning their homes into healthy-living havens, then you already know what a god-send it can be to simply sit down and share information with these people. On the other hand, if your family is going through this health-improvement venture alone, you're bound to face times when you don't know if a situation is cause for concern or a natural part of the process. You may need some outside help if:

- ✔ Your child is actually gaining weight despite her best efforts at low-fat eating and increased activity.

- ✔ Your child is exhibiting signs of anxiety and/or depression related to weight.

- ✔ Your child is exhibiting signs of an eating disorder (obsessing over food and weight, for example, or losing far too much weight too quickly and refusing to eat).

Keep your eyes open for any signs of your child's weight-loss efforts going askew. A teen who's desperate to lose weight may turn to weight-loss pills sold in a health-food store, some of which can have serious side effects and, in any event, aren't a long-term solution to her weight issue. Other, legitimate weight-loss medications are available by prescription but may have serious side effects. (We address the side effects of weight-loss medications in the section "Investigating medications for weight loss" later in this chapter.)

Exploring Your Options

When you're concerned enough about your child's weight-loss experience to discuss things with a third party, it's important to find a professional you're comfortable speaking with and who, in return, has great communication skills. You can't leave this issue hanging, with questions unanswered and miscommunications swirling about, so be prepared to do some research to find the right professional or support group for your child.

Talking with your child's doctor

Hopefully, your child's doctor has been in on your family's health-improvement goals from the beginning. If not, bring him in now. Not only is he most familiar with your child's health history, but he's also a source of knowledge on your family's health history. He can connect the dots between predisposing factors that may play a role in any unusual difficulty that your child is having with her weight loss. (If she's doing everything right and she's *gaining* weight, for example, your pediatrician may be able to shed some light on the cause.)

Some of the topics to discuss with your child's doctor include:

- ✔ Your child's refusal to adhere to a healthy lifestyle
- ✔ Lack of results despite a good effort from your child
- ✔ Self-esteem or social issues
- ✔ Weight-related health issues

Your child's pediatrician should be compassionate and sensitive to the issue of weight, especially if your child is shy and/or approaching the teen years. For introverted or self-conscious children (and most adolescents are nothing if not self-conscious, regardless of their weight), talking to an authority figure can be very difficult if they fear this person is going to lecture or somehow berate them for their shortcomings. Of course, if you talk with the doctor and get a sense of aloofness or condescension without having your concerns addressed, find someone who'll do a better job communicating with you and, in turn, your child.

You need solid guidance on these major issues. Any parent whose child is at increased risk for developing serious illnesses needs to know that she can make a call for advice and not feel as though she's intruding on the doctor's lunch hour. If your child's doctor either takes the issue of obesity too lightly or is far too judgmental about your family's lifestyle, you may be so uncomfortable asking for help that you just don't. We're not advocating a particular personality style that's ideal for a pediatrician; we're simply saying that your doc's way of doing business needs to gel with yours for the best results.

Investigating medications for weight loss

Can't your pediatrician just prescribe one of those weight-loss pills to help your child get down to a healthy weight? After all, given that obesity causes some serious health issues, isn't it best to lose the weight fast and then address lifestyle issues that may have contributed to weight gain? Well, if you've read through much of this book, you know that we advocate long-term lifestyle changes rather than quick fixes, but some situations may call for the help of medication.

Prescription medications

Some weight-loss medications on the market are considered safe for use in kids as young as 12 years old. (The one drug that has been shown to be safest is orlistat.) Studies indicate that children who used these medications had a reduction in their BMIs (body mass index), which translates into a decrease in weight-related health risks. Some concerns that surround the use of these medications, however, include:

✔ **Long-term effects:** Doctors simply don't know how effective these medications are at keeping weight off; they aren't quite sure if teens who use these drugs will have to use them for one year, two years, or for many, many years in order to maintain their weight. Along with weight maintenance, doctors aren't sure how long the health benefits will last.

✔ **Side effects:** Many of the less-than-pleasant side effects affect the gastrointestinal tract and may be embarrassing for teens.

✔ **Underlying factors:** A child must adhere to a healthier lifestyle for best results.

We advise you to explore every other avenue of weight loss with your child's doctor before putting your child on a weight-loss pill.

If your child is prescribed one of these medications, explain to him that he doesn't get a free pass to ease up on his healthy lifestyle. Medication isn't meant to be a quick solution to what is really a lifelong process. Weight-loss drugs should be used in conjunction with a healthy diet and regular exercise, not in place of them.

One weight-loss drug that has been used in teens, sibutramine HCl monohydrate, has been associated with some serious heart-related side effects.

Although weight-loss drugs are available by prescription, in this day and age, kids may be able to secure pills via the Internet or from a friend's parent's supply. Advise your teen that these drugs should *only* be used under a doctor's supervision.

Over-the-counter medications: Teen buyer, beware

Plenty of unregulated pills are widely marketed as cures for obesity. Some are sold in pharmacies (without a prescription, of course); others are on the shelves of "health" stores; some are advertised on TV; some are sold through magazines. School-age children aren't likely to fall prey to these ads because they're unlikely to have money at their disposal and because customers must be 18 years of age to purchase most of these over-the-counter products.

Teenagers, as a group, are risk takers. Talk to your teenager about taking any kind of pill or supplement that's touted as having weight-loss benefits. Tell him that if weight loss were as simple as taking a pill, everyone in the world would be skinny! Warn him about possible side effects, which may include:

✔ Heart palpitations

✔ Faintness

✔ Electrolyte imbalances (with use of diuretics)

The real problem with these pills is that they don't address the real issues that contribute to weight gain. As a result, even if your teen were to experience weight-loss success with these medications, he's very likely to put the weight right back on after he stops taking them if he hasn't modified his diet and exercise habits. And taking medications like laxatives and ipecac for weight loss are in a whole other category of danger, which we talk about in the "Weight loss gone too far: Eating disorders" section at the end of this chapter.

Weight-loss programs and support groups

Weight loss is sometimes easier, especially for teens, with the support of a peer group. Being surrounded by other kids dealing with similar issues often helps children work through their problems and realize that they aren't the only ones facing certain obstacles.

Despite the fact that there are more overweight children now than there have been at any time in history, hooking your child into a support network for kids may not be a snap. If you don't know of any organized groups in your area, ask your child's doctor for advice. Even if she doesn't personally know of any groups, she should be able to point you in the right direction, like suggesting you call the local hospital, a particular church, a social worker, or a group like Weight Watchers or Overeaters Anonymous.

 Weight Watchers has proven their program to be an incredibly effective means of modifying those lifestyle factors that contribute to being overweight and obese. However, a child under the age of 17 can't participate in meetings without a doctor's note. And if your teen is looking for a group filled with people her own age, you may need to look elsewhere.

In most groups, a moderator plays the role of referee, making sure that no bullying occurs or overly harsh judgments are tossed around the room. Your child should expect to encounter many different personality types and be ready to support others in their times of need — support groups are a two-way street, after all. Make sure that she understands that she won't always be the center of attention; also, make sure that a shy child knows that, at some point, she'll be expected to share her feelings.

Many support groups center around sharing personal experiences and advice, but a support group is only as good as the people who run it. Before you send your child off to a support group meeting, talk at length with the moderator to get a feel for what goes on in meetings. If you hear something about radical new therapies that involve a lot of yelling at each other, or if there seems to be an emphasis on shaming one another out of their unhealthy habits, you may want to move on and find a different group, one that underscores the importance of compassion, understanding, and guidance through experience.

Supporting the family

As you research support groups for your child, you may come across groups that focus on supporting the overweight family. Again, do your research and find out what these groups are all about. Get answers to these questions:

✔ How often does the group meet?

✔ How are age groups divided?

✔ Who moderates meetings?

✔ What are the ground rules for meetings?

✔ What are the goals of the meetings?

One big issue to know more about is the kinds of topics discussed. For example, do adults talk only about their children's weight-loss struggles, or is there a forum for talking about adult weight loss as well? Does the group discuss medical breakthroughs regarding obesity or legislation regarding obesity discrimination? In order for you to get the most out of any support group, it has to deal with issues that concern you. Keep looking until you find a good fit.

Obese children deal with enough discrimination out in the real world. A support group should be an oasis from that kind of cruelty.

In the end, your child may love being surrounded by other kids dealing with similar issues, or she may find that she isn't really digging the group interaction. Let her decide what's working and what isn't in terms of a support group, and if she wants to call it quits for a while, respect that decision.

Recognizing and Dealing with Severe Weight-Related Issues

When concern over your child morphs into the type of anxiety that haunts you day and night, you probably need to intervene in an entirely new way. Obviously, an obese child deals with issues that may stem mostly from her weight, and normal, age-related stress is made worse by the condition of obesity. Most teenage girls, at one time or another, worry about finding a date for the prom, whether they're popular, and how pretty they are compared to other girls. Teenage boys, meanwhile, are concerned with where they stand in the pecking order of high school males as well as how they're viewed by the opposite sex. Obese teens have these same worries, often coupled with a devastatingly low self-esteem. These circumstances can lead to chronic, severe depression, which in turn can make a weight issue even worse.

In this section, we talk about the kinds of worries that may be keeping you awake at night and advise you on how to find help for your child. These worries include:

- ✔ The need for therapy
- ✔ Surgical options
- ✔ Eating disorders such as binge eating, bulimia, and anorexia

Therapy for psychological problems

Years ago, the medical community believed that most obese people suffered some sort of psychological trauma that was the impetus for their overeating; essentially, they were attempting to silence their nerves with food. These days, doctors believe this theory holds little credence, at least for most people. The theory surrounding obesity today is not that it's *caused* by psychological issues, but that it certainly *can cause* psychological problems.

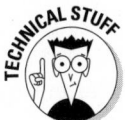

Doctors consider obesity the result of overeating, lack of exercise, and a predisposition toward becoming severely overweight. Although some childhood or even adult traumas can cause a person to seek out comfort foods, most often, this isn't the cause of true obesity.

If you believe that your child may benefit from the intervention of a therapist, she probably won't work to find some hidden, repressed trauma that may have caused him to begin overeating. Rather, she'll probably deal with the issues that are secondary to his weight gain, such as:

- ✔ Depression
- ✔ Feelings of isolation
- ✔ Anxiety or panic attacks
- ✔ Low self-esteem
- ✔ Eating disorders such as bulimia

To determine whether your child needs this type of help, first check with your child's doctor. He can give you his medical opinion on what kinds of therapy your child may benefit from and also recommend a psychologist, social worker, or psychiatrist.

You can also work the recommendation another way: Contact your medical insurer to find out about your mental health benefits. The insurance company should be able to provide you with a list of therapists who participate in your medical plan. You can then hand that list to your pediatrician, and he can give you his recommendations based on the names in front of him.

A bad therapist (or one who's completely unversed in dealing with obesity and its emotional effects) can end up doing more harm than good. Children are especially vulnerable to therapy, which is great if they're in the hands of a miracle worker and horrific if they're working with someone who's insensitive to the needs of obese children.

When you finally hook up with a qualified therapist, make sure you speak with her about her philosophies before you send your child in for a session. Ask about the following:

- ✔ What a typical session entails

- ✔ How many obese children she's worked with in the past

- ✔ What her goals are for your child

- ✔ How long she typically treats children

- ✔ How she handles emergencies (like if your child has a major panic attack when her office is closed)

A qualified therapist won't share with you any information that passes between herself and your child inside her office, but she's required by law to let you and the police know if your child is a threat to himself or to others.

Again, the wrong match between therapist and patient can do more harm than good, and whereas adults may benefit from some combative interplay in a therapist's office, depressed children generally fare much better with someone who's nurturing (at least on some level). Overweight children often end up working on accepting themselves, which, as you can imagine, is also a task best left to a nurturing, kind therapist.

Surgical options

You've no doubt heard about *gastric bypass surgery,* which is being hailed as a cure for many obese adults. Basically, in this surgery, a doctor goes in and reroutes the plumbing in the stomach. The alteration makes the stomach smaller and narrows the connection between the stomach and the small intestine. The person can no longer eat large amounts of food, and weight loss is the ultimate result of this surgery.

Gastric bypass is becoming more and more common among obese adults, and physicians are also performing the surgery in severely obese teenagers (those who have reached their full growth potential), but only after the teens have tried unsuccessfully for at least six months to lose weight.

Gastric bypass for teens isn't easy to come by. The surgery's only performed on teens in a handful of hospitals in the United States.

The screening process: Is your child a good candidate?

If you live near one of the few medical centers that perform gastric bypass on teens and you and your child are seriously considering this option, you can expect that your child will be put through a rigorous screening process, which will include:

- ✔ Evaluating his BMI to ensure he's actually obese enough to benefit from the surgery

- ✔ Evaluating any weight-related ailments such as diabetes or high blood pressure

- ✔ Evaluating his maturity level to assess whether he can handle modifying his lifestyle after the surgery

- ✔ Evaluating his home life to determine whether the family's willing to change its entire family's lifestyle in order to ensure the child's success

A child who suffers from serious health conditions such as diabetes or sleep apnea because of his weight is more likely to be approved for the surgery. If obesity merely causes your child embarrassment and difficulty performing everyday tasks, his case may not be considered serious enough for surgery.

Children have a long life ahead of them, and doctors want to make darn sure that the surgery is going to be a success. Collecting these assurances is a major part of the screening process for weight-related surgery. Doctors don't want to see your child back in the hospital in a year because he didn't change his eating habits. Failing to follow doctors' orders (like eating small, low-fat meals) after the surgery can lead to nausea, vomiting, and diarrhea.

The risks involved with surgery

Some serious risks and issues surround gastric bypass, so in the event that your child is considering gastric bypass, you both need to:

- ✔ **Realize that this is major surgery and, as such, it involves some major risks, including infection and death.** Complications can also extend a year or two after surgery, resulting in major nutritional deficiencies and (occasionally) death.

> ✔ **Acknowledge that the long-term effects of gastric bypass surgery done on teens aren't fully understood.** Your child may experience nutritional deficiencies or other problems related to the surgery when she reaches middle age, for example. The surgery is so new that there's just no telling what lies ahead.
>
> ✔ **Make sure that your child is prepared for the recovery process.** Gastric bypass isn't outpatient surgery; recovery is long, complicated, and involves sticking with a healthy diet and exercise.

One big complication of this surgery is that sometimes patients lose so much weight that they need cosmetic surgery to remove (or tuck) the excess skin they're left with.

Our point of view on this surgery is that it's a complicated procedure, and the recovery can be as complicated and dangerous as the operation itself. The long-term effects of gastric bypass haven't been fully evaluated in teen patients, so we're not comfortable recommending it as a weight-loss option. However, we present the information here so that you can make an informed decision if your teen is interested in this surgery.

Weight loss gone too far: Eating disorders

You want your child to lose enough weight to feel well, both physically and emotionally. However, obsessing over the number on the scale can be just as devastating to her self-esteem as being overweight in the first place, and it can lead to serious health issues, as well. This section informs you about some common eating disorders, why they happen, what their symptoms are, and what you can do to help in the event that your child seems to be slipping into this dark and dangerous realm of weight loss.

Exact numbers on eating disorders are unknown. These conditions carry a great deal of self-inflicted shame, so sufferers are more concerned with hiding the problem than with getting the appropriate help.

Talk to your teen if you're worried about the possibility of an eating disorder; however, because eating disorders involve considerable shame and secrecy, don't take her word for it that everything's fine. If you really suspect a problem, take her to see her doctor, and let the two of them talk alone. She's much more likely to open up to someone who effectively says, "I'm a medical professional, and I know what's going on here. Let's get you some help."

Binge eating disorder

One relatively new area of research in the area of eating disorders surrounds a condition called *binge eating disorder*. The main components of this eating disorder are:

- ✔ Frequently overeating (or "bingeing" on abnormally large amounts of food)
- ✔ A sense of being completely out of control while bingeing
- ✔ A deep feeling of regret or guilt during and after bingeing episodes
- ✔ Eating more quickly than usual during binges

Unlike bulimia, which involves bingeing and then purging oneself of the food, people who suffer from binge eating disorder don't vomit or use laxatives after a binge. For this reason, binge eating disorder often leads to obesity and all its related health issues.

Scientists are trying to determine if and how brain chemicals and normal bodily functions may play into this problem. It seems to affect more women than men and is associated with a history of depression (although depression may be the *result* of binge eating and not its cause).

Like other eating disorders, binge eating can wreak havoc on a teen's self-esteem and health. Because binge eaters feel as though they're unable to control themselves around food, they're often unable to stick with weight-loss efforts. They feel completely out of control where food is concerned and will do almost anything to secure forbidden foods (those not kept in the home); they may even binge on healthy foods. The guilt that they feel about bingeing can also result in severe depression, making them feel as though they'll never succeed in losing weight. This vicious cycle of depression and overeating continues to fuel itself on guilt.

The binge eater doesn't simply overeat. She eats abnormally large amounts of food and may eat it very quickly, feeling as though she can't get it in fast enough. So where one person may eat five slices of pizza and say, "I can't believe how I binged tonight," the true binge eater may eat an entire pizza, a half-gallon of ice cream, a bag of chips, a box of cookies, and wash it down with a gallon of milk. Obviously, that's more food than anyone should eat in one sitting, and it's the type of eating that's the hallmark of this eating disorder.

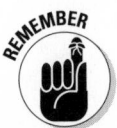

If you suspect that your teen has this disorder, don't try to handle it yourself. Therapy has been shown to be effective in treating this disorder. If you're concerned that your teen is a true binge eater, talk to her doctor to get a recommendation for a therapist who's well versed in eating disorders.

Bulimia

Like binge eaters, bulimics eat large amounts of food. However, bulimics purge themselves of the food by forcing themselves to vomit or by using laxatives. For this reason, bulimia is also called *binge-purge disorder.*

Girls are more vulnerable to bulimia than boys are, although the causes of this disorder are unknown. Bulimia is associated with some very serious physical side effects, including:

- ✔ Dehydration, possibly resulting in faintness
- ✔ Electrolyte imbalances, possibly resulting in an irregular heartbeat
- ✔ Damage to kidneys and liver
- ✔ Esophageal tearing and rupture
- ✔ Intestinal damage and upset
- ✔ Dependence on laxatives
- ✔ Damage to tooth enamel from repeated vomiting
- ✔ Severe depression

Unlike anorexics (see the following section), bulimics often maintain a normal weight; some are even overweight, so you can't look to rapid and unusual weight loss as a sign that something's amiss. Teens may become entangled in bulimia after they've lost weight because they know that they don't want to gain the weight back but feel powerless when faced with food. Bingeing and purging seems to work for a time, until they realize that they can't stop and experience a sense of hopelessness and depression.

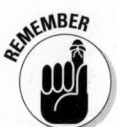

Bulimia isn't something that you can treat at home. If you think that your teen is struggling with bulimia, find a therapist for her to work with. She needs to regain a sense of control over her life in order for the bingeing to come to a stop.

Anorexia

Anorexia, an aversion to food and obsession with weight loss, usually isn't something that formerly obese teens struggle with; they seem to be more predisposed to the bingeing disorders addressed in preceding sections. However, because bulimia is occasionally linked to anorexia, we discuss the disorder briefly here.

Like other eating disorders, anorexia affects more females than males, and usually begins as a response to some sort of stress. Anorexics are usually characterized as perfectionists, so concerned about their physical appearance that they'll go to any lengths to make sure they don't gain an ounce. Symptoms of anorexia are usually easier to spot than bingeing symptoms, which are usually kept under wraps by the sufferer. Anorexia can result in:

✓ Extreme weight loss, to the point where the teen looks unwell

✓ Anemia

✓ Dehydration

✓ Dry skin and brittle hair

✓ Cold extremities and low blood pressure

✓ Irregular heartbeat

✓ Loss of teeth

✓ Cessation of menstruation

✓ A light, downy covering of hair over the body (called *lanugo*)

The anorexic truly believes that she is overweight, even after she's dropped down to a dangerously low body weight. Regardless of her size, she fears food and refuses to eat it.

Torn between food and the "perfect" figure

It's no wonder that eating disorders plague women especially. Society is obsessed not just with weight and appearance but also with food! Food is everywhere we turn, so you're supposed to eat food, love food, *and* maintain the perfect figure. What a confusing message for a teen to sort out! In addition to being hammered with these messages, by nature, teens are risk takers. They don't believe that the natural consequences of their actions (especially risks to their health) are going to catch up with them, so to a teenager, using laxatives to control or maintain her weight may seem like a great idea.

Chapter 15

Keeping the Weight Off

. . . .

In This Chapter

▶ Finding ways to keep up the good work

▶ Dealing with weight-loss related changes

▶ Praising children's weight-loss accomplishments

▶ Looking to the future

. . . .

*L*osing weight is a major accomplishment for an obese child. As she makes significant strides toward her goal weight, you can see the pride in her face as she starts to feel as though all the effort really *is* going to pay off.

However, keeping the weight from coming back full force takes equal effort. Obesity isn't a hit-and-run problem, where your child drops the weight and is home free for the rest of her life. Anyone who has lived a sedentary lifestyle with bad eating habits is at risk for falling back into those old routines because they're *easy.* It's so much easier for your child to sit and watch TV rather than go outside to play, just as it's easier for you to pick up pizza and wings rather than light up the grill for some fish and veggies for dinner. If scientists could come up with a way for every man, woman, and child to be fit by sitting on the couch and snacking, how many of us would bother to venture outside for some fresh air and exercise or wash the lettuce for a salad?

There's bound to be a period of time before your child reaches her goal weight when everyone in the household just gets bored with the healthiness. They want to go back to the way things were — the way they *should* be, in their opinion, and the way they're *going* to be when you come back to your senses (or so they think). Stand firm when faced with such dissension in the ranks. Just as you've led your child to the threshold of weight loss, you're going to see her (and the rest of the family) all the way — to an entirely new lifestyle.

Maintaining Positive Change

The hardest thing about losing weight and keeping it off is that the job never ends, especially for a formerly obese child. Think about what kinds of habits caused your child to become overweight in the first place: Eating large quantities of fattening foods, leading a sedentary lifestyle, and perhaps even feeling too far gone or too scared (or both) to do anything about it. Now put these habits and emotions into perspective: Isn't it much easier to grab a handful of cookies and a can of soda for a snack — especially when you're feeling blue or bored — than to prepare a veggie pita or munch a fibrous piece of fruit? Doesn't it feel good to settle in on the couch after a long day of sitting at your desk? (And doesn't the prospect of taking a walk seem like a real drag in comparison?) Isn't it simple to get tangled up in depression and to start feeling as though you can never begin to crawl out from what-ever trouble you've found yourself in, and isn't it easy to soothe those feel-ings with a hot fudge sundae?

The reason so many children (and adults) in this country are obese is because it's easy to get that way — much easier than it is to get healthy and easier than establishing and sticking with healthier habits. Formerly obese children may have an especially hard time maintaining good habits because they've come to associate food with so many other emotions: sadness, happi-ness, boredom, guilt, nervousness. And because these kids have been eating at all times of the day and night, it may be hard for them to accept structured meals and snacks. If your child has been settling down in front of the TV just before bedtime with a box of something for as long as you can remember, it's part of his nighttime routine. It gives him comfort and relaxes him before he heads off to dreamland. And changing that routine is like taking a pacifier away from a baby.

If your child has a hard time giving up his nighttime snack, replace it with something healthy like fruit or a whole-wheat bagel. If the swap doesn't work, change his whole bedtime routine so that the absence of his snack isn't so obvious — or heartbreaking. In fact, you can use this time to institute newer, healthier habits. For example, instead of spending the evening watching videos with your child, take a walk together or play outside just before bath time, or snuggle up together with a good book (rather than a tasty snack) at bedtime.

Taking things one day at a time

Weight loss for an obese child can go one of two ways:

- He may still be young enough so that the changes you've introduced into the house become second nature to him. He may never look back longingly on his former ways.

- He may be so set in his ways that, for him, keeping the weight off is like an alcoholic staying away from liquor. He has good days and bad days, but weight loss is something he can absolutely conquer.

Obviously, you hate to think of your child struggling with addiction, because being hooked on *anything* — whether it's booze or drugs or food — can be a living hell. And trying to give the addiction up, even though you know it's literally killing you, can be even worse, at least initially.

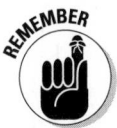

The hard thing about leaving an addiction behind (aside from any physical dependencies) is the realization that the habit gave you comfort and made you feel good (at least some of the time). Kicking a habit reminds people of their shortcomings — at least until they've been over their addictions for a good amount of time and can acknowledge how strong they are and how far they've come.

The worst thing about a food addiction is that your child can no longer eat the foods he's come to depend on (for comfort, to pass time, and so on), and he can't make a clean break from food altogether. You make all the difference in how well your child does in the long run; he needs you to be consistent on a daily basis. Sure, it's fine to celebrate a birthday with cake, and it's all right for the entire family to relax together and watch some TV now and then. But if you start to feel as though things are spiraling down into unhealthy territory again, you have to say, "Enough!" and pull everyone back up to where they should be. You need to regularly evaluate how his new, healthy routines are going and correct them as soon as you see them deteriorating. Clean out the pantry from time to time and toss out any unhealthy foods that have (somehow) found their way into your home. Encourage your child to make his own breakfast, lunch, and snacks while you stand by silently, ready to reeducate him on the finer points of nutrition if need be. Help him measure out portion sizes and/or decipher food labels, for example.

Keeping your guard up without going overboard

When it comes to your continued observations and corrections about your family's healthy lifestyle, you may start to feel like a sentry at the pantry door, and what's worse, you may start acting that way. Your kids may start to avoid the issue of food and weight when you ask, and you may start to resemble an unsympathetic drill sergeant rather than a concerned parent.

It's very easy to fall into compulsive behavior where weight loss is concerned: Counting calories, fat grams, and time spent exercising start out as necessities but can turn into obsessions. And the very last thing in the world you want to do is to turn your child into a nervous, obsessive weight-watcher. She's more likely to suffer from other eating issues (like anorexia and/or bulimia) when weight and food become the only things she's interested in and when she thinks she has to keep the weight off in order to please you.

Being the one in charge of maintaining your family's healthier lifestyle is a tough balancing act. You know that you couldn't have helped your child become healthier without getting tough, so how can she continue to succeed if you lose your edge? It's not really a matter of losing your edge but rather remembering that no matter how old your child is (from toddler to teenager), she's still a child who needs a consistent, balanced adult to keep her on the right track. Children tend to mimic what they see, so if you behave in an overly aggressive manner where your child's weight is concerned, you may get that attitude thrown right back at you. In the case of a teenager, you also may incite a rebellion, and then all the strides your child has made are for naught.

And what about the worry? Will you ever be able to look at your child and breathe a sigh of relief, thinking that she's completely free of the shackles of obesity? Probably not. You can be proud (and elated) that she's lost the weight, but you may never fully let go of those obesity-related concerns. Having those worries in the back of your mind shows that you're an educated and concerned parent; you're determined to do everything you can to keep your child from backsliding *because* of your concern.

If you toss all your worry out the window and assume that because your child has come so far, excess weight will never bother her again, you're less likely to recognize the early signs of backsliding. You're also more likely to allow bad habits to reenter the home.

Your child's weight loss should be about your child pleasing herself and keeping herself healthy. She's so much more than the number on the scale. When she successfully loses weight, help her find new interests and activities to take the place of her old bad habits. If she can fill her time productively, she's less likely to fall back into her unhealthy routines, and you're less likely to lose your mind worrying that she will.

Comparing the past and present

Feeling as though your child's weight loss is only a temporary respite from her weight problem is normal. Because you've been dealing with the obesity for quite some time, you're bound to think at one time or another that he's going to be a statistical failure. You want him to succeed so badly that it breaks your heart to know that he may not. Plus, this whole process is taking so long that you can't believe he'll ever reach his goal weight. And if *you* feel that way, you can't imagine that he's feeling much differently.

Keeping your chin up during these less-than-hopeful times is important because relaying a feeling of hopelessness or a "What's the use?" attitude to your child doesn't help him continue to succeed. Even if he's still a long way from his goal weight, things are going well as long as he's moving in the right direction.

Losing a substantial amount of weight takes a long time, and maintaining a high level of enthusiasm throughout the entire process is difficult. Just keep telling yourself — and your child — that slow weight loss is more likely to be permanent weight loss.

Compare your child now to the way he was several months ago (or whenever it was you adopted a healthier lifestyle). Note the significant differences between then and now. If he's made great strides in this healthy new lifestyle:

✔ He's feeling better about himself emotionally.

✔ He's feeling better physically.

✔ He may be doing better socially.

✔ His personality may have undergone a big change — for the better — because of all the other changes.

Remembering how far your child's already come when you know he still has a long way to go can be rough, and playing cheerleader every day for a year or more, especially when your new lifestyle starts to feel like just another routine, can be even worse. However, these are the times when you should look back on the family's old, unhealthy lifestyle and ask yourself if you're willing to go back. To regain your energy and motivation, recall everything you've learned about obesity and its health risks, and remember your child at his lowest point of self-esteem.

You can't take care of the family if you haven't taken the time to care for yourself. Your child is less likely to maintain his weight loss and continue with his healthy lifestyle if you don't stick with this program, also. It may not seem fair, but it's the truth. The family that sticks together keeps the weight off — together.

Evaluating what your child has learned

In order to maintain your child's positive weight-loss results, you have to remain on the ball as far as your family's lifestyle goes; you can't let down your guard to the point where you no longer take an interest in what your child eats or how she spends her time. However, she needs to take as active a role as possible in her own life, too. Now, you may think, "She's losing the weight; she's outside playing with her friends; of course she's taking an active role!" She's made a great start, but if you were to stop nudging her toward the right decisions, would she continue on in a healthy direction, or would she think to herself, "Hey, I'm free to do whatever I want now!"?

Because everyone in the household has to eat every day, asking your child questions about her choices in an appropriate context is a breeze. And because activity should also be a regular occurrence in everyone's lives, raising that issue shouldn't seem odd, either. You need to bring these topics up to your child in order to assess how much she's learned about healthy lifestyles and to make sure she's not just going through the motions. Now, don't get us wrong — the motions are great. Most kids begin the weight-loss process by doing what they're told. Eventually, however, as we discuss in Chapter 12, your child will be faced with outside influences and find herself in situations where she has to make important choices.

In order to gauge whether your child is developing the skills and knowledge she needs to maintain weight loss and an overall healthier lifestyle, look for the following sorts of behavior modifications:

✔ An increase in her intake of fresh fruits and veggies

✔ A decrease in her intake of high-sugar, high-fat foods

✔ An increase in her activity level

✔ A decrease in TV viewing or other sedentary activities

✔ An increase in interests outside of the home

✔ A decrease in her self-esteem issues

✔ An increase in the amount of positive communication between yourself and your child

✔ A decrease in tension between the two of you

Your child trots off to school each day to learn about science, math, and spelling. When she returns home, *you* become the teacher, imparting knowledge about living a life of wellness. And just as teachers in the primary grades have a higher-level involvement with their pupils, you have to hold your child's hand in the beginning of the program, but as she learns more, you can back off a bit and let her make her own decisions.

What if you realize that after months of effort, nothing has really sunk into this child's mind? What if your work and dedication has actually taken the responsibility out of her hands and made her dependent on you? As long as the numbers on the scale are headed in the right direction, she's playing a part in improving her health. You just need to reconstruct parts of your plan in order to get her more involved (and this goes for children of all ages). Here are a few recommendations for getting your child back on the learning track:

✔ **Instead of handing her an already-prepared snack, give her choices.** Even a toddler can decide whether she wants applesauce or a cut-up banana, pieces of bagel or pretzels. By providing choices, you let her know that she has options, that she can make choices between good foods and other good foods, and — most important — that you aren't going to make every decision in her life. An older child should be able to narrow healthy choices down for herself.

✔ **Let older children help out in the preparation of healthy meals so that they learn what's bad and what's good.** Explain to your child the differences between grilled foods and fried foods, for example, and why you've been preparing the family meals in a certain way. Show her that creating healthy foods isn't difficult. (So that she doesn't get overwhelmed and frustrated, choose easy recipes when she's starting out with you in the kitchen.)

✔ **When your child has a solid idea of what's healthy and what isn't, work together to create weekly menus.** Let her look through cookbooks and choose meals that pique her interest. Tell her that many not-so-healthy recipes can be modified into low-fat meals. (Chapter 9 is a good resource for ways to cut back on fat in your favorite recipes.)

Whether you do everything for your child or teach her to do it for herself, she's going to lose weight, at least initially. But if she has a deeper understanding of the process — for example, which foods are high in fat, which are better choices, and how and why you prepare her meals a certain way — she's more likely to carry that information into her daily decision-making process. It's never too late to start teaching her these things, but the sooner she learns, the better off she'll be in the long run.

The scoop on calories

Calories, calories, calories. You hear about them all the time, but do you know what they are? A *calorie* is a measure of the potential energy a unit of food contains. If you eat a banana containing 100 calories, you put a certain amount of stored energy into your body. In order for those calories not to be stored as fat, you have to use that energy through physical activity.

The body — especially a growing body — needs a certain amount of calories each day just to maintain its proper functioning, so you can't just say, "Well, we'll just cut out calories all together, and my child will lose weight easily." Caloric recommendations vary according to a person's age, body-frame size, and activity level. But healthy eating doesn't just mean taking in the right number of calories. There's also a difference in the type of calories a person can ingest. Calories that come from fatty foods are more dense and more easily converted into fat in the body than calories that come from other sources. The fact that not all calories are created equal is just one reason why counting calories can be misleading.

Even if you think your child is learning a lot about weight loss, avoid taking the topic too far by discussing and teaching her about calories (for a calorie lesson, see the sidebar "The scoop on calories"). Drilling calorie counts into a child's head often results in the replacement of one eating problem with another (usually bulimia or, in extreme cases, anorexia). This kind of information is also probably more complex than your child can understand. You'd think a calorie is a calorie, but there's a big difference between a calorie that comes from a protein-rich food, for example, and one that comes from a fatty source. You can ingest 200 calories from either type of food, but the calories from fat convert themselves into body fat much more easily, and that's bad news for someone on a weight-loss plan.

Being alert for signs of backsliding

Backsliding, falling off the wagon . . . call it whatever you want — it's when your child makes great progress in losing weight and then falters and starts putting weight back on. Backsliding, which we discuss further in Chapter 11, happens to adults and kids, even when you think you've done everything to prevent it. A backsliding child is at the mercy of parents who have put all kinds of effort into revamping the entire family's lifestyle. The kid probably feels bad enough already about putting a few pounds back on, but when his parents make him feel as though he's disappointed them personally, he has even more self-esteem issues to deal with.

If the numbers on the scale start going up again, *don't* freak out. You need to get to the bottom of what's happened in order to help your child get back on the losing track (and that's meant in only the most positive way). Some questions to ponder and issues to consider include:

- ✔ **How are things in the cafeteria?** If he's packing a healthy lunch, is he actually eating it or chucking it and purchasing cheeseburgers and chili fries every day?

- ✔ **What kinds of activities has he been involved in?** Losing weight effectively takes a combination of activity and healthy food choices. Perhaps he's not enjoying whatever activity he's been involved in and needs to explore other options.

- ✔ **How's his mindset?** Is he feeling hopeless or resentful of this new lifestyle? Is he longing for the old days of sitting around and eating in front of the TV? He may need some gentle reminders about the long-term health effects of obesity (see Chapter 3).

- ✔ **What do his friends have to say about his weight loss?** Is he being teased because he won't dive into the bag of chips at a pal's house? Peer pressure is a powerful force in a child's life. Reassure him that losing weight is the best thing for *him,* and his friends shouldn't enter this picture.

We understand how, faced with a child's backsliding, you can start to lose heart. After all, weight loss isn't the only thing going on in your busy life, and you can't follow your child around every minute of the day to ensure he's making the right decisions. But you have to remain a constant source of unconditional love and support for your child, even when you're feeling upset or scared or angry with him for not following through in every aspect of his weight-loss agenda. It may not be the only thing going on in your household, but weight loss is one of the most important things you'll ever be faced with correcting. We're talking about your child's health. You've got a limited window of opportunity to mitigate the damage his weight will eventually do to him and lead him *away* from a future filled with illness, such as heart disease and type 2 diabetes.

Childhood obesity experts recommend a weekly weigh-in session for kids on a weight-loss program. Fluctuations in weight over the course of a single day are common, but stepping on the scale every morning or evening can be a frustrating (and disheartening) experience for your child — and for you, too. Instead, let your child pick a specific time of day one day during the week for weigh-in. (Weighing in before breakfast one Monday and after dinner the following Monday won't give you the truest weight-loss readings.)

Do your best to be encouraging even when the scale doesn't help matters. And remember that permanent weight loss takes time. If your child acknowledges that he's made a couple of mistakes in judgment during the past week that have resulted in a backslide, that's *good*. He's learning what types of behaviors result in weight gain and seeing the results of bad choices, right in front of his eyes. Ensure him that he'll do better next time, and then drop it.

Seeing Your Child Through Major Change

Every stage of childhood has its downside. A kid in elementary school wants to be more independent, a high schooler often wants independence she's not ready for emotionally, and toddlers are simply ornery little people sometimes who just want everything.

Parenting children is hard enough without adding the stress of weight loss into the picture. When your obese child starts to drop pounds, you may sense that she's changing — for better or for worse. Of course, change is a normal part of growing up. Most children, at some point, struggle with their identity, test their parents' limits and try their parents' patience. Slimmed-down kids are faced with unique challenges, however. Formerly obese children may find themselves suddenly accepted by the very peers who have shunned them for so long. In addition, a child who's never had a social life is often ill equipped to jump into peer group settings and make all the right moves after she's lost a significant amount of weight. This section will give you advice on how to see your child through these types of major transitions without driving her — or yourself — crazy.

Dealing with a new identity

Now that your child has started to lose weight, you'll hopefully start to see a change in her personality for the better. She should be feeling better about herself physically and emotionally. She may be making new friends and branching out socially. In fact, she may seem like a different kid altogether (and that's not always a welcome sort of change when she seems a little full of herself).

To put these changes in perspective, think about what she's been through. Overweight people of any age are often subjected to cruel remarks and unkind behavior, and your child lived for several years (at least) with the burden of being grossly overweight. She wasn't able to participate in activities with her peers, and, as a result, she may have been an outcast. Now all of that is changing. She's being accepted — at last! With this acceptance, she's learning how to behave around other kids her age; what's more, she's trying to figure out how to *be* like other kids her age.

 An obese child who has spent years being shunned by her classmates may not know how to behave when they start accepting her. Give her time to figure out who she really is — but don't back down on rules you set for her own good.

Setting rules for their own good

You probably already have rules in place in your home, such as no swearing, no smoking, and no drinking. Maybe these activities were never an issue because your child never had contact with anyone else, and he certainly never went anywhere. Now that he's becoming more social and trying new things in his new body, stick to your guns and don't relax the rules. Losing an immense amount of weight, although it's a great accomplishment, can result in a scary change of identity for a child, and it won't help him adjust if he feels as though he's been tossed out into a new world of endless possibilities and no one's keeping watch. If it was heartbreaking for you to watch him be left out of dances and parties all these years, you may be very, very excited that he's finally going to have some sort of social life. Just keep everything in perspective: He's still a child, and like any child, he needs guidelines and rules.

 Here's one truism about children: They'll always try to push their limits and break your rules. Kids who don't have any rules to break are the ones who often end up in real trouble because they need something to rebel against (and they often end up fighting societal authorities, like teachers and cops, instead of parental ones).

Putting your child's change in perspective

Some of the change that a formerly obese child experiences is a normal part of growing up. Preteens and teenagers aren't always the easiest people to deal with. Their hormone levels are all out of whack, which makes them moody, and when you throw the emotional issue of weight and weight loss into the mix, you may feel as though you've created a monster.

No matter how your child is behaving at the moment, you can bet the farm that only *some* of it is related to his weight loss, which is why it's vital that you keep the lines of communication open. Imagine this scenario: Your preteen son was teased for years by a group of popular kids that he (naturally) came to hate. Now that he's lost weight, these same kids aren't being so mean to him; in fact, during lunch and gym class, they're actually being pretty cool, talking to him, letting him in on their jokes, and treating him like he's someone worthy of their attention.

Of course this switch confuses your child. He knows that these kids haven't always been nice to him, so now he doesn't know what to make of their attention. He may be so eager for their acceptance that he begins behaving in ways that he knows are wrong (like making fun of other kids who are obese, just like he used to be). But of course, he wants to have friends — every kid does. And almost every kid struggles with befriending bad influences at one time or another.

If he can talk to you openly, assure him that problems with peers are a normal part of growing up and that he'd probably feel the same confusion even if he didn't used to be obese. Remind him that overcoming obesity taught him to make good choices in his life and he can carry that lesson over into social settings now because he'll face more big decisions as his peers accept him as a "normal" kid.

Seeing a change in your child's body that results in a change in his social life is exciting — for him and for you. Just do your best to make sure that now that he's safe from the perils of obesity he doesn't get himself into other kinds of trouble.

Accepting newfound independence

As your child starts losing weight, the best situation you can hope for is a happy balance between your involvement in your child's weight loss and her independence in the same venture. It's a tough row for you to hoe when your daughter orders you to stop fixing her meals, to stop accompanying her to the scale on weigh-in day, and to stop talking to her about her weight. Period.

"Well!," you think. "That's a fine thank-you after all I've done for her!" Don't take it too personally. She needs to build this kind of self-confidence in her own abilities to take care of herself. Do you really want her hanging around your kitchen at age 30, waiting for you to make her lunch?

Girls and their mothers are particularly hard on one another where weight is concerned. Although your daughter may have desperately needed your help when she was obese, even then, the two of you may have had a hard time agreeing on a weight-loss plan. If you're also overweight (or if you've lost a large amount of weight), you may be communicating unspoken messages to your child without even realizing it. (Do you fret when she weighs in or wince when she opens the refrigerator door?)

Any parent who has a child with a health problem (and obesity falls into that category) tends to be a bit overprotective at times. You've been worried about this child for so long that you don't know when it's okay to stop. And with obesity, it's so easy for her to fall back into old habits. Some studies even suggest that obese children who lose weight may tend to gain it back more easily in the future.

So where do you draw the line? You have no intention of standing by and allowing her to undo all the good you've both worked so hard to achieve. Well, you have to back off a little or else you risk mutiny. Show her you trust her by easing up on the weight issue. You'll always be able to discuss food in some context (she has to eat, and someone has to shop for groceries), but for now, do your best to avoid specific questions like, "What did you eat for lunch today?" and "You haven't been drinking soda at Amy's house after school, have you?"

Your child may be very eager to put the past behind her. If she's conquered her weight problem, she doesn't want to associate herself with her former overweight self anymore. You need to recognize that and stop asking her questions that only make her feel that you're dragging her back into an emotional place that she doesn't want to even think about anymore.

Let her embrace her independence and her new self. She has a lot to be proud of and a lot to look forward to, so allow her to make her own choices and decisions. You'll *always* be watching out for problems with her weight, but you don't have to voice those concerns. If she starts putting the weight back on, then it's time to actively step in and be encouraging, not disparaging. Until then, let go and let her find her own way. She may just surprise you.

Celebrating Your Child's Accomplishment

What kind of celebration is appropriate when your child reaches her goal weight? Is it wrong to make a big deal out of her success? What if she backslides? Will a big acknowledgement now only make her feel worse if she puts the weight back on?

Yes, make a big deal out of her accomplishment because it's worth celebrating! She's on her way to a happier, healthier, brighter future unencumbered by the burden of extra weight and all the miseries (both physical and emotional) associated with it.

Obviously, you don't want to center this celebration around food, so get creative and do something that your child will enjoy. Encourage an activity that has somewhat healthy benefits, whether they're social or physical. For example, don't send mixed messages by renting five videos for her to watch in one weekend. Avoid promoting her old habits, which are so easy to slip right back into. Consider the following celebration ideas (and reshape them as needed to suit your own child).

✔ **Let loose with friends:** Has she been bugging you to have a big sleepover? Now's a great time for it. She's feeling more comfortable in her own skin and may need opportunities to strengthen her social skills. Be sure to supply plenty of healthy snacks, and limit the videos to one or two. Encourage other activities, like crafts or games.

✔ **Get sporty:** Has she been asking for a ski pass or a new bike? Awesome. If her sporting heart's desire is too expensive, encourage her to join local sports games or other activities. You want her to enjoy and pursue social *and* physical activities.

✔ **Try some new clothes:** Is there some article of clothing she's wanted for a long time and could never wear when she was heavy? Maybe she was never comfortable in jeans, and now she's asking for a stylish pair. She's starting to feel like a regular kid now, and she wants to look the part, too, so take her on a shopping trip.

✔ **Have a mini-makeover:** Does she want to try a new hairstyle or pierce her ears? These minor cosmetic alterations are often rites of passage for kids. In addition, your child may want to leave her old self behind as much as possible. Let her do it on the condition that any changes she makes are gradual. She's undergone a lot of physical changes during the past several months and should take things slowly whenever possible.

Let your child know how proud you are of her determination to stick to the program, and then take time to congratulate yourself. Plenty of parents don't recognize the signs or seriousness of childhood obesity (even when the signs are obvious to everyone else). You've done your absolute best by this child, and that's the mark of a truly great parent.

Your family has learned so much throughout this weight loss process, and you're all now well educated in the finer points of losing weight and keeping it off for good. As we say in the "Being alert for signs of backsliding" section earlier in the chapter, backsliding does happen, but children whose parents are involved in establishing and enforcing healthy rules around the house do much better in the long term than children whose parents don't do these things.

Looking to a Happier, Healthier Future

Realistically speaking, what measure of long-term success can you expect from your child's weight loss? Because childhood obesity is such a common health problem these days, you'd think an abundance of information would be available. Shockingly, few studies have been done on how obese children fare in the long term where weight loss is concerned. As we discuss in

Chapter 3, doctors are very concerned about the health effects of obesity on children as they grow into adults, but so far, that concern hasn't trickled down into funding studies examining how successful obese children are at keeping the weight off.

However, Dr. Leonard H. Epstein, an expert in the field of childhood obesity, has conducted several studies on the role that parents play in their child's weight loss. He's found that children whose parents join them in some sort of educational weight-loss program are more likely to lose the weight to begin with *and* to keep it off years down the line.

Years ago, pediatricians spoke directly to obese children about losing weight and eating healthy foods, gym teachers talked to them about increasing physical activity, and teachers took special interest in their social needs. Nowadays, most adults who deal with children realize that in order to get a message through to a child, they have to go through the parent. Parents usually have more of an influence on their children than any other authority figure in that child's life.

You have more power over your child's long-term weight-loss success than you may realize; recognize that fact and use it to her advantage. To do this, you can't simply be involved. You have to commit to leading a healthy life. Learn about nutrition (see Chapter 7 for help); know how to plan a menu (check out Chapter 8 for menu planning tips, Chapter 9 for cooking information, and Appendix A near the end of this book for meal ideas); and have a solid plan in place for getting and keeping everyone active (read Chapter 10 for exercise tips).

Above all else, remember that you have a tremendous amount of power and influence over your child. You largely control how well (or how poorly) your child eats. Your encouragement has a tremendous impact on how she feels about exercise. Become your child's primary source of information and support by keeping yourself interested and educated on the subject (by reading up on the latest studies and trying out new recipes and activities). If *you* can stick with it, your child will be more likely to succeed — by simply following along with your plan.

Part IV
The Part of Tens

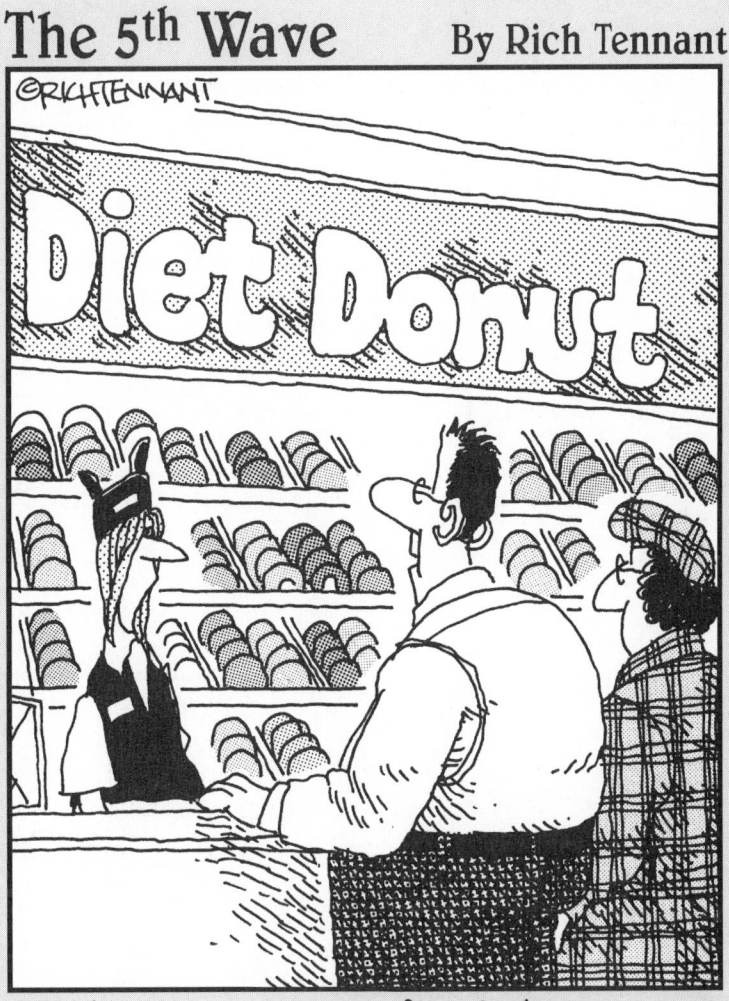

The 5th Wave   By Rich Tennant

"I'll have two lettuce filled, three carrot glazed, five celery frosted,..."

In this part . . .

Want to know ten good ways to get everyone off the couch, or ten different ideas for cutting back on fat? They're in this part, along with some other fun lists that will help you keep your family's health lifestyle on track! This part is a fun, easy read — just the type of thing you'll have time for on a crazy-busy night when everyone's headed in different directions. Take a peek at these lists whenever you need an idea, some inspiration, or a reminder about why you changed the family's way of life in the first place!

Chapter 16

Ten Reasons Lifestyle Changes Will Make a Difference

. . . .

In This Chapter

▶ Enjoying better health

▶ Letting go of old routines

▶ Discovering new personality traits and abilities

▶ Looking to a healthy future

. . . .

When you first begin changing the way you shop, the way you cook, the way your family eats, and the ways in which everyone in the household spends their time, it seems like you have a long, long road ahead and that permanent change and its positive effects are light years away. Well, they aren't. Now, don't get us wrong; we're not saying that any of this is going to be easy. But when the family makes significant strides in beating back old habits, you'll probably be amazed at how happy you all are to have left the old ways behind. Yes, it takes a lot of hard work and dedication to get there, and at times it may seem as though you'll never reach that point. This chapter gives you a glimpse into the great changes you can expect to see for your child in the future.

Increasing Self-Esteem

An obese child has a hard time fitting in with her peers; she may be the subject of teasing and cruel comments at school or in public. When she starts losing weight and feeling better both physically and emotionally, you'll see a change in her mood. She may become more outgoing and show interest in activities you never would have dreamed she'd want to try! At the very least, her attitude about things in general will be markedly improved when she feels good about herself. If you've spent years worrying about this child, this change in her outlook on life will be a relief — like letting go of a deep breath you didn't even know you were holding.

Getting Rid of Aches

Excess weight has a tremendous negative effect on bones and ligaments. Obese children can suffer from aches and pains that prevent them from partaking in physical activities. This problem can be so serious, in fact, that the shinbones in obese children can become deformed from the amount of weight they bear (see Chapter 3 for more). If permanent damage like this hasn't already occurred, then a child will feel her orthopedic aches and pains start to subside when she starts losing weight. The better she feels physically, the more active she can become. And the more she *can* do, the more she'll *want* to do.

Elevating Energy

An overweight child may have a hard time getting involved in any kind of activity because he has no energy. The foods he's been eating probably provide little in the way of significant nutrition, and his body just isn't up to the task of being active — at least not yet. It takes time, but leading a healthy lifestyle results in an increase of energy. It's only natural: Vitamins and minerals *work* inside the body; their job is to make us feel well. (For the scoop on nutrition, check out Chapter 7.) Being active may wear your child out at first, but as his muscles become accustomed to regular exercise, you should see a definite change — a decrease in the panting and huffing and the ability to play for longer periods of time. And the very best part of increased energy levels — the desire to get outside and *move*.

Opening the Lines of Communication

Enforcing the no-eating-in-front-of-the-TV rule in your household may just encourage everyone to actually — gasp! — talk to each other at mealtimes. Even if you don't sense any major communication gaps in your family unit, you'll probably be surprised by how sitting down to a meal together really makes everyone feel connected, just by *being* together for a period of time. You discuss problems and share happy times, and everyone feels as though they belong to something solid — the family. And if the kids help out with the preparation of the meal, that's a great time to subtly educate them on the finer points of healthy eating. (Chapter 11 has lots of ideas for initiating enjoyable family mealtimes.)

Looking for New Adventures

When your family's looking for new ways to eat and new opportunities to become active, new worlds open up to you. For example, places you never would have thought of visiting before are now your family's weekend stomping (and hiking) grounds, and you're regularly cooking foods you never tried before! When overall health improves, energy increases, and life seems brand new. You won't believe all the things your family has been missing. Don't fight it; get out there and explore, explore, explore! (Read Chapter 10 for tips on getting the whole family involved in exercise, and see the Appendix A for some interesting low-fat menu options.)

Finding Hidden Talents

In addition to discovering places that you never knew existed, by increasing your activity levels, your whole family is likely to uncover abilities that they may not have known they had. After all, your son probably won't discover that he has an aptitude for ice skating if he's sitting in front of the TV every day, and your daughter may never know that she's a great swimmer if she never tries it. And as for you, you may find out that, contrary to everything you've believed all these years, you're a great cook! In order to learn about yourselves, you have to try out as many activities as you're capable of . . . and see what happens.

Inspiring and Helping Others

Your child is likely to have great sympathy and empathy for other overweight kids. When he's down to a healthy weight range, he may feel as though he wants to help everyone overcome their weight problems! Although it may not be a great idea to let him set up a soapbox in the yard, if you find some sort of weight-loss advocacy group in your area, he may make a great peer counselor for an overweight child who truly needs a pal and a role model.

He Loses, You Lose (The Worry), Everyone Wins

Here's a simple way to look at your child's weight loss: When he's at a healthy weight and he knows all about making healthy choices, he's at lower risk for a lot of health problems. He's also at lower risk for feeling like an outcast among his peers, and he's more likely to have the confidence to go out and develop his natural talents, which translates into a better chance for a happy, secure future. Now, we're not saying that losing weight is a cure-all for every problem your child will ever encounter, but let's face facts: Growing up is hard enough without the added burden of being obese. If your child can get rid of the weight, he'll have licked a significant problem, which will only bolster his confidence when he's faced with other dilemmas. And when he can successfully deal with anything life throws his way, *you'll* sleep better at night. Honestly.

Achieving Better Long-Term Health

It's almost inconceivable to think a young adult in his 20s could be at high risk for heart disease and stroke, but that's the case more and more as the youth of this country become heavier. An obese child is at risk for developing type 2 diabetes, high blood pressure, asthma, sleep apnea, and a myriad of other health problems and dealing with these problems for the rest of his or her life. (Flip to Chapter 3 for more on obesity-related health problems.)

Dropping weight improves both short- and long-term health. Your 8-year-old could be laying the groundwork in his body *right now* that will contribute to future health problems. Changing your family's lifestyle can prevent and sometimes even correct health issues that are related to excess weight.

Looking Good!

Of course, a healthy lifestyle is primarily about health. But when the family is eating healthy foods, being more active, learning about their hidden talents, and feeling better about life in general, you'll start to see more smiles more often. You'll catch a little twinkle in your son's eyes, and your daughter may suddenly start paying more attention to her appearance as she gets ready for school. These changes are in addition to the physical changes associated with weight loss, and all the changes add up and make your child feel better both emotionally and physically. You're sure to see the glow that a person gets when he's comfortable in his own skin — and that's what's really important.

Chapter 17

Ten Tips for Maintaining Weight Loss

As you well know, changing your family's lifestyle is no easy feat, and it's not as though you can circle a day on your calendar when you expect to be "finished" with the task. A healthy lifestyle is a lifelong goal and an ongoing process. Stressful events or boredom may knock your child off the healthy-living track, and he may want to revert right back to his old ways. After your child loses weight and is feeling and looking healthier, how can you help him maintain his enthusiasm and energy level so that you never have to start this whole process over again? This chapter provides some useful tips for keeping everyone in a healthy state of mind and body.

Turning Away from Temptation

To keep your child on track with his healthy lifestyle, teach him to walk away from tempting situations — literally, if possible. There's nothing weak or cowardly about removing oneself from a potentially harmful situation. If your adolescent sees a cake in a bakery window, for example, all he has to do is make his feet take him somewhere else. Teach your school-age child how to say no politely but with conviction so that when he has to make the right decision, like when he's offered an ice cream sundae at a friend's house, he isn't pressured into accepting the treat by a well-meaning adult. (Chapter 12 offers more advice that you can give your child on how to resist temptation.)

Keeping Moving

Teach your child that *all* activity counts, whether it's 10 minutes or 30 minutes at a time. The point is to move more *throughout* the day, and the goal is to fit 30 minutes of at least moderate activity (such as walking, biking, or playing tag) into every day. (Check out Chapter 10 for activities that are appropriate for every age group.)

Suppose your high-schooler doesn't have time for structured exercise every single day. Tell her to park her car at the farthest point of the school parking lot and walk the extra distance. Instead of driving her to her friend's house, let her hoof it down the street. Encourage her to think about making the choice to be the most active that she can be, in every situation, and activity will become second nature to her. (And she'll never waste time looking for a close parking spot again!)

Weighing In

You don't want your child to become obsessed with the scale, but he does need to check in with it every now and then, just to make sure that everything is proceeding as it should. A once-a-week weigh-in is plenty. Weighing in every day is too frequent and may frustrate your child because weight can fluctuate from day to day; weighing once a month is too seldom because any backsliding may be difficult to correct if it has gone on for several weeks. Encourage your child to choose a weigh-in day, and advise him to weigh in at the same time each day.

Enforcing the House Rules

At the very least, the rules in a healthy house should include the following:

✔ No eating in front of the TV

✔ Family dinners several times a week

✔ No distractions during meals (meaning no TV, laptops, books, newspapers, and so on)

For more on household ground rules, check out Chapter 11.

Getting Everyone Involved

When the entire family is subject to the same set of standards regarding meals and activity, enforcing health-promoting rules (like no eating in front of the TV, shutting the TV off altogether on nice days, and taking everyone on a bike ride) is a lot easier. A child of any age will have a hard time accepting that her mom, dad, or siblings can do and eat whatever they want while she has to give up her favorite treats and nonactivities. Your child stands a better chance of long-term success if the entire family switches to a healthier lifestyle, regardless of who's thin and who needs to lose a few pounds.

Junking the Junk Food for Good!

When the initial enthusiasm over replacing sugary or fat-laden snacks with healthy foods in your household dies down, or after your child has shown significant strides in losing weight and increasing her activity level, you may be tempted to start buying your family's old favorite snacks — just enough so that everyone can have a little, but not so much that anyone will start gaining weight. What's life without a treat now and then, you ask?

You're entering very dangerous territory with this kind of thinking. Sure, an occasional treat is fine, but bringing junk food into the house — even in small quantities — can undo everything your child has worked so hard to achieve. Remember, one of your goals in making healthier choices is to change your child's craving for sweets and other treats — the foods that, by the way, made him overweight in the first place. To offer these foods to him is just confusing and counterproductive. And completely unnecessary. A piece of cake at a birthday party isn't the end of the world, but if you bring home a cake and he eats the whole thing, he may feel like a failure. Save yourselves the confusion and just stick to a no-junk policy.

Sacking Mealtime Snacks

Letting the kids help out when you're preparing healthy meals is a great way for them to learn about healthy living, and it's also a chance for you to connect with them after a busy day spent doing your own things. However, make sure that they're not snacking throughout the meal prep. Even if it's healthy food, if your child overeats, he's going to gain weight. That's the simple truth. It's possible to eat the equivalent of an entire meal while preparing a meal, so keep an eye out for this kind of behavior and nip it in the bud. Mealtime snacking is just a bad habit to get into.

Kissing Off Bad Habits

Be vigilant about not allowing your child to slide back into her old ways after the weight has come off. For example, when she's feeling healthier and you can see a major difference in her energy and happiness levels, she may forget that her love of watching TV contributed to her weight gain in the first place; and because she isn't obese anymore, she may figure that she's in a kind of "safe zone." She may believe, for example, that she can watch TV to her heart's content *because* she isn't heavy anymore. That kind of thinking is just the first step toward cutting corners in other areas, too. (Maybe she'll just take a walk twice a week rather than every day, and maybe she can have cookies every day as long as she doesn't also have a cheeseburger.) Encourage her to cling to her new, healthy habits and leave the past where it belongs. (Chapter 15 offers tips on catching this type of backsliding and correcting it before it goes too far.)

Getting Support

If you know of a support group in your area for overweight children and their families, check it out (even if you're not normally a "joiner"). Knowing that you aren't the only parent to face a child's weight problem can be a tremendous relief in times of stress. And letting your child know that he isn't some sort of unusual specimen — that there are other kids out there who are also changing their lifestyles and trying to lose weight — may just be the boost he needs to continue on this path when he's gets a little tired of the whole thing. (Chapter 14 has tips on when and where you might look for some outside help.)

Seeking Out New Information

Even if you consider yourself pretty well informed, there's always more to discover about healthy living and weight loss. Dedicate some time each week to finding new recipes and investigating new activities for your child and the rest of the family to try. Experts devote their entire careers to finding ways to improve and maintain weight loss, so don't let their hard work go unnoticed — become an expert yourself by doing regular research on these topics. As we say throughout the book, healthy living isn't synonymous with leading a boring, bland life. The more you know about healthy options (both for eating and exercising), the more likely your family is to stick with this healthier lifestyle.

Chapter 18

Ten Ways to Cut Fat and Calories from Your Family's Diet

In This Chapter

▶ Doing away with hidden fat

▶ Preparing your kitchen for healthy cooking

▶ Making healthy substitutions

When you begin the process of turning your family's lifestyle around, you have so much to consider that it's easy to miss a major thing or two. If you ban fast food but continue to bring home sugary drinks, you've done *half* the job well. If you prepare a healthy sandwich for your teenager and watch him heap gobs of mayonnaise on top . . . again, that's only partially healthy. To help you go all the way, this chapter is filled with reminders for cutting out the hidden sources of fat and calories in your family's diet.

Skip Fast Food

One of the best things you can do for both your child's weight loss and your entire family's health is declare a moratorium on fast food. Don't just cut back to once or twice a week — cut it out completely and start cooking healthy meals at home. Most fast food contains an enormous amount of fat; some items even contain more fat than an adult's recommended daily allowance! So if the kids are clamoring for shakes and burgers, pretend your car just won't make the turn into the parking lot anymore and head for the safety — and healthfulness — of your own kitchen.

Say Fry-Bye

Before you do anything else in your kitchen, toss your deep fryer into the trash. If you use a frying pan for your deep-fried foods, stop! Frying is hands down the worst form of cooking as far as your family's health is concerned. Fried foods absorb so much fat that even healthy foods like veggies can't offer anything in the way of nutrition after they've been crisped to within an inch of their lives. Plus, research indicates that eating fried foods not only contributes to heart disease but may also lead to the development of certain types of cancer.

Choose Snacks Wisely

You don't have to cut snacks out of your kids' lives in order to keep their fat consumption low. Let them have low-fat yogurt, pretzels, animal crackers, skim-milk string cheese, fruit, whole-wheat toast, low-sugar cereal, veggies . . . there's plenty out there to choose from. Just remember: An entire bowl of low-sugar cereal with skim milk and fruit is far better nutritionally and fat-wise than *half* a doughnut.

Hey, Hey! Ho, Ho! Condiments Have Got to Go!

We're talking high-fat condiments, such as high-fat dressings, regular mayonnaise, and cheese- or butter-based sauces. Condiments are one of those food items that people tend to think don't really count because they're added to other foods. Make sure that you read the nutrition labels on condiments, and teach your kids to do the same. Your child may make a beautiful veggie wrap and then douse it with blue cheese dressing, not realizing that she's adding fat to her otherwise extremely nutritious meal.

Vinegar, mustard, salsa, hot sauce, plain yogurt, salt, pepper, and various herbs (dried or fresh from the garden — experiment with different tastes!) are good low-fat, low-calorie, all-purpose toppers to food.

So Long, Sweet Drinks

Sugar-sweetened juices and sodas are among the worst beverages you can keep in the house. Sugary juice contains almost no nutrients to speak of, and soda contains absolutely *nothing* that a growing child needs. Kids who drink these beverages tend to drink *a lot* of them (in other words, they don't stop at one 8-ounce serving), which means they take in vast amounts of excess sugar, which is then converted into fat. Rather than sugar-sweetened drinks, keep skim or 1 percent milk in the fridge, and encourage kids to drink lots of water. The body actually needs and can use certain elements contained in those liquids. If your kids absolutely must eat something sweet, give them some fresh fruit.

Prep Your Kitchen

Get more comfortable in a well-stocked kitchen, and your meal planning will be a snap. Instead of falling back on your old, timeworn (but not very healthy) recipes, you'll be eager to try new things and repeat new favorites. You're less likely to fall into old ways if you've made things as easy as possible for yourself, so if you need new kitchen equipment — sharper knives, a food processor, a steaming basket for veggies, and so on — to handle your veggies and lean cuts of meat, go stock up!

Know Your Substitutes

Did you know that you can use applesauce rather than vegetable oil in many cooking recipes, or that you can use low-fat ricotta cheese in place of cream cheese? Skim milk replaces whole milk in almost any recipe, and frozen yogurt can stand in for whipped cream topping. You really can make almost any recipe healthier by knowing how to replace high-fat ingredients with healthier substitutes. After you make a switch here and there, you get the hang of it, and you may even come up with your own favorite substitutes!

Prepare for Busy Days

Your family is far less likely to fall prey to the lures of fast food or ordering in if the freezer holds a week's worth of healthy meals. Double or triple the recipes when you cook, and freeze the extras for days when you just don't have the time to lay out a freshly prepared meal.

Go Skimmy Dipping

Everyone needs dairy in their diets. The USDA food pyramid recommends two to three servings daily, and kids, especially, need calcium for their growing bones and developing teeth. But your family does *not* need whole-milk products; their high fat content doesn't make them healthier. Skim dairy products provide your family with all the vitamins and minerals they need without all the fat. (And plain low-fat yogurt, by the way, is a great substitute for sour cream!)

Make Healthy Even Better

When you make a healthy meal, make it the best it can be. Rinse cooked lean ground beef with hot water after draining it to get more fat out. Separate your gravy, and skim the fat off the top of your homemade soups (just stick the container in the fridge and wait for the fat to congeal on the top). Trim the fat from cuts of meat before cooking them. Don't drown salads in high-fat dressings. Keep butter out of your skillet when you stir-fry. Always ask yourself, "Is there a way I can make this meal even better for my family?" and then *do* it.

Chapter 19

Ten Fun Ways to Fit Exercise Into Your Child's Day

*W*hen you get to be a certain age, it's exhausting to even consider putting an exercise DVD on and jumping around your living room for an hour. However, you know that in order to help your child lose weight, you have to play a part in getting her moving. You set an example for your child, so if *you* hate exercise, why *shouldn't* she? How on earth are you going to get motivated past your own feelings on exercise, anyway?

We've got good news for your whole family: Exercise doesn't have to be a structured, timed activity. It can include almost any type of movement. And the more fun the activity, the better the chance your child — and you — will want to do it again and again! This chapter gives you some fun and easy exercise ideas to get everyone moving.

Walk

Walk with your child wherever and whenever you can. Walk to the store, to the park, to Grandma's, and to friends' homes. Don't let the weather be an excuse to drive wherever your feet can take you. Invest in some rain- and cold-weather gear, and hop to it! Walking is one of the easiest exercises to do, even for a child who is significantly overweight. Chat him up while you walk to take his mind off the fact that he may be getting tired. Make it fun, and he'll want to do it again.

 If your child is older and independent enough to travel on foot alone, don't drive him to a destination that's within walking distance. He needs to start thinking of the healthiest ways to get through his day, which start with being as active as possible.

Bring the Dog

A child who is less than eager to take a walk, play in the yard, or explore a nature trail may be persuaded to do so if a little four-legged friend is allowed to come along. If you don't already have a pet, borrow a friend's dog (as long as it's kid friendly). If your child sees the activity as doing something nice for a lovable animal, he may be more excited about moving his feet down the street or through the park.

Tag!

Play games in the yard that involve running. Tag, Capture the Flag, Ghost in the Graveyard, Manhunt . . . remember these from your own childhood? There's no reason you can't get outside with your kids and instigate a little fun. Some kids really need that kind of extra nudge from Mom and/or Dad to get the game going. If they're ready to take things to another level, try a game of kickball, flag football, or soccer. It's good for the kids, and it's good for you, too.

Dust Off the Bikes

Biking is a fun, easy, low-impact way to get your family exercising. Ride around the neighborhood, or find parks or bike trails to explore. Make sure everyone is outfitted with a helmet, including yourself. (We know it gives you helmet head, but you're setting a good example, remember?) If your child is reluctant to pedal his way around the block, think about adding some bells and whistles to his cycle. Sometimes having a cool bike to show off to his friends is all it takes to get a kid off and burning some rubber.

Racers, Take Your Marks

Encourage your kids to race each other, either on foot in the yard or around the block on their bikes (as long as it's safe to do so, of course). Make sure the competition is fair — you can't put your overweight youngster up against an older, more active child and expect a fair race. If you can't find an even match, race your child yourself (and don't try too terribly hard to come out the winner). You can also let him compete against himself by investing in a stopwatch and timing how long it takes him to get from one point to another. When his time starts to drop, you'll see him put in more and more effort to get that time even lower.

Visit Mother Nature

One way to introduce your child to hiking trails is to make a game out of it. Nature is always changing, so pick a theme for the day, like, "Who can find the most interesting rock?" or "How many different kinds of leaves can we find today?" It may sound silly, but kids love to have a mission, and it keeps them busy for a long, long time. Don't forget to bring along a bag so that your child can carry her treasures home if she wants to (and if it's appropriate — you don't want her to pick rare flowers when a posted sign says not to).

Introduce Something New

Being active is a lifelong goal. You want your child to be active every day, so from time to time, he may become bored with whatever he's doing. When things start getting a little stale — you've taken 100 nature walks together, he's played soccer in the yard 87 times, and his bike's tires have gone flat from all the riding he's done — help him look for something new. Take him golfing. Sign him up for tennis lessons. Maybe he'd love rollerblading. Skiing may be a blast for him. With so many activities out there, he's sure to find one he likes. Whatever he wants to try, encourage him. If it doesn't work out, try something *else*.

Work Those Kids

Yard work or other household chores can be pretty labor intensive, so stop doing everything yourself, and let your child help out with the chores. Have her rake the leaves and haul them back to the edge of your property, mow the lawn, or wash the car. Of course, some kids don't consider this kind of work fun, but others can't wait to start building leaf piles and sudsing up the minivan.

Try not to have high expectations of the quality of work, especially if your child is still young. The point is getting her to move her muscles, not create a perfectly manicured lawn.

Dance, Baby, Dance!

Turn up the radio and start grooving with the kids. They'll never even know what hit them, but when you're all through, everyone will be sweaty and laughing. Encourage creative moves, and show them a few steps from back in your day. (The Bus Stop? Electric Slide? Macarena?) Your kids won't believe their eyes when they see you showing off your expertise.

Make a Kid-Safe Playroom

When it's raining or all of 4 degrees outside, you may have some trouble getting your child involved in activities. So create a kid-safe room in the house where he can run, jump, and somersault to his heart's content. (Young kids, especially, need room to roam.) Consider putting a small climber somewhere in your house for your child to play on in inclement weather. Have an old couch sitting around? Let your child use its cushions for jumping and rolling (and throwing). Just remember, if you have kids, your house is never going to look perfect until they move out, anyway — you may as well let them have a safe, padded space of their own to get a little crazy in.

Part V

Appendixes

The 5th Wave — By Rich Tennant

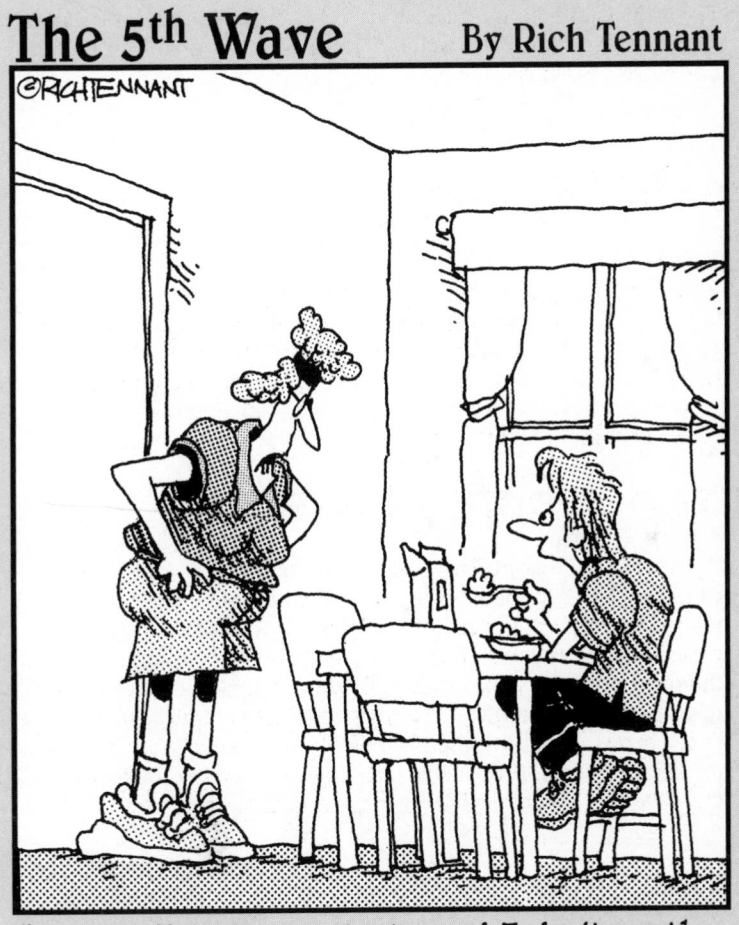

"I know I walk regularly and I do it on the street, but if anyone asks, I'm a fitness-walker, or a power-walker, NOT a street-walker."

In this part . . .

You'll find over 30 tasty and healthy recipes to pull out when you're stumped for new snack and meal ideas. We also include an exercise log and a weight loss chart.

Appendix A

Recipes

*L*earning to eat well isn't about sacrificing every food your family has ever enjoyed. We assure you, healthy meals can go way beyond plain greens and bland chicken breasts. In this Appendix, we've compiled tasty, out-of-the-ordinary, low-fat, healthy recipes to cover the day from sunup to sundown. One thing you should know — and your family should learn — is that cutting the fat out of your diet doesn't mean that you have to eat the same foods prepared the same ways all the time. What a bore that would be for your taste buds! Unfortunately, many families never get beyond this misconception, and their attempts at healthy eating end before they've done much in the way of culinary exploration. We're sure that you'll find something of interest and a few new favorites here!

In addition to recipes provided by this book's coauthors, this Appendix includes contributions from several professionals in the healthy-eating arena: Megan Brenn-White, a chef and author who has worked in New York City and California and is a frequent contributor to the Food Network Web site; Julie Negrin, Director of Culinary Arts at the JCC in Manhattan, who has appeared on the Today Show; and Cindy Guirino, RD, LD, CDE, ACE Personal Trainer, and founder of UB-Fit, LLC Medical Nutrition Therapy.

Breakfast

Everyone should clear a few minutes to kick-start their day with a healthy meal. Not only do children who eat breakfast regularly perform better in school, but you can also use this time as a way to connect with each other and discuss (and prepare for) your plans for the busy day ahead. Toss those high-sugar cereals in the trash can and send everyone off fortified with a nutritious meal.

Egg White Omelet

For a nutritionally complete start to the day, serve this tasty and colorful omelet with toast, fresh fruit, and juice.

Preparation Time: *10 minutes*

Yield: *1 serving*

2 eggs	*¼ cup fresh spinach*
¼ cup skim milk	*1-ounce slice nonfat cheese*
½ tomato, diced	

1 Spray a medium skillet with cooking spray and heat for 2 minutes over medium heat.

2 Separate the egg whites from the yolks, and beat the whites in a bowl with the skim milk. Discard the yolks.

3 Pour the egg mixture into the skillet, tilting the pan so that the egg covers the bottom. Add the veggies and cheese to one half of the egg, and fold the other side over top. Remove from skillet when egg is set. Season to taste.

Per serving: *Calories 117 (From Fat 4); Fat 0g (Saturated 0g); Cholesterol 7mg; Sodium 439mg; Carbohydrate 7g (Dietary Fiber 1g); Protein 20g.*

○ Apple Carrot Muffins

These muffins combine a fruit and a veggie into one tidy, portable package. And they're moist enough that you and your kids won't be tempted to slather them in butter — trust us! (This recipe comes from Megan Brenn-White.)

Preparation time: *40 minutes*

Yield: *12 muffins*

1 cup whole-wheat flour	3 eggs
1 cup white flour	½ cup sugar
1 tablespoon baking powder	½ cup vegetable oil
Pinch of salt	1 cup grated apple (unpeeled)
½ teaspoon cinnamon	1 cup grated carrot (peeled)

1 Preheat the oven to 350 degrees.

2 In a large bowl, mix the whole-wheat flour, white flour, baking powder, salt, and cinnamon.

3 In a separate bowl, blend the eggs, sugar, and vegetable oil until well combined. Stir in the grated apple and carrot.

4 Pour the wet ingredients from Step 3 into the bowl containing the dry ingredients from Step 2, and mix thoroughly.

5 Fill the muffin cups three-quarters full with batter, and bake for 25 minutes.

Per serving: *Calories 216 (From Fat 98); Fat 11g (Saturated 1g); Cholesterol 53mg; Sodium 126mg; Carbohydrate 26g (Dietary Fiber 2g); Protein 4g.*

🍎 Oatmeal with Stir-Ins

Oatmeal is a warm, nutritious start to a child's day. Unfortunately, children who love oatmeal are usually accustomed to the super-sweetened varieties that offer up more sugar than anything else. This recipe starts with basic rolled oats and sweetens the bowl naturally.

Preparation time: *5 minutes*

Yield: *1 serving*

½ cup old-fashioned oats	½ cup sliced fresh fruit
1 cup water or 1 percent milk	

1 Prepare oats according to package directions. Use milk in place of water for creamier oatmeal.

2 Stir your child's favorite fresh fruit into the oats before serving.

Per serving: *Calories 185 (From Fat 27); Fat 3g (Saturated 0g); Cholesterol 0mg; Sodium 1mg; Carbohydrate 37g (Dietary Fiber 5g); Protein 6g.*

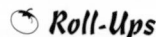 *Roll-Ups*

Kids will love this breakfast because it's tasty and fun in a finger-food kind of way. You'll love these roll-ups because they're so easy, quick, and healthy. (This recipe comes from Cindy Guirino, founder of UB-Fit in Dayton, Ohio.)

Preparation time: *5 minutes*

Yield: *1 serving*

One 8-inch whole-wheat tortilla	*1-ounce slice low-fat or nonfat cheese*
1 medium apple	*Cinnamon to taste*

1 Wash the apple and cut it into thin slices.

2 Lay the tortilla flat on your work surface, and place the apple slices down the center of it. Top with the cheese, and sprinkle with cinnamon.

3 Fold the sides of the tortilla in toward the center, and then roll the whole thing up.

4 Microwave the roll-up for 15 to 30 seconds before serving.

Per serving: *Calories 204 (From Fat 27); Fat 3g (Saturated 1g); Cholesterol 6mg; Sodium 345mg; Carbohydrate 42g (Dietary Fiber 6g); Protein 10g.*

Lunch

Resist the urge to hand your child's nutritional needs over to the school cafeteria. Some schools provide healthy meals, but many others don't. Fast food, soda, and ice cream are the rules rather than the exception in some school lunchrooms. The good news is that you can teach your child to prepare her own healthy, delicious lunch to take with her. And you can bet your bottom dollar that, unlike junk food, the following meals will provide her with the long-lasting energy she needs to see her through the rest of the school day!

Turkey Pita

Who says a healthy lunch can't also be delicious and fun to make? Pita bread looks just like a pocket when you cut it in half and separate the two layers, so it's not surprising that kids love it. They're sure to get a kick out of stuffing the pocket with food — just make sure the filling's healthy!

Preparation time: *5 minutes*

Yield: *1 serving*

½ pita

3 ounces precooked white-meat turkey

3 lettuce leaves

2 tomato slices

1 tablespoon mustard

1 Carefully separate the two sides of the pita pocket.

2 Trim any fat from the turkey slices. If you're using cold cuts, make sure it's breast meat.

3 Arrange the turkey, lettuce, and tomato inside the pocket. Top with mustard.

Tip: Serve this pita sandwich with carrot sticks, and offer animal crackers or fresh fruit for dessert.

Per serving: *Calories 222 (From Fat 15); Fat 2g (Saturated 0g); Cholesterol 71mg; Sodium 380mg; Carbohydrate 21g (Dietary Fiber 2g); Protein 30g.*

☼ Fruit Pizza

What better way to get your kids to eat fruit than to put it on a pizza? Everybody loves pizza! This recipe is quick and fun because it allows everyone to get creative with their favorite fruits.

Preparation time: *25 minutes*

Yield: *4 servings*

Pizza crust mix (preferably one made with whole-wheat flour)

½ cup natural applesauce

2 cups fresh or thawed frozen fruit of your choice (allow fruit to drain well)

1 Mix crust according to package directions and spread onto a baking sheet. Bake the crust at the oven temperature listed on the package until it's golden brown, and then remove it from the oven.

2 Spread applesauce on top of the partially cooked pizza crust.

3 Place the fruit on top of the pizza and put it back into the oven for 10 minutes.

Per serving: Calories 191 (From Fat 15); Fat 2g (Saturated 0g); Cholesterol 3mg; Sodium 244mg; Carbohydrate 40g (Dietary Fiber 4g); Protein 5g.

☼ Fruit-Filled Spring Rolls

If your family's clamoring for Chinese, spring this recipe on them! These rolls go over well with kids because they have a lot of different fruits in them and are especially tasty dipped in low-fat yogurt.

Preparation time: *10 minutes*

Yield: *12 servings*

2 bananas, thinly sliced into rounds

1½ cups strawberries, cut lengthwise into quarters

2 peaches, peeled and sliced

1 cup raspberries

1 cup blueberries

¾ cup low-fat strawberry yogurt

12 large square sheets rice paper

Chopped mint for garnish (optional)

2 cups low-fat strawberry yogurt for dipping (optional)

1 Place 1 sheet of rice paper into a bowl of warm water and press down gently to submerge it. Allow the paper to sit in the water for 1 minute, and then remove it carefully, taking care not to tear it. Place the rice paper sheet flat on a plate.

2 Spread 1 tablespoon of yogurt over the top, and spread slices of fruit down the middle of the sheet.

3 Fold 2 sides of the rice paper in over the fruit, and roll up the rest of the paper.

4 Cut the roll in half diagonally. Repeat Steps 1 through 3 to make 12 spring rolls.

5 Garnish the rolls with mint and serve with yogurt for dipping (if desired).

Tip: In place of fresh peaches, raspberries, and blueberries, you can use thawed frozen fruit.

Per serving: *Calories 93 (From Fat 3); Fat 0g (Saturated 0g); Cholesterol 0mg; Sodium 37mg; Carbohydrate 25g (Dietary Fiber 3g); Protein 2g.*

☺ Walking Fruit Salad

When you're heading out the door for a hike or a day in the park, you need a healthy, portable snack. These fruit-filled apples certainly qualify, and they provide lots of energy, too!

Preparation time: *15 minutes*

Yield: *Four ½-apple servings*

2 medium apples, any variety

¼ cup grapes, halved

¼ cup raisins

¼ cup crushed pineapple, drained

1 cup low-fat cottage cheese or low-fat yogurt

¼ cup low-fat granola

1 Core each apple, and cut it in half.

2 Fill each apple with ¼ cup of the cottage cheese or yogurt.

3 Add grapes, raisins, pineapple, or your favorite fruit. Sprinkle with granola.

Per serving: *Calories 185 (From Fat 13); Fat 1g (Saturated 1g); Cholesterol 5mg; Sodium 200mg; Carbohydrate 39g (Dietary Fiber 5g); Protein 7g.*

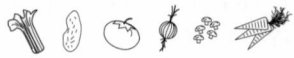

☞ Crunchy Veggie Wraps

Serve this veggie-filled wrap for lunch or a light dinner.

Preparation time: *5 minutes*

Yield: *4 servings*

½ cup salsa	1 red tomato, chopped
4 low-fat flour tortillas	¼ cup sliced red onion
⅔ cup shredded romaine lettuce	⅓ cup grated carrots
1 red or green bell pepper, chopped	¼ cup crumbled nonfat or low-fat feta cheese
½ cucumber, chopped	1 cup alfalfa sprouts

1 Spread 2 tablespoons of salsa over one side of each tortilla.

2 Divide the remaining ingredients evenly among the tortillas, sprinkling the veggies and cheese down the center of each tortilla.

3 Roll up each tortilla, and cut it in half diagonally.

Tip: You can substitute your favorite vegetable for any of the ones in the ingredient list.

Per serving: *Calories 163 (From Fat 18); Fat 2g (Saturated 0g); Cholesterol 0mg; Sodium 542mg; Carbohydrate 32g (Dietary Fiber 4g); Protein 7g.*

Snacks, Drinks, and Frozen Treats

Snack time may be when your best intentions break down. While you're scrambling to put together a healthy meal for dinner, the kids are clamoring for chips, microwave popcorn, and soda, and you consider letting down your guard just because it's the easiest thing to do — or so you think. Healthy snacks can be convenient and delicious; the key is to prepare them ahead of time.

☞ Veggies and Yogurt Dip

This dip is a great way to work more veggies and dairy (from the yogurt) into your child's diet. Serve it as a side dish with lunch or dinner, or enjoy it as a snack all by itself.

Preparation time: 10 minutes

Yield: 2 servings

8 ounces low-fat plain yogurt

1 tablespoon powdered ranch or Italian dressing mix, or to taste

½ cup baby carrots

1 red, green, or yellow bell pepper cored and cut into strips

2 celery stalks, cut into 3-inch strips

1 cup cucumber slices

1 In a small bowl, stir together the yogurt and powdered dressing mix. Serve with veggies.

Per serving: *Calories 64 (From Fat 10); Fat 1g (Saturated 1g); Cholesterol 3mg; Sodium 241mg; Carbohydrate 10g (Dietary Fiber 1g); Protein 4g.*

☞ Black Bean Dip

Beans are a great source of protein and fiber. You can use this quick dish either as a dip, a side dish, or an excellent burrito filling. The yogurt isn't necessary if you're avoiding dairy; it adds creaminess, but the beans themselves yield a fairly smooth purée. (This recipe comes from Megan Brenn-White.)

Preparation time: 10 minutes

Yield: Six 1½-cup servings

Two 15-ounce cans black beans, drained

½ cup plain low-fat yogurt

1 jalapeño, seeded and roughly chopped

1 garlic clove, roughly chopped

½ cup roughly chopped red or yellow onion

1 tablespoon lime juice

1 tablespoon cumin

2 tablespoons olive oil

Salt and freshly ground pepper to taste

1 Combine all ingredients in a food processor and process until smooth. Season with salt and pepper to taste.

Vary It! *For extra spice, retain all or some of the jalapeño seeds and add them to the food processor with the vegetables.*

Tip: *You can make this dip in a blender, but you may have to add a bit more yogurt or lime juice to keep the ingredients liquid enough to blend.*

Per serving: *Calories 142 (From Fat 52); Fat 6g (Saturated 1g); Cholesterol 1mg; Sodium 283mg; Carbohydrate 16g (Dietary Fiber 6g); Protein 7g.*

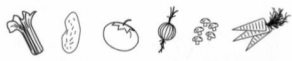

☉ Fruit Smoothie

This smoothie tastes great anytime — as a snack, beverage, or dessert!

Preparation time: *5 minutes*

Yield: *1 serving*

4 ounces skim milk

4 ounces plain or vanilla nonfat yogurt

4 ounces orange juice

½ frozen banana, peeled

½ cup frozen strawberries

1 Combine all ingredients in a blender, and blend on high until smooth.

Per serving: *Calories 231 (From Fat 8); Fat 1g (Saturated 0g); Cholesterol 5mg; Sodium 148mg; Carbohydrate 46g (Dietary Fiber 4g); Protein 12g.*

☉ Mango-Pineapple Salsa

Looking for the perfect, fresh topper for fish or whole-wheat crackers? This salsa blends fruit and vegetables together deliciously — and nutritiously!

Preparation time: *10 minutes*

Marinating time: *1 to 4 hours*

Yield: *About 3 cups*

1 cup finely chopped pineapple

¾ cup finely chopped mango

⅔ cup finely chopped red bell pepper

½ cup finely chopped seeded tomato

⅓ cup finely chopped seeded English hothouse cucumber

⅓ cup finely chopped red onion

3 tablespoons chopped fresh cilantro (optional)

2 tablespoons chopped fresh mint (optional)

2 tablespoons fresh lime juice

1 Combine all ingredients in a medium bowl, and cover the bowl with plastic wrap.

2 Refrigerate for 1 to 4 hours to let the flavors blend, tossing occasionally.

3 Serve as a salsa-type dip with Melba toast or over grilled or broiled fish.

Per serving: *Calories 19 (From Fat 1); Fat 0g (Saturated 0g); Cholesterol 0mg; Sodium 1mg; Carbohydrate 5g (Dietary Fiber 1g); Protein 0g.*

Frozen Yogurt Pops

When it's warm outside, nothing is easier or tastes better than these cool, healthy pops.

Tools: *8 small paper cups (approximately 2 inches in size), 8 wooden ice-pop sticks*

Preparation time: *5 minutes*

Yield: *8 servings*

Two 8-ounce containers of your favorite low-fat yogurt

1 Pour yogurt into the paper cups, filling them almost to the top.

2 Stretch a small piece of plastic wrap over the top of each cup. Poke an ice-pop stick through the plastic wrap and into the center of each yogurt cup.

3 Put the cups in the freezer until the yogurt is frozen, about 30 minutes.

4 Hold the stick and tear the cup off the frozen pop before serving.

Per serving: *Calories 59 (From Fat 4); Fat 1g (Saturated 0g); Cholesterol 5mg; Sodium 27mg; Carbohydrate 12g (Dietary Fiber 0g); Protein 2g.*

☺ Frozen Fruit Icy

Kids love this slushy, fruity treat any time of the year. It's an easy-to-prepare, healthy alternative to high-fat snacks like ice cream.

Preparation time: *30 minutes (including thaw time for frozen berries)*

Yield: *6 servings*

2 cups frozen strawberries	*¼ cup honey*
1½ cups water	*2 tablespoons lemon or lime juice*

1 Partially thaw frozen berries about 20 minutes; retain the juice for flavoring.

2 Combine berries (and juice), water, honey, and lemon or lime juice in a blender. Blend for about 1 minute or until smooth. Pour into a bread pan, cover with foil, and freeze until firm, about 20 to 30 minutes.

3 Remove the pan from the freezer and use a spoon to scrape the ice into bowls.

Per serving: *Calories 59 (From Fat 2); Fat 0g (Saturated 0g); Cholesterol 0mg; Sodium 1mg; Carbohydrate 15g (Dietary Fiber 1g); Protein 0g.*

☺ Fruit and Yogurt Parfait

This parfait is just like a sundae, but healthier. And it's fun for kids to make!

Preparation time: *10 minutes*

Yield: *1 serving*

1 cup vanilla low-fat yogurt	*¼ cup sliced or chopped peaches*
¼ cup strawberries	*¼ cup crushed pineapple*
¼ cup blueberries	

1 Spread ¼ cup yogurt in the bottom of a 10- or 12-ounce glass.

2 Layer the strawberries on top of the yogurt.

3 Spread ¼ cup yogurt on top of the strawberries.

4 Layer the blueberries on top of the yogurt.

5 Spread ¼ cup yogurt on top of the blueberries.

6 Layer the peaches on top of the yogurt.

7 Spread ¼ cup yogurt on top of the peaches.

8 Layer the crushed pineapple on the yogurt as the final layer.

Vary It! *Top the parfait with low-fat granola for a tasty crunch.*

Per serving: *Calories 240 (From Fat 30); Fat 3g (Saturated 2g); Cholesterol 12mg; Sodium 164mg; Carbohydrate 42g (Dietary Fiber 2g); Protein 13g.*

○ *Strawberry Sorbet*

You can make this quick sorbet with a blender or food processor, but I recommend a food processor because it doesn't require as much liquid as the blender. You end up with something very close to what you would get from an ice cream maker. (This recipe comes from Megan Brenn-White.)

Preparation time: 5 minutes (plus 30 minutes thaw time)

Yield: 6 servings

10-ounce bag frozen strawberries (about 2 cups)

2 tablespoons lime juice

3 tablespoons maple syrup

1 Allow the frozen strawberries to thaw slightly, about 30 minutes. (Alternatively, you can use your microwave to thaw the berries for 3 to 4 minutes on medium power.)

2 Place the strawberries in a food processor along with remaining ingredients. Pulse until you achieve a smooth texture, scraping down the sides occasionally.

3 Scoop into serving dishes. If the sorbet's too soft, place the dishes in the freezer for about 10 minutes.

Tip: *To make this sorbet even creamier, throw some frozen bananas into the food processor with the other ingredients.*

Per serving: *Calories 44 (From Fat 1); Fat 0g (Saturated 0g); Cholesterol 0mg; Sodium 2mg; Carbohydrate 11g (Dietary Fiber 1g); Protein 0g.*

⌔ Creamy Hummus and Crunchy Pita Chips

Hummus and pita chips are a delicious, healthy alternative to the standard potato chips-and-dip fare. They're also quick and easy to prepare. (This recipe comes from Megan Brenn-White.)

Preparation time: *20 minutes*

Yield: *4 to 6 servings*

Hummus

15-ounce can chickpeas

½ cup tahini (Middle Eastern sesame paste)

5 tablespoons lemon juice

1 garlic clove

1 teaspoon salt

½ cup water

3 tablespoons extra-virgin olive oil

Freshly ground black pepper, to taste

1 Put all the ingredients into a food processor and process until smooth.

Vary It! *You can add more water to achieve a creamier consistency. You can also add more lemon juice, olive oil, salt, or pepper to adjust the flavor to your taste.*

Pita Chips

3 whole wheat pitas

Olive oil

3 tablespoons of dried mixed herbs (oregano and basil)

1 teaspoon salt

Dash pepper

1 Preheat the oven to 350 degrees.

2 Slice the pitas in half, separating the pocket, so that you have 6 circles.

3 Brush the pitas liberally with olive oil, and sprinkle them with the herbs, salt, and pepper.

4 Cut each circle into 6 or 8 pieces, as you would a pizza, and spread them on a baking sheet.

5 Bake for about 8 minutes or until golden. Allow the chips to cool before serving them with hummus.

Per serving: *Calories 347 (From Fat 187); Fat 21g (Saturated 3g); Cholesterol 0mg; Sodium 866mg; Carbohydrate 32g (Dietary Fiber 5g); Protein 10g.*

◯ Banana Ice Cream

Who's screaming for ice cream? You and the kids can follow this recipe to make a naturally sweetened frozen treat without adding an ounce of fat to the mix. (This recipe comes from Julie Negrin.)

Preparation time: *5 minutes (plus overnight freezing time and 20 minutes thaw time)*

Yield: *4 servings*

4 ripe bananas   ½ cup apple juice (or more if needed)

1 Peel the bananas, break them into thirds, and freeze them in an airtight bag for at least 12 hours.

2 Thaw the bananas at room temperature for 20 minutes before pureeing them in a food processor or blender with apple juice until soft ice cream consistency is achieved.

Tip: *Serve this ice cream plain or topped with naturally sweetened chocolate chips.*

Per serving: *Calories 116 (From Fat 5); Fat 1g (Saturated 0g); Cholesterol 0mg; Sodium 2mg; Carbohydrate 30g (Dietary Fiber 3g); Protein 1g.*

Dinner

Studies have shown that families who eat dinner together several times a week are less likely to have weight problems. Dinnertime is an *excellent* opportunity for everyone to talk about healthy eating options. It's also a great time to get your child involved in the preparation of the meal and to explain why and how you've cut the fat from the meal. We've included lots of options in this section so that when everyone is ready, you can try out some really interesting new tastes. Healthy eating is *not* boring, and these recipes prove it!

☁ Summer Squash Stir-Fry

Stir-fry lets you serve your family all kinds of different veggies at one sitting. And because stir-fry is relatively easy to prepare, it allows you to experiment with different tastes and textures. Start with their favorites, and then play around with the recipe, adding some interesting newcomers to the dish.

Preparation time: *30 minutes*

Yield: *Five ½-cup servings*

1 bag or box of brown, long-grain rice (enough for 6 to 8 servings)	*1 medium onion, chopped*
	1 large ripe tomato, peeled and chopped
½ cup chicken or vegetable broth	*1 tablespoon Worcestershire sauce*
1 garlic clove, crushed	*2 tablespoons tomato paste*
2 medium zucchini, sliced	*1 teaspoon salt*
2 medium yellow squash, sliced	

1 Boil water for rice or prepare rice in the microwave according to package instructions.

2 Preheat a large skillet or wok for about 1 minute at medium heat, and then add the broth and garlic. Stir it around for 1 minute.

3 Add the zucchini, yellow squash, and onion. Stir-fry for 3 to 4 minutes.

4 Add the remaining ingredients, and reduce the heat to simmer. Stirring occasionally, simmer 3 or 4 minutes or until the vegetables are cooked but not limp. Serve over brown rice.

Per serving: *Calories 64 (From Fat 8); Fat 1g (Saturated 0g); Cholesterol 1mg; Sodium 610mg; Carbohydrate 13g (Dietary Fiber 4g); Protein 3g.*

☁ Grilled Veggies

When you're looking for a healthy side dish at dinnertime, veggies win hands-down. These grilled vegetables are a delicious alternative to raw or steamed, and they're so quick and easy to prepare that you'll want to have them every night!

Preparation time: *15 minutes*

Yield: *2 to 4 servings*

1 medium zucchini

1 medium yellow squash

3-ounce portabella mushroom, whole

1 red, green, or yellow bell pepper

Cooking spray

1 tablespoon allspice

1 Slice the zucchini and yellow squash into spears. Cut the pepper in half, and remove the core. Cut the pepper halves in quarters.

2 Lightly spray the veggies with cooking spray, and sprinkle them with allspice or a seasoning blend.

3 Grill the veggies either directly on your grill or wrapped in foil approximately 25 to 30 minutes.

Per serving: *Calories 52 (From Fat 4); Fat 0g (Saturated 0g); Cholesterol 0mg; Sodium 5mg; Carbohydrate 11g (Dietary Fiber 4g); Protein 2g.*

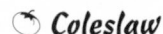
⌒ Coleslaw

If your family is accustomed to their coleslaw served up with loads of mayo, here's a great low-fat alternative that uses buttermilk as a substitute.

Preparation time: *5 minutes*

Yield: *Four 1-cup servings*

4-cup package of shredded coleslaw mix

1 cup plain low-fat yogurt

¼ cup low-fat buttermilk

1 tablespoon cider vinegar

1 teaspoon Dijon mustard

Pinch of cayenne pepper

Salt and freshly ground white pepper to taste

1 medium carrot, peeled and shredded

1 Place the shredded coleslaw mix in a salad bowl. In a separate bowl, combine the yogurt, buttermilk, vinegar, mustard, cayenne pepper, salt, and pepper, and whisk until smooth. (You can also prepare the dressing in a food processor or blender.)

2 Combine the coleslaw mix and dressing, toss together, and allow the mixture to marinate in the refrigerator for 2 to 3 hours or overnight.

3 Serve chilled, garnished with shredded carrots.

Per serving: *Calories 65 (From Fat 13); Fat 1g (Saturated 1g); Cholesterol 4mg; Sodium 249mg; Carbohydrate 9g (Dietary Fiber 2g); Protein 5g.*

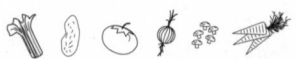

Chicken Fajitas

Instead of visiting a Mexican restaurant drive-thru, make your own fajitas at home. They're relatively quick and easy to prepare, even for a novice in the kitchen.

Preparation time: *20 minutes (plus 2 to 3 hours for marinating)*

Yield: *4 servings*

½ cup balsamic vinegar

¼ cup soy sauce

2 cups brown rice

1 pound boneless, skinless chicken breast

1 large green bell pepper

1 large red bell pepper

1 medium onion

½ cup grated low-fat cheddar cheese

½ cup plain low-fat yogurt

4 soft tortilla shells

1 Combine the vinegar and soy sauce in a bowl. Cut the chicken breasts into cubes or strips, and marinate them in the vinegar and soy mixture for 2 to 3 hours in the refrigerator.

2 Prepare the rice according to package instructions.

3 Cut the peppers and onion into strips.

4 Spray a nonstick pan with vegetable spray. Add the peppers and onions to the pan, and sauté over low-to-medium heat for 8 to 10 minutes until vegetables are soft. Add the chicken to the peppers and cook uncovered, stirring occasionally, until the chicken's cooked through (no pink remains).

5 Place one-fourth of the chicken and vegetable mixture in one tortilla shell, and add ⅛ cup each of cheese and yogurt. Serve with a ½ cup of rice on the side.

Per serving: *Calories 427 (From Fat 94); Fat 11g (Saturated 5g); Cholesterol 35mg; Sodium 1,293mg; Carbohydrate 61g (Dietary Fiber 5g); Protein 21g.*

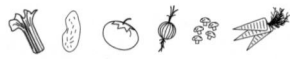

Taco Salad

Salad doesn't have to be boring! Add some life to lettuce by serving it up Mexican-style. This recipe substitutes baked tortilla chips for the traditional taco shells, which are usually deep-fried and very high in fat and calories.

Preparation time: *20 minutes*

Yield: *4 servings*

1 pound ground turkey breast	1 cup shredded nonfat cheese
1 packet taco seasoning	1 cup crushed baked tortilla chips
8 cups torn lettuce	8 ounces plain nonfat yogurt
2 red tomatoes, chopped	2 cups salsa (optional)
1 cup kidney beans	

1 In a skillet, brown the ground turkey over medium heat until it's no longer pink. Drain any fat from the skillet.

2 Add the taco seasoning and water according to directions on the seasoning packet.

3 Place lettuce in large bowl. Top with meat, tomatoes, beans, cheese, and crushed tortilla chips. Add nonfat yogurt to taste and salsa (if desired).

Per serving: *Calories 326 (From Fat 22); Fat 2g (Saturated 0g); Cholesterol 81mg; Sodium 1,021mg; Carbohydrate 33g (Dietary Fiber 7g); Protein 44g.*

Fish Tacos with Mango-Jicama Salsa

We all know that fish is a great source of lean protein that cooks up quickly, but it can be easy to get in a rut with how we prepare it. Fish tacos are a very simple (and different) way to give nearly any piece of grilled, pan-seared, or broiled piece of fish a Mexican flavor. The mango-jicama salsa adds crunch and a sweet and spicy flavor to your taco, but guacamole or other salsas work equally well. (This recipe comes from Megan Brenn-White.)

Preparation time: *25 minutes*

Yield: *4 servings*

Fish Tacos

Four 5- to 6-ounce fish fillets (red snapper, salmon, flounder, or your favorite)

Salt

Pepper

Olive oil

Juice of 1 lime

8 small corn tortillas

1 Wash the fish, and dry it with paper towels. Rub it with a little bit of olive oil, and sprinkle it with salt and pepper.

2 Preheat a nonstick pan over medium heat, and cook the fish until it flakes easily (for most fish, that's about 3 to 4 minutes per side).

3 Sprinkle cooked fish with lime juice. Divide each fillet in half, and place 2 pieces in each warmed corn tortilla. Flake the fish a bit with a fork, garnish with mango-jicama salsa along with hot sauce and/or additional cilantro to taste, and serve.

Mango-Jicama Salsa

½ small jicama

1 ripe mango

1 small bunch fresh cilantro

1 jalapeño, seeded and finely chopped

Juice of 2 limes

2 teaspoons chili powder

1 tablespoon extra-virgin olive oil

Salt and pepper to taste

1 Peel the jicama by cutting it in half, laying one half flat on the cutting board, and cutting ⅛-inch strips of peel off all the way around.

2 Repeat Step 1 with the other half, and then chop the jicama into ¼-inch pieces. Place the chopped jicama in a medium bowl.

3 Cut the mango into 2 large slices alongside the pit, score the flesh into ¼-inch squares with a paring knife, and then cut the fruit away from the peel. Add the diced mango to the jicama.

4 Finely chop the cilantro (you need about 3 tablespoons), and add it to the jicama along with the rest of the ingredients. Mix well before serving.

Tip: The acidity of the lime juice preserves the mango-jicama salsa fairly well, so it will keep at least 2 days covered in the refrigerator.

Tip: If you have leftovers, serve the fish for lunch the next day on a bed of mixed greens with a citrus dressing and some of the mango-jicama salsa for extra crunch.

Per serving: *Calories 341 (From Fat 63); Fat 7g (Saturated 1g); Cholesterol 50mg; Sodium 452mg; Carbohydrate 39g (Dietary Fiber 7g); Protein 32g.*

Grilled Cilantro-Lime Chicken Tacos

The grilled chicken used here as a taco filling is equally delicious on top of a healthy salad. The fresh cilantro and lime juice make this dish taste authentic and extremely flavorful. (This recipe comes from Megan Brenn-White.)

Preparation time: *15 minutes*

Yield: *6 servings*

2 tablespoons extra-virgin olive oil	2 large boneless, skinless chicken breasts
3 tablespoons finely chopped fresh cilantro	2 lime wedges
1 garlic clove, minced	6 small corn tortillas
1 jalapeño, seeded and finely chopped	Mixed greens
1¼ teaspoons hot sauce (Mexican is preferred, but others work just as well)	Soy cheese
Juice of 2 limes	Salsa
1 teaspoon salt	Pickled jalapeño peppers
½ teaspoon pepper	Guacamole
	Fresh cilantro

1 Mix the olive oil, cilantro, garlic, jalapeño, hot sauce, lime juice, salt, and pepper in a medium bowl. Set aside.

2 Place the chicken breasts between two layers of plastic wrap, and pound them with a mallet or rolling pin until they're about 1- to ¾-inch thick. Add them to the marinade, rub the marinade into the chicken a bit, and allow it to marinate for at least 20 minutes in the refrigerator.

3 Preheat a grill pan or grill, and grill the chicken for about 5 to 7 minutes or until no longer pink. Remove the chicken to a cutting board, and let it rest for another 2 to 3 minutes. Slice it into thin strips, and sprinkle with additional lime juice.

4 Divide the chicken among the corn tortillas, and dress the tacos with any combination of the remaining ingredients. Serve immediately.

Per serving: *Calories 277 (From Fat 81); Fat 9g (Saturated 2g); Cholesterol 165mg; Sodium 246mg; Carbohydrate 3g (Dietary Fiber 1g); Protein 44g.*

Turkey Burgers

These delicious burgers taste enough like meatloaf that you can eat them without buns. Using low-fat turkey cuts some of the saturated fat normally found in burgers, and packing them full of tasty vegetables and fresh herbs increases their general goodness. (This recipe comes from Megan Brenn-White.)

Preparation time: *20 minutes*

Yield: *4 servings (4 large patties or 8 small ones)*

2 tablespoons pine nuts	*9 medium basil leaves, finely chopped*
1 tablespoon olive oil	*¼ cup finely chopped parsley*
½ medium onion, finely chopped	*1 egg, lightly beaten*
2 cups fresh chopped spinach	*Pinch each of salt and pepper*
½ red bell pepper, finely chopped	*Olive oil for cooking*
1½ pounds lean ground turkey	

1 Heat a small sauté pan over medium heat, and toast the pine nuts, stirring frequently. When they're slightly golden, remove them from the pan, and allow them to cool. Finely chop the nuts and set aside.

2 In a medium sauté pan, heat the olive oil over medium-high heat, and add the onion. Stir frequently until the onion begins to soften, and then add the spinach and bell pepper. Cook for 2 to 3 minutes until the spinach has wilted and the peppers also begin to soften. Remove the vegetables from the pan, and allow them to cool.

3 Place the turkey in a large mixing bowl, and with your hands or a utensil (being careful not to overmix), gently incorporate the pine nuts, vegetables, fresh herbs, egg, salt, and pepper. Form into patties and place on a sheet pan or tray.

4 Heat a large nonstick sauté pan or grill coated with a little bit of olive oil. Cook the patties for about 3 to 4 minutes on each side, or until they're done to your liking.

Per serving: *Calories 277 (From Fat 81); Fat 9g (Saturated 2g); Cholesterol 165mg; Sodium 246mg; Carbohydrate 3g (Dietary Fiber 1g); Protein 44g.*

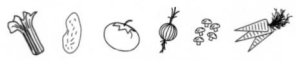

⚘ Creamy Carrot Soup

Creamy soups don't have to be unhealthy; adding oats, arborio rice, or other grains and then blending well produces a thick, creamy texture that's sure to please calorie counters. This carrot soup is quick and delicious, and your family will never guess that the creaminess comes from standard breakfast oats. (This recipe comes from Megan Brenn-White.)

Preparation time: *20 minutes*

Yield: *Six 1-cup appetizer servings; three 2-cup main course servings*

2 tablespoons extra-virgin olive oil	5 cups vegetable or chicken stock
1 large onion, chopped	¼ cup rolled oats
½ teaspoon sea salt	1 teaspoon fresh lemon juice
2 pounds carrots, peeled and cut into ½-inch rounds	Pinch of grated ginger
	2 tablespoons chopped fresh dill

1 In a medium pot, heat olive oil over medium heat, and then add the onions and salt. Cook until the onions are softened and translucent (about 5 to 8 minutes), stirring often to prevent browning.

2 Add the carrots, cover the pot, and cook over low heat for 5 to 6 minutes, stirring occasionally to prevent browning.

3 Pour the stock into the pot, and add the oats. Raise the heat and bring to a boil. Reduce heat to low and simmer for 25 minutes, covered, until the carrots are very tender.

4 Using an immersion blender, blend the soup until creamy, adding additional stock until it's your desired consistency. If you use a countertop blender, blend the soup in small batches, taking care to vent the top of the blender to avoid an eruption of hot soup.

5 Add lemon juice and grated ginger, adjusting seasoning to taste. Garnish the soup with dill, and serve.

Per serving: *Calories 148 (From Fat 50); Fat 6g (Saturated 1g); Cholesterol 0mg; Sodium 1,104mg; Carbohydrate 23g (Dietary Fiber 5g); Protein 5g.*

⚘ *Spicy Napa Cabbage Salad*

This quick salad is a great accompaniment to Asian meals. The dressing is nice on all types of greens, but it works particularly well with the mild-cabbage flavor of the napa cabbage. (This recipe comes from Megan Brenn-White.)

Preparation time: *10 minutes*

Yield: *8 servings*

1 medium napa cabbage	1 tablespoon mirin or rice wine
1½ tablespoons sesame seeds	1 tablespoon rice vinegar
1 tablespoon soy sauce	1 teaspoon lime juice
½ teaspoon toasted sesame oil	¼ teaspoon crushed chili flakes

1 Clean the cabbage, and chop it into strips. Place the chopped cabbage in a large bowl.

2 Toast the sesame seeds in a small pan over medium heat until they're golden, stirring frequently. Set aside to cool.

3 Mix the remaining ingredients well in a small bowl.

4 Add the dressing to the cabbage, toss, and top with the toasted sesame seeds.

Per serving: *Calories 30 (From Fat 9); Fat 1g (Saturated 0g); Cholesterol 0mg; Sodium 123mg; Carbohydrate 3g (Dietary Fiber 1g); Protein 1g.*

Salmon Patties

Salmon is a great source of omega-3 fatty acids and is considered to be one of the most beneficial sources of animal protein. These patties are a beautiful addition to a brunch, but they also work as appetizers or a light lunch or dinner. (This recipe comes from *Conscious Cuisine* by Cary Neff (Sourcebooks).)

Preparation time: *15 minutes*

Yield: *6 servings*

1 small potato	*¾ teaspoon freshly ground black pepper*
½ pound fresh salmon filets without skin or bone	*¼ cup chopped scallion*
1 large egg white	*1 tablespoon chopped fresh chervil, parsley, dill, or cilantro*
½ teaspoon sea salt	*½ cup chopped seedless grapes*

1 Preheat the oven to 350 degrees.

2 Peel the potato and finely chop it. Blanch the chopped potato by boiling it in water until tender and then removing from the heat. When the potato is cool, drain the water off, and dry the chopped pieces on a kitchen towel.

3 Place the salmon in a food processor and pulse until roughly chopped (3 pulses or so). Add the egg white, salt, and pepper. Process until smooth. Transfer the mixture to a bowl, and fold in the scallion, herbs, grapes, and potato.

4 Heat a griddle or sauté pan over medium heat, and coat it with cooking spray or olive oil. Using a ¼-cup measure, form 6 patties and place them in the pan. Brown the patties on both sides (approximately 3 minutes per side).

5 Place the patties on an ungreased baking sheet and bake until cooked through, about 5 minutes.

Tip: Be sure to make fairly thin patties if you plan to skip Step 5 (baking in the oven). Heat the sauté pan or griddle with a bit of oil to a fairly high heat and brown on both sides. Turn the heat down to medium and continue to cook the patties, flipping them once, until they're cooked all the way through. You may want to cover the pan to speed the cooking time.

Per serving: *Calories 74 (From Fat 14); Fat 2g (Saturated 0g); Cholesterol 22mg; Sodium 231mg; Carbohydrate 6g (Dietary Fiber 1g); Protein 9g.*

Orange Beef and Vegetables

Here's a recipe that combines your standard stir-fry with an unexpected treat: fruit juice! Kids love this meal because of the tangy and crunchy combination. Add low-fat meat for protein, and you have a complete and nutritious meal.

Preparation time: *10 minutes*

Yield: *4 servings*

2 medium seedless oranges	12-ounce beef top round steak, thinly sliced across the grain
1 package brown rice	
1 tablespoon canola oil	10-ounce bag frozen stir-fry vegetables

1 Grate the peel off one orange, and set aside. Juice both oranges, and set the juice aside.

2 Prepare the rice according to package instructions.

3 Heat the oil in a nonstick skillet. Add the sliced beef, and stir-fry until no longer pink. Remove to a bowl.

4 Put the frozen vegetables in the skillet with the orange peel and juice. Cook for 4 minutes.

5 Add the beef back in, and stir-fry for 1 minute, or until the beef is heated through. Season with salt and pepper to taste.

Vary It! *If your family isn't particularly fond of rice, you can serve this dish over whole wheat noodles. Prepare 6 to 8 servings according to package instructions.*

Per serving: *Calories 230 (From Fat 88); Fat 10g (Saturated 3g); Cholesterol 48mg; Sodium 44mg; Carbohydrate 15g (Dietary Fiber 5g); Protein 20g.*

➂ Mini Black Bean Burgers

Tired of the same old burgers? Want to try something vegetarian? These mini bean burgers are great for a quick dinner and also provide lots of protein. Their small size appeals to kids, but you can make them any size you like! (This recipe comes from Julie Negrin.)

Preparation time: *30 minutes*

Yield: *6 to 8 servings*

2 tablespoons olive oil	*Coarse salt and ground pepper*
2 scallions, finely chopped	*2 yams, baked and peeled*
2 garlic cloves, crushed	*1 large egg, lightly beaten*
Two 15½-ounce cans black beans, drained and rinsed	*½ cup plain dry breadcrumbs*
	1 package mini burger buns or dinner rolls

1 Heat broiler, and brush a baking sheet with 1 tablespoon of oil.

2 In a small skillet over medium heat, heat 1 tablespoon oil, and then add the scallions and sauté 1 minute (until softened). Add the garlic and sauté 30 seconds. Transfer to a large bowl.

3 Add approximately three-quarters of the beans to the bowl, and mash them with a fork or potato masher. Add in the remaining beans, and season the mixture generously with salt and pepper.

4 Fold the yam, egg, and breadcrumbs into the beans. Divide the mixture into small balls of equal size, and flatten them into patties. Place the patties ½ inch apart on the baking sheet. Broil 4 inches from the heat 8 to 10 minutes.

5 With a thin metal spatula, carefully turn the burgers over. Put them back under the broiler for 2 to 3 minutes more, until they're crisp. Top the burgers with salsa, and serve them with guacamole.

Per serving: *Calories 238 (From Fat 63); Fat 7g (Saturated 1g); Cholesterol 27mg; Sodium 404mg; Carbohydrate 35g (Dietary Fiber 6g); Protein 8g.*

Appendix B

Weight Chart and Exercise Log

*Y*ou can use the weight chart provided on the following page of this appendix to keep track of your child's progress as he or she loses weight. Filling in the chart and recording progress is an excellent motivator. Just photocopy the weight chart page that follows so that you're not limited to the one page in this book. Here are a few sample entries:

Day, Date	Time of Day	Weight	Previous Weight	Weight Loss	Total Weight Loss
Monday, 1/2	Morning	152			
Monday, 1/9	Morning	151	152	−1	−1
Monday, 1/16	Morning	150.5	151	−.5	−1.5

With the exercise log, which comes right after the weight chart, your child can record the amount of physical activity he or she is participating in. As with the weight chart, you should photocopy the exercise log page because, with any luck, your child will be logging pages and pages of activities. Here are a few sample entries:

Date	Time of Day	Activity	Duration	Comments
1/12	3:30 p.m.	Walk in park	30 minutes	I felt tired at first, but halfway through I started feeling more energetic.
1/14	10:00 a.m.	Shovel snow with Dad	25 minutes	It's hard work! I'm tired.
1/15	4:00 p.m.	Walk around neighborhood	30 minutes	I wish the rest of our neighbors had shoveled their sidewalks.

Weight Chart

Day, Date	Time of Day	Weight	Previous Weight	Weight Loss	Total Weight Loss

Exercise Log

Date	Time of Day	Activity	Duration	Comments

Index

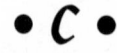

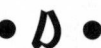

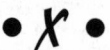

● *X* ●

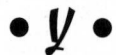

● *Y* ●

BUSINESS, CAREERS & PERSONAL FINANCE

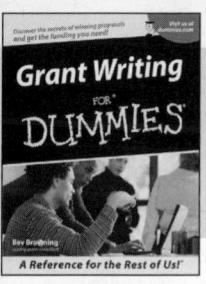

0-7645-5307-0

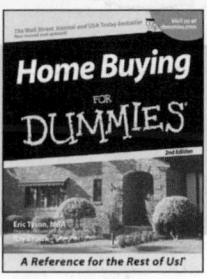

0-7645-5331-3 *†

Also available:
- Accounting For Dummies †
  0-7645-5314-3
- Business Plans Kit For Dummies †
  0-7645-5365-8
- Cover Letters For Dummies
  0-7645-5224-4
- Frugal Living For Dummies
  0-7645-5403-4
- Leadership For Dummies
  0-7645-5176-0
- Managing For Dummies
  0-7645-1771-6

- Marketing For Dummies
  0-7645-5600-2
- Personal Finance For Dummies *
  0-7645-2590-5
- Project Management For Dummies
  0-7645-5283-X
- Resumes For Dummies †
  0-7645-5471-9
- Selling For Dummies
  0-7645-5363-1
- Small Business Kit For Dummies *†
  0-7645-5093-4

HOME & BUSINESS COMPUTER BASICS

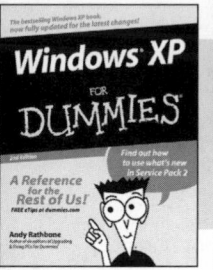

0-7645-4074-2

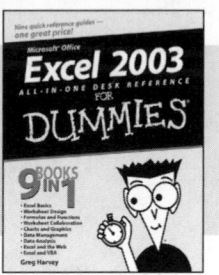

0-7645-3758-X

Also available:
- ACT! 6 For Dummies
  0-7645-2645-6
- iLife '04 All-in-One Desk Reference
  For Dummies
  0-7645-7347-0
- iPAQ For Dummies
  0-7645-6769-1
- Mac OS X Panther Timesaving
  Techniques For Dummies
  0-7645-5812-9
- Macs For Dummies
  0-7645-5656-8

- Microsoft Money 2004 For Dummies
  0-7645-4195-1
- Office 2003 All-in-One Desk Reference
  For Dummies
  0-7645-3883-7
- Outlook 2003 For Dummies
  0-7645-3759-8
- PCs For Dummies
  0-7645-4074-2
- TiVo For Dummies
  0-7645-6923-6
- Upgrading and Fixing PCs For Dummies
  0-7645-1665-5
- Windows XP Timesaving Techniques
  For Dummies
  0-7645-3748-2

FOOD, HOME, GARDEN, HOBBIES, MUSIC & PETS

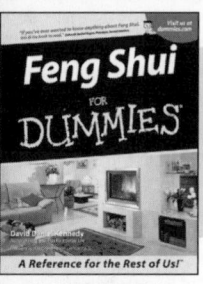

0-7645-5295-3

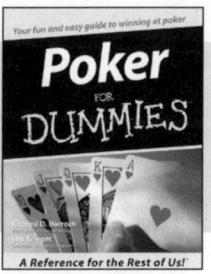

0-7645-5232-5

Also available:
- Bass Guitar For Dummies
  0-7645-2487-9
- Diabetes Cookbook For Dummies
  0-7645-5230-9
- Gardening For Dummies *
  0-7645-5130-2
- Guitar For Dummies
  0-7645-5106-X
- Holiday Decorating For Dummies
  0-7645-2570-0
- Home Improvement All-in-One
  For Dummies
  0-7645-5680-0

- Knitting For Dummies
  0-7645-5395-X
- Piano For Dummies
  0-7645-5105-1
- Puppies For Dummies
  0-7645-5255-4
- Scrapbooking For Dummies
  0-7645-7208-3
- Senior Dogs For Dummies
  0-7645-5818-8
- Singing For Dummies
  0-7645-2475-5
- 30-Minute Meals For Dummies
  0-7645-2589-1

INTERNET & DIGITAL MEDIA

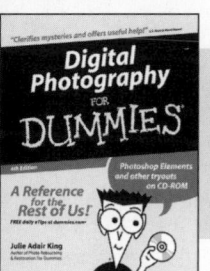

0-7645-1664-7

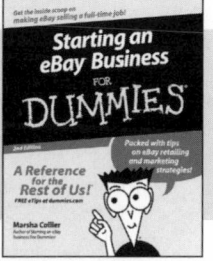

0-7645-6924-4

Also available:
- 2005 Online Shopping Directory
  For Dummies
  0-7645-7495-7
- CD & DVD Recording For Dummies
  0-7645-5956-7
- eBay For Dummies
  0-7645-5654-1
- Fighting Spam For Dummies
  0-7645-5965-6
- Genealogy Online For Dummies
  0-7645-5964-8
- Google For Dummies
  0-7645-4420-9

- Home Recording For Musicians
  For Dummies
  0-7645-1634-5
- The Internet For Dummies
  0-7645-4173-0
- iPod & iTunes For Dummies
  0-7645-7772-7
- Preventing Identity Theft For Dummies
  0-7645-7336-5
- Pro Tools All-in-One Desk Reference
  For Dummies
  0-7645-5714-9
- Roxio Easy Media Creator For Dummies
  0-7645-7131-1

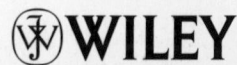 **WILEY**

SPORTS, FITNESS, PARENTING, RELIGION & SPIRITUALITY

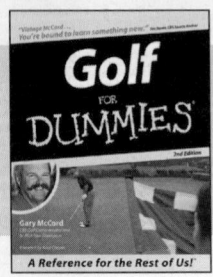

0-7645-5146-9

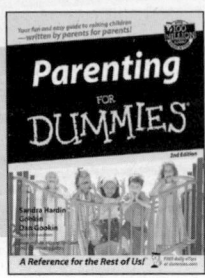

0-7645-5418-2

Also available:

- Adoption For Dummies
  0-7645-5488-3
- Basketball For Dummies
  0-7645-5248-1
- The Bible For Dummies
  0-7645-5296-1
- Buddhism For Dummies
  0-7645-5359-3
- Catholicism For Dummies
  0-7645-5391-7
- Hockey For Dummies
  0-7645-5228-7

- Judaism For Dummies
  0-7645-5299-6
- Martial Arts For Dummies
  0-7645-5358-5
- Pilates For Dummies
  0-7645-5397-6
- Religion For Dummies
  0-7645-5264-3
- Teaching Kids to Read For Dummies
  0-7645-4043-2
- Weight Training For Dummies
  0-7645-5168-X
- Yoga For Dummies
  0-7645-5117-5

TRAVEL

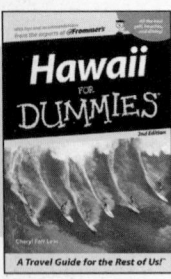

0-7645-5438-7

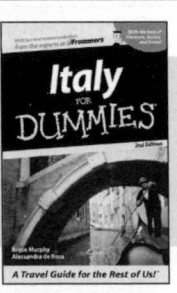

0-7645-5453-0

Also available:

- Alaska For Dummies
  0-7645-1761-9
- Arizona For Dummies
  0-7645-6938-4
- Cancún and the Yucatán For Dummies
  0-7645-2437-2
- Cruise Vacations For Dummies
  0-7645-6941-4
- Europe For Dummies
  0-7645-5456-5
- Ireland For Dummies
  0-7645-5455-7

- Las Vegas For Dummies
  0-7645-5448-4
- London For Dummies
  0-7645-4277-X
- New York City For Dummies
  0-7645-6945-7
- Paris For Dummies
  0-7645-5494-8
- RV Vacations For Dummies
  0-7645-5443-3
- Walt Disney World & Orlando For Dummies
  0-7645-6943-0

GRAPHICS, DESIGN & WEB DEVELOPMENT

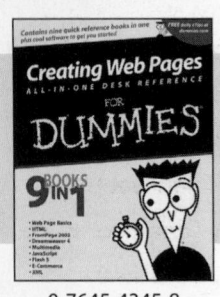

0-7645-4345-8

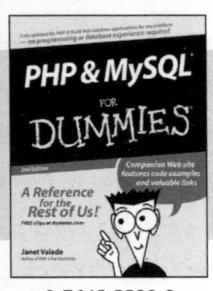

0-7645-5589-8

Also available:

- Adobe Acrobat 6 PDF For Dummies
  0-7645-3760-1
- Building a Web Site For Dummies
  0-7645-7144-3
- Dreamweaver MX 2004 For Dummies
  0-7645-4342-3
- FrontPage 2003 For Dummies
  0-7645-3882-9
- HTML 4 For Dummies
  0-7645-1995-6
- Illustrator CS For Dummies
  0-7645-4084-X

- Macromedia Flash MX 2004 For Dummies
  0-7645-4358-X
- Photoshop 7 All-in-One Desk Reference For Dummies
  0-7645-1667-1
- Photoshop CS Timesaving Techniques For Dummies
  0-7645-6782-9
- PHP 5 For Dummies
  0-7645-4166-8
- PowerPoint 2003 For Dummies
  0-7645-3908-6
- QuarkXPress 6 For Dummies
  0-7645-2593-X

NETWORKING, SECURITY, PROGRAMMING & DATABASES

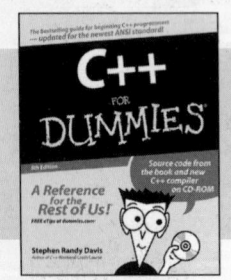

0-7645-6852-3

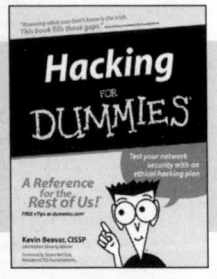

0-7645-5784-X

Also available:

- A+ Certification For Dummies
  0-7645-4187-0
- Access 2003 All-in-One Desk Reference For Dummies
  0-7645-3988-4
- Beginning Programming For Dummies
  0-7645-4997-9
- C For Dummies
  0-7645-7068-4
- Firewalls For Dummies
  0-7645-4048-3
- Home Networking For Dummies
  0-7645-42796

- Network Security For Dummies
  0-7645-1679-5
- Networking For Dummies
  0-7645-1677-9
- TCP/IP For Dummies
  0-7645-1760-0
- VBA For Dummies
  0-7645-3989-2
- Wireless All In-One Desk Reference For Dummies
  0-7645-7496-5
- Wireless Home Networking For Dummies
  0-7645-3910-8

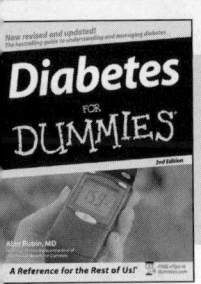
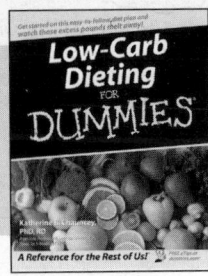
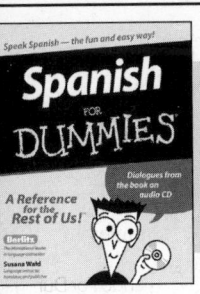
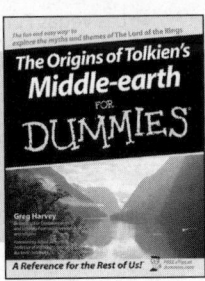
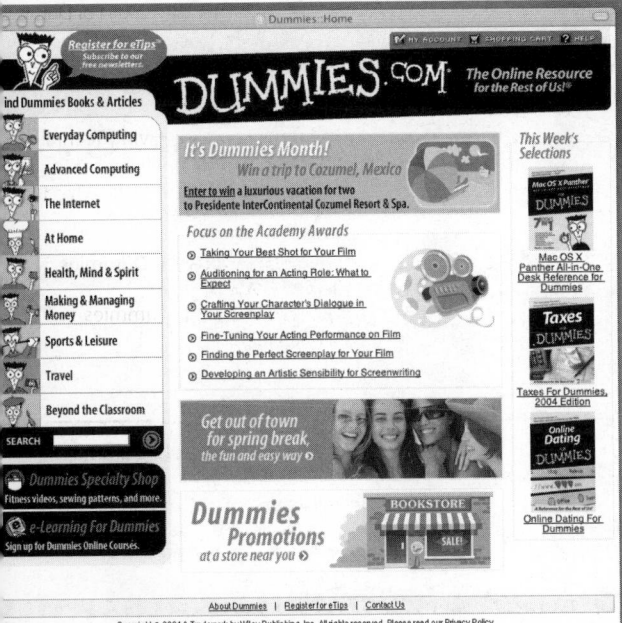
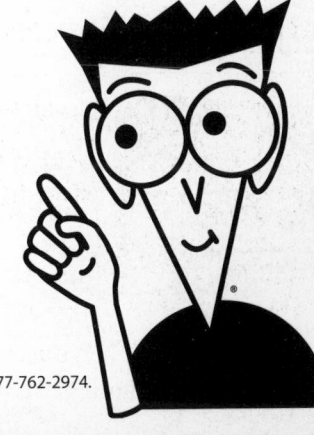

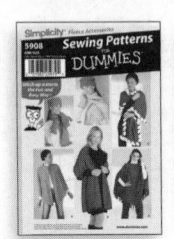
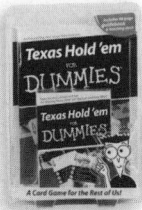
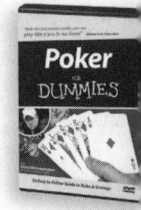
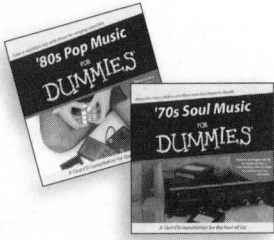
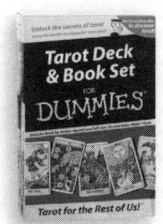
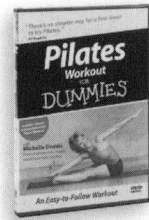
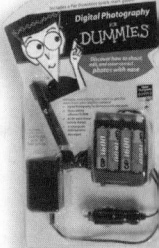
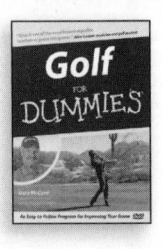
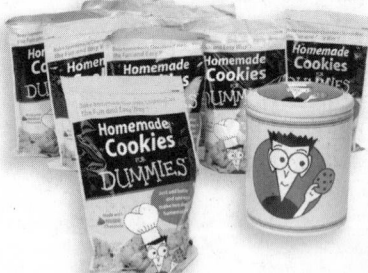
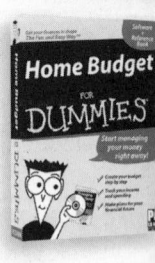
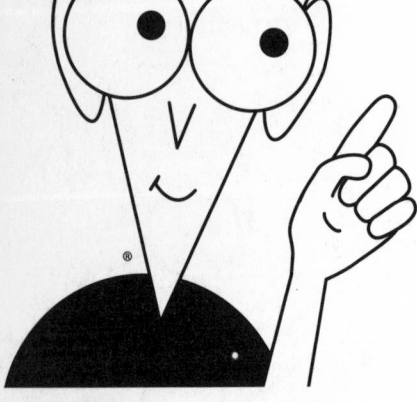